# PERSONAL WELLNESS
## HOW TO GO THE DISTANCE

*The Wellness Educator's Guide*

**Al & Carol Bacchus,** MT (ASCP), BS, MA, PhD

*with*
Daniel McCready, MD
E. Gnanaraj Moses, PhD, PhD
Debbie Rose, RN, MS
F. Carl Schneider, MD

*Edited by*
**Margaret Savage, MD, MPH**
Member, American College of Preventive Medicine
Former Medical Program Director,
The Koop Foundation, Inc.

**meduwell.com publishing**
**Frederick, MD**

*meduwell.com publishing*
**An Imprint of Engineering Systems Solutions, Inc.**
*5726 Industry Lane*
*Frederick, MD 21704*
**Dedicated to Publishing Excellence**

**Personal Wellness: How to Go the Distance**

First Edition
**Book Design:** James Arkunsinski
**Cover Design:** James Arkunsinski, Carol Bacchus and Gina Morfino
**Editor:** Margaret Savage, MD, MPH
**Proofreader:** Nita Congress

Permission from The McGraw-Hill Companies for the use of the anatomy drawings in the color section of this book is gratefully acknowledged. The drawings were originally published in the *Student Study Art Notebook* which accompanies the textbook, *Hole's Human Anatomy and Physiology*.

The information and suggested applications in this book are intended for educational purposes and should not be construed as medical, legal or financial advice. Please consult licensed professionals in medical, legal and financial matters that require expert guidance in implementing your personal plans.

*Library of Congress Catalog Card Number: 99-91054*

**Subject Headings and Key Words:**
Wellness, Self-Care, Wellness Education, Health Philosophy, Whole-Person Healing, Personality, Mental Health, Relationships, Spirituality, Integrative Medicine.

**Authors**: Bacchus, A; Bacchus, C; McCready, D; Moses, E.G; Rose, D; Schneider, F.C.

ISBN 0-9674834-0-9

*Printed in the United States of America on acid-free paper.*

# Dedicated to

**Gerald and Enid Bacchus, Al's parents**

*You did the best you could with what you had.*


**To our children, Michael, Annette, David & Debby**

*Thanks for hanging in there as we grew together.*


**To our granddaughter, Kaitlyn**

*You are so precious!*


*(Chapter dedications pay special tribute to people who
made a major difference in our lives.)*

# Foreword

Each year in the United States, approximately 500,000 people require emergency room treatment as a result of attempted suicide. More people in the 15-24 age group die from suicide than from cancer, heart disease, AIDS, birth defects, stroke, pneumonia and influenza, and chronic lung disease combined. From 1980 to 1996, the rate of suicide in the 10-14 age group increased by 100%.

The above statistics are part of *The Surgeon General's Call To Action To Prevent Suicide*, issued on July 28, 1999. This is one response to the World Health Organization's 1996 call to prevent suicide. The problem is worldwide in scope.

A blueprint for addressing the problem was introduced in the Surgeon General's report. The approach is referred to by the acronym AIM — Awareness, Intervention and Methodology.

As an educator for the past thirty-eight years, I have had the privilege and responsibility to study and respond to this major mental health problem in the college-age population. Leading honor students on the campus of the University of Maryland, College Park, in discussions of these issues, in contemplating the root causes and the possible solutions, has been the most rewarding part of my career. In a course titled "The Self-Examined Life," I attempt to challenge students to reach beyond book knowledge and know themselves well enough to be prepared to handle success and failure.

The following true stories illustrate aspects of the root causes of suicide.

## Gus, the Mayor

As an honor student and physics major, Gus was a perfectionist. Always serious about life, Gus felt that when he took on a task, he should finish it. And the task should be done right. Moreover, Gus felt when he took on a project his entire worthiness was on the line. Highly motivated, Gus was very successful. In time he became mayor of Annapolis, Maryland. And by all accounts he was one of the best mayors in the city's history.

During his term as mayor, Gus took on the task of balancing the budget without raising taxes — a task that many said would be difficult even for God. But with eleven days to go before the decision about raising taxes had to be made, Gus called his staff together to say: "I have bad news and I have good news. The bad news is that it looks as though I am not going to be able to balance the budget. The good news is that if I can't, I am going to kill myself." People laughed.

Those who knew Gus well said that the suicide note told the truth: He killed himself because he couldn't balance the budget. Perfectionists believe that you are what you do. And if you can't accomplish the goals that you set for yourself, then you are no longer worthwhile — no longer lovable. Gus never understood that one's work could be excellent without being perfect.

## Jason, in search of "the molecular Holy Grail"

An outstanding graduate student at Harvard, Jason was in his sixth year of graduate study in the Chemistry Department. Jason was by all accounts one of the most promising students in one of the most outstanding programs in the country. His advisor was a Nobel Prize winner.

For his dissertation, Jason was attempting to synthesize a very complex molecule. Indeed, it was said that Jason's project was chemistry's equivalent of "the Holy Grail." But Jason took it on and worked around the clock. But the task was too big, and so with his worthiness on the line, Jason killed himself. His lab mate said there was no doubt in his mind that what killed him was the molecule. When you are a perfectionist, you are what you do, and if you don't accomplish your goals, you are no longer worthwhile — no longer lovable. Excellent work is not enough when you are a perfectionist. For Gus it was the budget; for Jason, the molecule.

## Kathy, the super-champion athlete

Both an outstanding student and an outstanding athlete, Kathy received all A's in high school and held three state records in track. She was so outstanding that the county school system declared a day in her honor during her senior year.

Kathy was the kind of student all universities seek to recruit. As an honor student at North Carolina State, she was very successful in college. As an athlete she was running in the NCAA championships of a 10,000-meter race that she was expected to win. But with 3,200 meters left in the race, Kathy found herself running in eighth place. And so, Kathy turned away from the stadium and jumped off a bridge. As far as Kathy could see, you either accomplish the goals you set for yourself, or you are no longer worthwhile — no longer lovable. For a perfectionist, just being outstanding is not enough. For Gus it was the budget; for Jason, the molecule; for Kathy, the championship.

## Bruce, the best baseball pitcher of his day

An outstanding student at the University of Southern California, Bruce seemed to have it all — handsome, articulate and an accomplished musician. Bruce was also an outstanding athlete. As a pitcher on the USC baseball team, his record was forty wins against five losses. In his senior year, he won the award for the NCAA Outstanding Collegiate Pitcher of the Year. After his senior year, he signed a contract with the LA Dodgers. But Bruce injured his arm, and at age twenty-five the best collegiate pitcher in America was washed up.

So Bruce climbed the fence of his beloved baseball stadium at USC, and went out near the pitcher's mound. Placing his USC diploma on his left and his Pitcher of the Year award on his right, he shot himself. As far as Bruce could see, you are what you do. And if you can't accomplish the goals you set for yourself, you are no longer worthwhile — no longer lovable. If you are a perfectionist, it is not enough to be an outstanding student and musician. You must have it all.

## Emily, the "A" student

As close to perfect as most elementary students ever get, during the first six grades of school, Emily got all A's. She was a beautiful child who was loved by her teachers and classmates. Then one day when she was thirteen years old, she got a B. The next day she killed herself. Psychiatrists at Menninger said it was a classic case. Emily never learned the difference between what you do and what you are as a person. As far as Emily could see, if you didn't get all A's you were no longer worthwhile — no longer lovable. Excellent grades were not enough. Emily needed to be perfect.

• • • • •

Add to the problem of suicide the recent incidents of tragic homicides in schools, colleges, at the workplace and in communities across the country. Add to these problems the mortality and morbidity caused by chronic, preventable diseases in our society and the world at large. Add to those conditions the expressed lack of general fulfillment in life, the dissatisfaction of consumers with our healthcare system and the insatiable appetite for acquiring things, and we can see a need for wellness education.

Wellness education must be defined in terms of the effect on people's lives, not in terms of information to be committed to memory or even to be regurgitated to earn grades in school. The problems to be addressed may all be lumped under the heading "suicide prevention." The sudden ending of life may be acute suicide. The premature death and disease from preventable lifestyle causes may be prolonged suicide. The lack of meaning and fulfillment in life may be spiritual suicide.

The goal of wellness education is also captured in the AIM slogan of the Surgeon General's report. Wellness education must foster Awareness, and must address Intervention and Methodology.

In this *Wellness Educator's Guide*, Dr. Bacchus and colleagues present one approach to wellness. This personal application of the principles of wellness, along with an educational model that is a framework for teaching wellness, is the result of fifteen years of classroom interaction on the campus of the University of Maryland.

It was my pleasure to have helped to lay the foundation for this work back in 1983 in heart-to-heart discussions with Al. Since then, we have kept up our philosophical exchanges, and it is specially gratifying to see these principles being disseminated to help bridge the consumer and health professional audiences. The principles of self-examination, self-understanding, self-acceptance, self-management and self-realization are applicable to all.

As his self-disclosures reveal, Al has challenged himself to apply to his own life what he teaches. His struggle with perfectionism and specialness has been part of the drive to produce this work.

Scattered throughout this book are strategies to deal with "Life's Givens." As I have summarized for my students in the honors course "The Self-Examined Life," an awareness and contemplation of life's givens help to protect against suicide and a lack of achievement in life. It helps as motivation to live a healthy lifestyle, prevent disease, fulfill our potential and find real happiness.

To live fully, we must each find a way to cope with life's givens, which are:

1. To be mortal and thus at risk of death during every moment of life,

2. To make all decisions on the basis of only partial knowledge, thereby rendering ourselves fallible and constantly open to the risk of being wrong,

3. To be susceptible to disease and genetic disadvantage, thereby jeopardizing the plans that we make for each new day,

4. To arrive in the world with no inborn meaning, thereby rendering a personal search necessary,

5. To carry within us a capacity for bad will toward others, thereby rendering us capable of inflicting harm upon others,

6. To be characterized by behavior that is constantly vulnerable to persuasion from pleasure and pain,

7. To be susceptible to tolerance and addiction, thereby placing ourselves at risk, and

8. To enter the world as a separate entity and to stand responsible for our personal connectedness and/or aloneness.

May the use of this guide promote wellness on an individual and a universal level.

*John Burt, EdD*
*Former Dean, College of Health and Human Performance*
*University of Maryland*
*College Park, MD*

*August 1999*

# Acknowledgments

It gives us great pleasure to thank those who played an active role in helping to get this work published. More than the support and encouragement, we want to acknowledge the health-promoting level of intimacy we have experienced from each relationship. Along with those who are listed on the title page for their review of content, and those to whom chapters are dedicated, we want to express deep gratitude to:

*John Burt* — your inspiration and influence will go with us forever. Thanks for the Foreword and all the time you take to share philosophy for living.

*Glen Schiraldi* — your advice, help and intimate discussions will always be a source of joy for us. Thanks for introducing Al to yoga in 1983.

*James Dotson* — your vision for "Center Point" and "Managing Life Successfully" was an inspiration to us.

*Bill Loveless* — our reconnection at World Med '98 as we met for our private conference, and later the pleasure of introducing you, was spiritually uplifting.

*Bob Feldman* — your positive comments after reading our very first concept paper in 1986 was great encouragement.

*Marc Micozzi* — your stimulation of my interest in integrative medicine research, and in the field of complementary and alternative medicine on a whole, were steps in the right direction for getting to do the educational programs I envisioned. Thanks for introducing George and Lee to me.

*George Haynes* — your thoughtfulness and emotional strength are much appreciated.

*Lee Lipsenthal* — you are blessed with the capacity to brighten any day. Thanks for partnering in labor for the transformation of healthcare and medical education.

*Bill Neely and family* — your restorative ministry has touched our lives deeply. (Bill G., thanks for questioning the original subtitle.)

*Galina and James Arkunsinski* — your help, personally and professionally, has been most timely and greatly appreciated.

*Debbie Dick* — your friendship will always be treasured.

*Michael Gayle* — your music, your family and heart-to-heart conversations have been inspiring. Thanks for helping with the indexing and final proofing.

*Janet and Lee Kanter* — you were there just in time. We look forward to the programs we'll do together both in continuing medical education and spirituality and emotional growth.

*Zorita and Al Thomas* — thanks for prayer warriors and sound advice.

*Merle and Terry Burkett and family* — your friendship has been very supportive and timely.

*Carol and Bob Colacurcio* — thanks for introducing us to the incorporation of the healing power of cross-cultural music into wellness education.

*Ron Lynch* — your continued collaboration will always be treasured, and thanks for the introduction to Celebration Health.

To *Tin and Ana, Whit and Syl, Gerry and Marlene, Hetty and Afzal, Vet and Godfrey, Harold and Anne, Danny, Janelle and Michael, Janet and Norb, Donna, Joy, Norman, Julie and their families,* thanks for your expressions and specific acts of support and concern. We are now getting to do what we set out to do eighteen years ago.

To the many individuals and families, too numerous to list individually, who have been a part of our ups and downs over the many years we sought for our niche, we express appreciation. To the SAAA, AFI, RFLF, Sligo Choir and Inner-Visions families, we say a hearty thank you.

To the *Sam Koilpillai* family we tender special thanks for the privilege and pleasure of being involved in the Anantha Ashram project in Hosur, India. (Sam Uncle, we hope to assist in a much larger way and look forward to spending some time helping out at the homes for abandoned children.)

To *Starlet and Jaysingh Vedamuthu*, your kindness at the time in 1983 when we were homeless will never be forgotten. It was the time when the spark for this synthesis was generated.

To *Rob Abraham*, CEO of Health Management, Inc., and President of Integrative Medicine Research Institute, Inc., and the staff (*Rajan, Ponraj, Nigel, Stephanie* and *Julie*), thanks for a place to wait for the dream and for help during the wait.

Finally, heartfelt appreciation and a million thanks to *Margaret Savage* for assuming the editorial responsibilities; to *Jay Nathan* and *Dan Campbell* of Engineering Systems Solutions, Inc., for seeing the potential of Wellness Education; and to *Steve Winkelstein, Kim McCurry* and *Venice Mundle-Harvey* of Balmar Printing and Graphics, Inc., for expert guidance in the production process.

There are three people we want to give special recognition to, since without their active input this book, at this time, would not be published: *Mr. I. R. Thomas, James Arkusinski*, and *Jay Nathan*, President & CEO of Engineering Systems Solutions, Inc.

We have been touched by many lives and we are the richer for it.

Carol & Al

# Contents

# Preface

Once upon a time, a young woman left her village in the deep interior of her country to find a path to the eastern shore. She wanted to see the sunrise at its very beginning. She had never seen a full sunrise for herself. Legend told how beautiful, majestic and colorful a sunrise could be, but no one who had left in search of that experience had ever returned to share the story.

In the heart of the jungle, the dawning of a day was rather sudden as the sun came over the tall mountains surrounding the village. On most days, the rain clouds and the thick fog hid the sun altogether. The young woman longed to see the early dawn and experience the beauty of a full sunrise.

The trails leading away from her village ended in the fields where the villagers grew their crops and raised cattle. There were no maps for her to follow so she had to make her own path through the forests. As she encountered fallen trees, deep ravines, swollen rivers and other obstacles, she would make the necessary detours. But always, she would find her bearings and head towards the east.

After several days of lonely travel, she emerged from the forests onto a grassy plain where she could see many people heading in the same direction. There were small groups and large groups. Many groups and individuals continued to forge their own paths while some used the paths and trails left by those ahead of them.

As she thought about the choice of trails now open to her, the young woman felt inspired to experiment with the rest of her journey. She decided to join a group for a while. She sometimes traveled alone, stopping to examine life in the villages on the plain. Sometimes she needed rest for her blistered feet.

Her short-term adventures stretched into years and many times she felt comfortable enough to forget her original quest. She was seeing more sunny days, longer days, more colorful sunrises and more beautiful sunsets. Maybe this was all she needed. All she wanted.

Then one night, she heard the strains of music, beautiful music, soul-inspiring music like she had never heard before. It came from the hut of an old man playing a simple reed flute. As she listened, she knew that she must learn to play such music. Now her quest had another purpose. She must see the sunrise at its beginning and celebrate it with her own music.

She went to the tent the next day and asked the old man many questions. Questions about how he got to the plains; where he came from; how did he make the flute; would he be going on to the seashore; was he happy; were there any other musicians on the plains.

After several visits to the old man, the young woman started asking similar questions to everyone she met on the plains. New questions; old questions; simple questions; complex questions. A few people offered answers. The young woman concluded, "There are more questions than there are answers."

Then, unnoticed and without ceremony, she disappeared from the plains.

• • • • •

Over the last fifteen years, I have had the privilege and pleasure of facilitating a one-semester course at University of Maryland University College. The discussions and shared life experiences contributed by over three hundred individuals helped to clarify the questions and the search for answers.

This has been the most satisfying academic experience that I have had. So this book was written because the questions were worth sharing, the search for the answers had a positive effect on students and facilitator, and there seems to be a need to keep on asking questions about every aspect of life as we face a new century.

I asked my wife, Carol, to be co-author for this book because she inspired the theme of the course, she was a discussion leader at several sessions, she has a way of putting my complex and sometimes confusing ideas into simpler language, and she played an active role in every academic degree I earned.

This is my way of acknowledging her soul-mate partnership and her dedication to taking care of the family as I pursued graduate work.

I was very fortunate to get to know Dr. John Burt when he was Chairman of the Department of Health Education at the University of Maryland. His mentorship and encouragement gave me the freedom to design the course, which continues to be offered through that department. It is a distinct honor to have him write the Foreword for this book.

The other contributors are friends who gave of their time and of themselves to make this a better work than it would have been without their input. They are, in order of the length of their collaboration:

**E. G. Moses, PhD, PhD**, a clinical psychologist and educator, who has been a friend, confidante and counselor. Dr. Moses has been a professor at Howard University for over twenty years, and is the only person I know with two earned PhD degrees.

**Debbie Rose, RN, MS,** a registered nurse who entered the field of wellness in the early eighties by completing the Masters in Exercise Science at George Washington University. Debbie is a Health Promotion Director certified by the Cooper Institute for Aerobics Research. She currently directs the Wellness program at the Pentagon. Her expertise in fitness and wellness promotion brings a special perspective to her critique. She has contributed to this work from the wealth of her experience in establishing wellness programs. It was a particular pleasure to get her to teach a section of the course at the Shady Grove campus of University College. She is a good racquetball player who invited me for my first game at the Pentagon courts.

**F. Carl Schneider, MD,** a physician in pediatrics and fitness evaluation. For several years, he served as medical director of a program for prescribing and monitoring health promotion and fitness for the US Secret Service, the FBI and Firefighters.

**Margaret Savage, MD, MPH,** became a collaborator when she worked as Medical Program Director for The Koop Foundation, Inc. We shared the challenge of putting together a consortium for a $1.3 million grant application to the National Cancer Institute. Margaret has a passion for preventive medicine and electronic means of educating both consumers and practitioners. It was our good fortune that she was available to do the final editing of this work. Her critical reading of the whole manuscript in one week was a feat that reminded us of the all-nighters we had to pull to get the grant proposal in on time!

**Daniel McCready, MD,** a family physician in Virginia Beach, VA. Dan and I became friends during a two-day workshop in which I presented the educational model that forms the basis of this book to executives and physicians of the Sentara Health System. The reception there led us to believe that mainstream medicine is ready for integration of complementary and mind/body approaches to healthcare. Dan and I connected strongly on the vision of how wellness may impact the healthcare of the future.

The audience for this book is the adult population, both laypeople and healthcare professionals: all of those who are experiencing the struggle to balance job, family and career development as they strive to provide the best possible life for their loved ones and themselves. Many in this group, particularly the age bracket 32-56 (the baby-boomers plus or minus three years), are looking for growth in their career, seeking financial stability, and have serious questions about health promotion, disease prevention, happiness, fulfillment and meaning in life. They have seen enough of conventional healthcare to realize that each individual is unique, the individual has to take charge of health and well-being, and the present healthcare system is a sick-care system.

The examples shared throughout this book are all real experiences of real people (used with permission where it was needed). Details have been changed to preserve privacy. Some of the stories used are old fables or original fictional illustrations.

The recommended uses of this book are for personal study, group discussion where practical applications to life are a desired outcome and as a text for a course similar to "Personal Wellness & Self-Realization" offered at the University of Maryland University College. It is not designed for speed-reading or as a reference book.

It is my hope that the ideas shared here may find some practical application to life's challenges. To go the distance, one needs fuel for the body, mind and spirit.

**AB**

# Carol's Preface

I met Al in Lamson Hall, the women's dormitory at Andrews University, at two o'clock one morning in early October 1969! Since then, I have had the adventure of a lifetime.

Despite the predictions of failure in our marriage because of our intercultural differences, we have survived, raised three children, had our share of ups and downs and still believe the best has just arrived.

When Al asked me to co-author this book, I declined on the basis that I did not finish college (I did a two-year radiology technician program, and went to work). My greatest ambition was to be the best possible mother and wife that I could be, and I really couldn't write for publication. He persuaded me that all I had to do was to share some stories from our experience as illustrations of how we are going the distance.

I had helped Al with the research and typed his master's thesis at Andrews University. I did the graphics and typed the several drafts of his doctoral dissertation at Michigan State University. I helped him take care of his research animals during his post-doctoral fellowship at the University of Virginia. I graded his tests (I think he was using me to help keep departmental costs down by not having a teaching assistant) when he was an assistant professor of biology at Columbia Union College. I helped gather the materials for his course at the University of Maryland, and drew the first versions of the illustrations as he described the framework he had in mind. He asked me to think about his academic degrees as if I had earned them with him. That put things into a new perspective, and I accepted his offer.

I made a few presentations in his "Personal Wellness & Self-Realization" course over the years, and the student feedback was encouraging. One semester when Al had to make two trips to the Philippines, I was the substitute facilitator, and the student evaluations for that semester were not only on par with the other semesters but he says they were better. By writing and rewriting (maybe ten times altogether), with each of us editing and rewriting any part of the whole, we have arrived at a joint composition that reflects our combined effort.

Now I feel that I am really a part of the work and Al was not just giving me a shallow token of appreciation by persuading his publisher to put my name on the book cover. For the first time in my life, I feel comfortable about myself as a person, as a wife, mother, and contributor to meaningful thinking about life's challenges. I offer opinions and insights based on my experience. I am not an expert in any field.

My role in this work is mainly to tell the story of how this book was produced; tell how the practical applications of the principles of health promotion have affected my lifestyle, my health status and my level of satisfaction with my life; and share insights from twenty-nine years of marriage.

In this, we have become comfortable in sharing our personal experiences. These self-disclosures were not easy for me at first. However, as the course went on, and as we saw how they served the group discussions, I became more comfortable with them. By sharing personal life experiences, we connected better with each group. Members of the group quickly established a good comfort level of self-disclosure while maintaining privacy and dignity. The health promotion effects of social support became more than theory.

Our stories served to trigger similar memories and incidents, especially for the personal writing, which is a large part of the course. One of the aims of the exercises is to get beyond the usual facade of outward behavior and examine the core beliefs about life and life's experiences.

It has been fun and rewarding for me to contribute to this work. It was a special joy to do the several rough drafts and the original illustrations.

However, there is a greater joy in being a full partner. I hope that as you study this book individually or as part of a group, you will find some encouragement to do the things you know you can do.

Does anyone ever get to a point of perfection where no more growth is possible? I doubt that. In my case, I know the wide swings between failure and accomplishment, despair and hope, depression and motivation, and spiritual death and rebirth. As I re-write this preface, I know there is a major hurdle for me to face, but I have renewed strength and purpose to face it. Life is a journey and I will keep on trekking, one step at a time.

This book is really about how we are going the distance.

CB

# Introduction

"Success in the knowledge economy comes to those who know themselves — their strengths, their values, and how they best perform." So says Peter Drucker in the *Harvard Business Review* (March-April 1999).

This book is the summary of a college level course titled "Personal Wellness & Self-Realization," the goal of which is to help people know themselves. After fifteen years of asking and responding to questions from adults in the age range 20-60, I feel it is time to move out of the classroom. Part of what I understand my contribution in this life to be, is to ask and respond to questions from as many people as possible.

This introduction gives a brief overview of the contents of the book, the way in which the subject matter is dealt with in the class, and the exercises for practical applications to personal life. This is more of a self-study course than another health book to give information for the sake of information.

At the first session in the course, students are given an opportunity to express why they enrolled in the class, what they expect to achieve in the course, and how they expect to use what they learn, if anything. The ground rules set in the beginning are these:

1. Everyone has the right to his or her opinions, views and beliefs.

2. There are no bad questions. The only bad questions are those not asked.

3. There are no wrong answers to any question. There may be insufficient information or differing viewpoints, but all responses are worthwhile.

4. The scientific method is an excellent way of gaining new knowledge, but it is not infallible, it cannot be applied to all areas of knowledge, and it is not the only way of knowing.

5. As opposed to giving a body of facts, figures and research studies, we are more interested in ways of applying what is known, and experimenting in our own lives with making changes within the "safe" zone.

6. The method of classroom interaction is more of a facilitator/guide leading a search for usable knowledge, than of an expert pouring into "empty vessels" a body of information that they must memorize and regurgitate in order to squeeze an "A" out of the stingy hands of "the professor."

7. If you choose to share personal experiences or private details of your life, think ahead to what purposes they serve. Strive to maintain honesty and integrity in self-disclosure but, at the same time, protect privacy. Some self-disclosures need to be in a one-on-one format. Yet, sharing with a group engenders a social support atmosphere that is health promoting. Members of the group agree to confidentiality and privacy of information shared in self-disclosures.

The above ground rules create an atmosphere of cooperative learning and a shared search for personal growth.

A strong emphasis is placed on practical applications and opportunities for personal experimentation with real-life situations. As a personal study guide, this book may serve best if the user approaches the material as a self-taught course over several weeks or months. This is not a quick fix, self-help course. You really can't zoom into optimum well-being in eight weeks after thirty-something years or more of neglect. It takes time to understand the self, plan for desirable change and practice new habits.

In fact, as Peter Drucker says in the article cited above, "The conclusion bears repeating: do not try to change yourself — you are unlikely to succeed. But work hard to improve the way you perform." The most important conclusion from our classroom discussions is that getting to a comfortable understanding of the self is hard work — and long-term work.

This guide is an exploration into the core of one's being, to stimulate the mind to generate its own healing and growth.

At the center of the material in this book is a conceptual framework built on analogies. The reasoning went like this: human physiology can be organized into the following seven dynamic processes:

1. Homeostasis — the maintenance of balance.

2. Nutrition — the use of externally supplied foodstuff to support body chemistry.

3. Stress Adaptation — the response of the body to meet internal and external demands in excess of normal "wear and tear."

4. Work — the use of energy to effect changes in the internal and external environments.

5. Rest — the reduction of work and energy use to allow rebuilding and renewal.

6. Growth — the process of change over time to achieve maximum functional potential.

7. Reproduction — the process of creating offspring to continue the species through the individual.

So H-N-S-W-R-G-R is a summary of all of human physiology! Homeostasis, Nutrition, Stress adaptation, Work, Rest, Growth, and Reproduction — How Nancy Sings With Rick's Great Recipes. Part of the joy of learning is creating mnemonic aids that help to fix concepts.

Besides physiology, three other dimensions of human function can be described. These are:

1. The Mental Dimension — the functions of the mind dealing with information processing based in the biochemical and bioelectrical functions of the brain. This dimension of function gives humans the capabilities of learning, reasoning, decision-making, memory, creativity and imagination.

2. The Psychosocial Dimension — the processes of the mind dealing with definition of the self, the value of the self and the perceived effect of interaction with others.

3. The Spiritual Dimension — this function of the mind is the universal human desire for meaning, purpose and satisfaction in life. In this dimension, the drive to live a full life with joy, hope and fulfillment is integrated. This is the dimension that searches for a sense of connectedness with a larger whole.

The seven dynamics of the physiological dimension can be applied to the other three dimensions by analogy. This creates a four-by-seven Matrix of Integrated Human Function.

With the Matrix of Integrated Function as a framework for organizing discussions and knowledge, a five-step process is used to guide the personal application. These steps are:

1. Self-Examination — several instruments such as the "Inventory of Personal Interests" and "A Subjective Personality Profile" are used to elicit introspection and private inquiry with the individual setting the comfort level as to the extent of use. However, we discuss standardized assessment tools such as the Myers-Briggs Type Indicator and measures of human stress.

2. Self-Understanding — theories are subjectively applied through retrospective analysis to promote insight into "how I became who I am, and who I am becoming."

3. Self-Acceptance — through the above processes, the individual draws subjective conclusions regarding personal feelings of accepting the self "as is" and making decisions to effect desirable changes.

4. Self-Management — several theories of behavioral self-control are examined briefly, and techniques for practical applications are recommended.

5. Self-Actualization — an attempt is made to define this state based on the several theories of personality and happiness, and to promote a subjective evaluation of personal growth.

Finally, the definition of happiness is discussed, and a review of the current research on happiness is summarized.

The aims of this book are:

1. To present personal growth and personal health promotion as a pleasurable, desirable, practical pursuit.

2. To reinforce the desire of individuals to make changes in their health behaviors in the areas of nutrition, physical fitness, stress management, relationships, spiritual health and quality of life. This contributes to the final end of "the greatest happiness for the longest time."

3. To promote happiness, a sense of heightened fulfillment and peace of mind, within the chosen belief system.

4. To describe how an individual may take a personal path to integrate self-care, alternative therapies and mind/body medicine for optimum health and success.

5. To provide a package of material, that can be used by those who want to lead, teach or facilitate "Personal Wellness" for other people, be it an individual or a group.

The original subtitle for this book was "A Healthy Pleasures Approach to Total Well-Being." My thinking on this subject began in discussions with Dr. Burt back in 1983 when he shared one of his essays with me.

It is a purported letter from the general public to health educators, health promotion specialists and preventive medicine experts. This was part of a chapter titled "Metahealth: A Challenge for the Future" in the book *Behavioral Health: A Handbook of Health Enhancement and Disease Prevention*. The entire chapter is a stimulating discussion of the core reasons for the pursuit of health. The excerpt here is of the letter, used with permission of the author.

•  •  •  •  •

"To Those Concerned with Health Enhancement and Disease Prevention:

I am writing a single letter to all of you who are closely connected with my physical, mental, and spiritual health. Through this letter I hope to explain why I am, like millions of others in the world, so utterly desperate. You have advised me to put a curb on my pleasures, to resist the desire to engage in behaviors that will jeopardize my health and spiritual rightness. But I do not believe that you are fully aware of the implications of your well-intended advice. That is why I am writing to you.

Let me begin by reminding you of a fact that you seem to have forgotten: I am not the maker of my own temperament which unceasingly invites me to pleasure, an invitation that is more compelling to every sense than your invitation to longevity and spiritual enlightenment. For as long as anyone can remember, those of you in health enhancement and disease prevention have deflected and dispirited people through your teachings and promotion campaigns. I feel certain that this is not your intention. Nonetheless, when you go down the list of pleasures known to or available to most people, and one by one attach a risk to each and thereafter offer a strategy whereby behaviors can be changed to avoid that risk, it is tantamount to saying that pleasure and health are necessarily at odds with each other. Thus, in attempting to promote health you have simultaneously promoted an attitude—you must choose between health and pleasure—this thwarts that very health you seek to enhance.

Intentionally or not, you have caused most of us to think that ill health and bad luck are punishments for pleasure seeking; that it is only just that those who indulge the pleasures of eating should come to look funny (fat funny) and have their arteries clogged; that those who drink too much should be rendered impotent as a warning and develop cirrhosis of the liver if the practice continues; that those who smoke should develop emphysema and lung cancer; that those who have many sex partners should have herpes for life and syphilis and gonorrhea as short-term punishment; that those who eat sweets should have bad teeth; that those who gamble should end up broke, and those who drive fast should have accidents.

What I am trying to tell you is that the health problems of today's world do not result as much from an ignorance of risk factors or an ignorance of strategies to change behavior as from an ignorance of pleasure options that are not attended by a snag. In the battle for control of the human will—persuader vying against persuader—those of you in health enhancement and disease prevention have not been much of a factor. You have no sensitivity to the positive side of health: you don't understand the affirmative emotions. You don't understand the human will.

To prevent your getting off on another wrong track, let me hasten to add that although my temperament unceasingly invites me to pleasure, this does not negate my free will. This point is worth emphasizing: the invitation from my temperament is in every sense an invitation, nothing more. But I must tell you, with complete honesty, that as a free agent I am interested in pleasure. In truth, I weigh all my options to determine their pleasure content. You seem to have a bias against pleasure, but it is a bias that I do not share. At my very best, I am an intelligent consumer of pleasure options, and a major portion of my mental life is spent evaluating invitations to pleasure. Moreover, I somehow have the feeling that I am far more skillful at this matter than you give me credit for. Because you are preoccupied with promoting longevity and spiritual rightness, you have a tendency to judge my choices as stupid.

They are not really. You would understand if you stood in my shoes. The trouble is that being just a common person, my invitations to pleasure constitute only a short list, and due to your extensive research and teaching, nearly every pleasure on my list is now marked: "caution—this may be dangerous to health or spiritual rightness." What I desperately need is an invitation from someone who really understands health enhancement—an invitation to pleasure without a snag, without a caution sign. But it never comes. I have waited and waited—watching you destroy the few pleasures that I have discovered while remaining totally insensitive to my real problem. Don't you care? Can't you see that humanity places little value on longevity and spiritual rightness that is devoid of pleasure? What do you have against pleasure?

I know that you are very busy discovering new risk factors, teaching about old ones, propounding new models of health behavior, and writing books about health enhancement, but would it be asking too much to request that the next time you shoot down one of my pleasure options that you replace it with a new one—one without a snag? That is, unless it is true that health and spiritual rightness must forever be at odds with pleasure. In which case, I will just continue weighing pleasure options against longevity options, pleasure against spiritual rightness. Continue asking myself what, if not to enjoy pleasure, is health good for. And wondering—wondering if you are really trying to help me.

Let me end my letter with this observation. The English humorist Josh Billings once suggested that no person who lived to break one hundred years was famous for anything except living to be a hundred. This is not entirely true, but it points to an important presupposition held by people like me: health is something to be used for the accomplishment of goals, and pursuing self-selected goals represents one of the highest forms of pleasure seeking. So you must understand that health is a means; the end is pleasure. And if pleasure and health conflict, so much the worse for health. I know that you don't see it that way, but most of us do.

Sincerely,
An Unhealthy Citizen"

• • • • •

The new subtitle for this book keeps the concept of healthy pleasures but focuses on how it works over the long-haul. Health is the most important asset for going the distance. The distance is a satisfied life, having made a contribution. Quality counts more than quantity.

I must explain my wife's role in this work. She reads and rereads my writing to make it understandable. Without her, this book would have ended up being a compilation of the principles of physiology, psychology, religion and health statistics from the US Public Health Service.

With this in mind, she shares her ideas at the end of each chapter. I read and reread her contributions, and it leads to many stimulating discussions. The work was accomplished over a fifteen-year period.

Was it worth it? I don't know about worth. We just had to do it. It was our task, for this place, at this time. It is one of the assets that help us to go the distance. It is particularly satisfying to be making the final revisions today, our twenty-ninth wedding anniversary, knowing that all the rejections are behind us.

We are going the distance, and the journey now takes us into the exciting realm of answering and asking questions among consumers of health and wellness products, practitioners of conventional and alternative medicine, and the corporate workforce. Wellness education has become mainstream.

· · · · ·

# Carol's Introduction

As I look back on the years leading to the publication of this summary of the course "Personal Wellness & Self-Realization," I see why Al proposed the course and where the framework for organizing the course-work came from.

1983 was a very stressful year in our lives. My health was rather poor, and we were in the midst of a major financial disaster. We were just beginning to recover from the effects of the economic recession of 1981-82. These were circumstances that led to Al's change in career from medical research and teaching college biology to health promotion.

I can always tell when Al has a major creative period. He has many nights of restless sleep. Or, he awakes fully rested long before the alarm goes off.

During the time of idea capture for this book, he began to keep a notebook beside the bed, and most days I had notes to transcribe and illustrations to draw. He obtained a copy of a computer graphics package and the illustrations such as the "Functional Components of a Person," "Universal Relationships of a Person," "Wellness and Health States over Time" and "Evolution of the Healthcare Model" in Chapter 1, were first drawn on version 1.0 of Harvard Graphics.

I think that the seven dynamic processes used in the Matrix of Integrated Function came from the seven areas of physiology in which Al had to take doctoral comprehensive exams. (He failed the reproductive physiology exam and had to take it a second time. This, in the year our third child was born!)

His reading the C.S. Lewis classic, *The Four Loves*, and Leo Buscaglia's *Love* influenced the "four dimensions" part of the concept. Other books that influenced him at the time included Viktor Frankl's *Man's Search for Ultimate Meaning* and *My Experiment with Truth — The Autobiography of Mahatma Gandhi*.

On the personal level, I saw Al struggle to work through some difficult problems, and become addicted to racquetball. I had my own struggles with low resistance to infections and what we call "a severe case of genetic obesity." Through the years of preparation of this material, we had personal incentives to make it practical and applied.

Sometimes we gave up the project because we felt we were not good enough examples of what we were teaching. We had all the information necessary to teach a good program. We saw students who used the suggested activities and obtained good results. But somehow, we couldn't sustain the motivation and put in the work required to demonstrate that it worked for us. And that, in very significant areas of our lives. This led to the later chapters on cognition, emotions and motivation, reasons for procrastination and the personal pursuit of happiness.

Use of this book offers no guarantees of miraculous changes in health behaviors. It is my hope that it may be another tool and a little spark of encouragement to provide a push in the right direction.

I tried to capture a summary of this concept of a total person with hope and positive motivation breaking through obstacles to enjoy the beauty of life. This came out of a class assignment given early in the course as listed at the end of Chapter 1.

The assignment was to draw a personal symbol of total well-being. The concept that appealed to me was to capture the body, mind and heart of the individual connected to the rest of humanity as represented by the world, with the bright rays of early morning sunrise dispelling the dark clouds of obstacles in life.

Al and I refined this symbol over the last fifteen years, and then asked our graphics artist friend, James Arkusinski, to add his expert touch. He drew a computerized version, which has become the book cover.

My verbal summary to accompany the symbol is "love in all dimensions of function is the ultimate experience of health, wellness, self-realization and happiness."

The idea to have students compose a personal symbol of total well-being came from Viktor Frankl's concept of logotherapy. Used in a classroom situation, this activity has been a lot of fun. I hope that this book brings you a good combination of work and pleasure. It has given me such a combination to share in its development from conception to full-term birth.

It is great pleasure to go the distance with a soul mate.

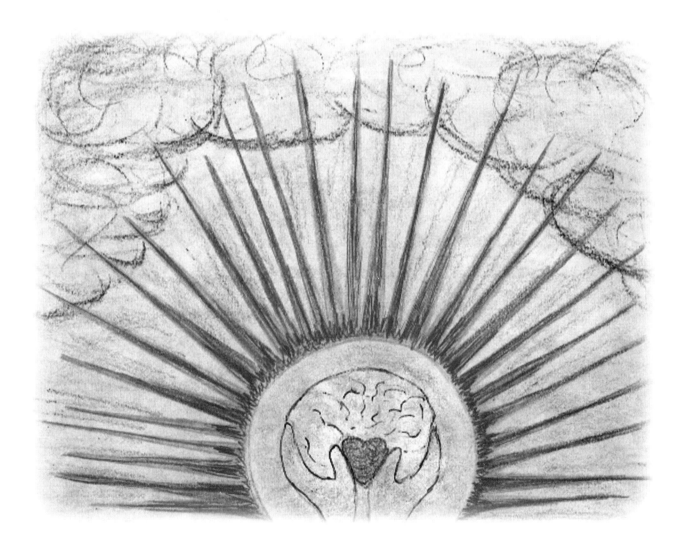

# Understand the Self and Whole-Person Healing

*"As one's sleep-smothered consciousness wrestles with a nightmare in its efforts to awake, so the submerged self struggles to free itself from its complexities and come out into the open."*

Rabindranath Tagore

One*1*

*Dedicated to*

**Columbia Union College**
**Takoma Park, Maryland,**

*where my quest for participation in wellness promotion began,*

*and to*

**The Department of Health Education**
**University of Maryland, College Park,**

*where that quest found focus and direction.*

The first house I helped to build was completed in three days. We gathered all the materials needed from the land around the building site. We dug the holes for the support pillars, built the frame, nailed on the lattice support for the roof and laid the grass roof in one day. The walls were woven in place and plastered with mud mixed with straw the next day, and on the third day we put up the inner partitions and moved the owner into his new home.

That was an unforgettable experience for a thirteen-year-old. Seeing someone's home being constructed and made livable in such a short time made a strong impression about building and framing for a building.

For a house, the foundation and framework are the most important parts of the structure. For personal wellness, the foundation and framework are also the most important parts of the structure. The foundation for wellness is a clear understanding of the self. The framework for wellness should be a model of healthcare that enables and empowers the individual to pursue optimum well-being.

## Defining and Understanding the Self

Thinking about "self" leads to several definitions. Each one contributes some understanding of parts where the whole is much greater than the sum of parts.

In biology, we say that the immune system is programmed to detect self from non-self. That is, the mechanism that protects us from foreign or invading organisms can seek out and kill bacteria, viruses and cancerous cells, while sparing the body's normal tissue. But when this mechanism or self-recognition fails, we develop "autoimmune" diseases. This is when the immune system cannot differentiate self from non-self, and destroys the normal tissue.

Another aspect of self emerges from how our mental functions operate. As the brain processes information, the way we deal with information, the way we learn, how we communicate with other people, use our knowledge and acquire wisdom helps to define a self. This self we call the "intelligent self." The variation of intelligence led to the concept of an intelligence quotient, the IQ. Fairly, and sometimes unfairly, this measure of intelligence has led us to label people as of high or low value with respect to their intelligent selves.

However, most of the common meaning of self connects to a third concept — what we have come to know as "the psyche." The self here is defined as the unique expression of what a person is, has been and will be. This is the essence of a person which gets programmed through the interplay of genetics, biological function, life experiences and the sense of value perceived in interaction with other people.

The psyche holds within it a description of several aspects of the self. These are the private self, the public self, the cognitive self and the emotional self. That is why we all seem to display different personalities under different circumstances.

Extremes of these differences may be dysfunctional or pathological. But even the most stable and consistent of us display

*The foundation for wellness is a clear understanding of the self.*

variations of our selves according to the environment in which we function.

The private self only the self knows. The public self is created by feelings of pleasure or pain in what we reveal of the private self. It is the image of the private self that we strive to display. The cognitive self is the mental picture we have of who we are and our modes of controlling that picture. The emotional self is the feeling and expressive self.

A fourth concept of self takes into account the individual's beliefs and values. The basis of deriving meaning and purpose in life is related to the essential beliefs and values of the individual. This is connected to the spiritual side of human nature.

Any definition of self must be related to body and mind. The body, the physical structure of a human being, is like the hardware of a computer system. The mind, the functional controlling mechanism of a human being, is like the software.

It has become necessary to health and wellness to know or discuss these definitions of self. They are important to understand whole-person healing, self-care and wellness. They are not just psychological constructs anymore.

Putting all this together in a simple schematic has been a topic of discussion with lay-people and professionals over the last fifteen years. The project was to merge the concepts and knowledge of body, brain, mind, self and spirit into one schematic that would help to clarify their relationships. What we arrived at after many revisions is shown in Figure 1-1. An attempt was made to include as much symbolism as may add meaning and insight to the illustration.

About three hundred students, seven hundred wellness workshop attendees and a dozen professionals offered critique and insights that were captured in this illustration.

Let us examine this schematic. Keep in mind these two major principles:
1. The foundation is the viewpoint that a person is not just a composite of body and mind but an integrated whole.
2. Integration focuses on function instead of parts or compartments.

Take your time to examine Figure 1-1 and see whether you agree with the following:
1. The body refers not only to the physical mass of flesh and bones but also to their functions which are based on the principles of biology, chemistry and physics.
2. The body is not as important as the mind, but without the substance of the body, mind function is not possible. That is why the body is shown at the bottom of the diagram and is smaller than the mind.
3. The shape of an octagon is used because the octagon is the universal "stop sign." It is a symbol for rules. The body and the functional parts of mind operate on rules and principles, some of which we understand, and some of which we don't understand.
4. Brain substance is part of body. All body functions are termed "physiologic functions."
5. The mind refers not to the physical brain but to the functions of the brain. Mind exists because of brain function. These functions are based on the computer-like

*The framework for wellness should be a model of healthcare that enables and empowers the individual to pursue optimum well-being.*

# Functional Components of a Person

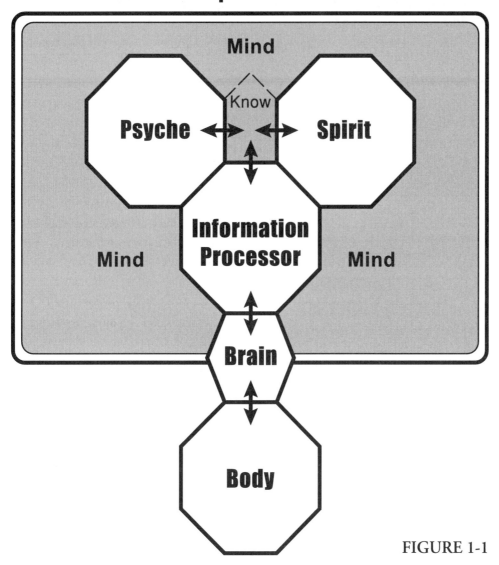

FIGURE 1-1

information processing capabilities which involve the brain and sense organs. These are "mental functions" and deal with information gathering, processing, storage, retrieval and use.

6. The mind has the capacity for conscious recognition of self as separate from others. This gives a person an identity, a unique knowledge of being a person. The personal value of the self is affected by interaction with others. These are "psychosocial" functions. They are in-corporated in the term "psyche" and are part of the mind.

7. The mind has the capacity to search for and recognize meaning, purpose and satisfaction with life. These functions provide the desire to live; give an interpretation of past, present and future; and reach for connection to and understanding of that which is beyond this world. These are "spiritual" functions. They are part of the mind and referred to as spirit — the human spirit.

The flow of information among these functions overlaps and intertwines so that a distillation of all information sets up a core of knowledge. This knowledge consists of facts and figures about the individual, other people, places, processes and things; a unique record and interpretation of all of life's experiences; and a set of beliefs and values that act as a guide to the desire to live with purpose, meaning and high quality.

## Defining and Understanding Human Function

In the process of integrating all the functions of body and mind, we experience emotions — conscious feelings and sensations generated by information interacting in the brain. Thus, a whole person with all the dimensions of function fully engaged is an emoting person with connections to other people and the rest of the universe.

This concept is depicted in Figure 1-2 which is intended to capture the viewpoint that the physiologic level of function is the most basic (and best understood), and that the spiritual level of function is the highest level, and probably the least understood and most individualized.

Figure 1-2 is a schematic of the relationship of the four dimensions, and their contribution to the integrated whole person. Each dimension contributes drives, emotions and capabilities which are integrated in the mind. The result of integration of the capacity to process information and emotion is IQ (Intelligence Quotient) and EQ (Emotional Intelligence Quotient).

As you examine this schematic, note the following:

1. The body of knowledge about how the four dimensions work is illustrated by the listing of items beneath each dimension. Most of our knowledge is about the physiologic dimension. The range of knowledge and relationships goes from the smallest subatomic particle to the largest entity, represented by the term "cosmos."

2. With reference to the cosmos, each of us defines a higher power according to our beliefs and experiences in life. Some beliefs personalize that power and use the name God or other appropriate term. Some beliefs depersonalize that power and call it "random events" or "the evolutionary force." This most distant relationship for some people may become most intimate spiritually. Since neither of these extremes can be proven scientifically, the spiritual dimension of humans remains the most mysterious.

3. The life sciences and conventional medical education emphasizes the study of the physiologic dimension. The social and behavioral sciences put emphasis on the mental and psychosocial dimensions. We used to leave the spiritual dimension to religion and philosophy. But all of this is coming together with the understanding that to practice whole person healthcare on an individual as well as professional level, we must understand the whole person and how all functions are integrated.

The above treatment of human function in four dimensions does not imply that these are physical compartments, that the functions occur separately or that there are no other functions. The implications are:

# Universal Relationships of a Person

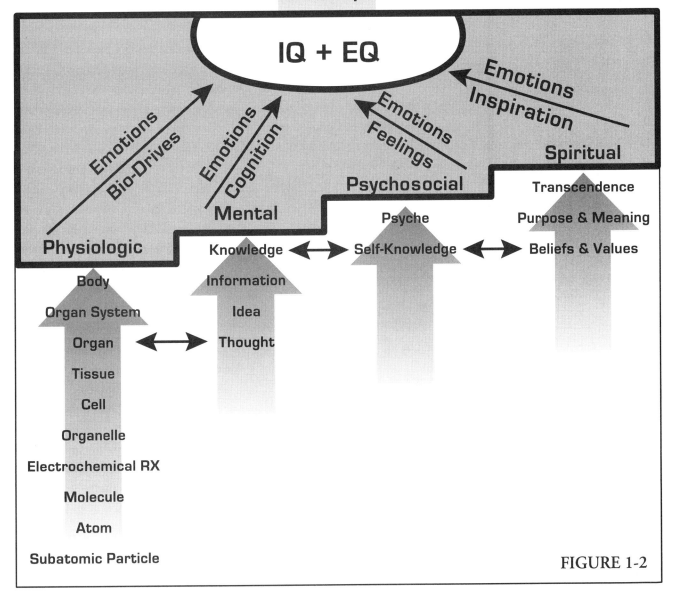

FIGURE 1-2

1. All functions are interrelated.
2. Physiologic function is the most basic level and the substrate for all other functions.
3. When physiologic function ceases to exist, all other functions quit.
4. It is in the highest level of function, the spiritual level, that humans define the final quality of life and judge satisfaction and fulfillment.

Let us explore in more depth what this all means to the way we are, the way we live and behave.

The physiologic dimension, which is the foundation, the substrate of the person, is the biology, chemistry and physics of the body. The integration of the biochemistry of body functions can be understood in seven dynamic processes.

These are:
1. *Homeostasis*, which means the maintenance of balance. This term was first used by the Harvard physiologist, W. B. Cannon, to refer to the mechanisms that keep the conditions that support life constant.
2. *Nutrition*, which refers to the processing of food material to extract energy and raw building materials for physiologic function. Since humans cannot produce needed chemicals from water, air and sunlight as plants do, they must break down complex food material into smaller chemical components that can move into the cells and be used in the chemical reactions of homeostasis.
3. *Stress adaptation*, which is the body's response to demands that push its mechanisms towards levels that increase the "wear and tear" beyond the normal process of aging.
4. *Work*, which is use of energy to produce changes in the environment, both internally and externally.
5. *Rest*, which is reduction in use of energy for conservation and replenishment of resources. This includes removal from awareness — a reduction of stimuli into the brain.
6. *Growth*, which is the process of maturation towards a state of optimal function and, eventually, the decline or loss of functional abilities.
7. *Reproduction*, which is the process of self-perpetuation for continuation of the species.

These dynamic processes of the physiologic dimension can be used to describe the other dimensions by analogy. Thus, we can speak of "mental nutrition," which can be defined as the process of supplying and using information — "food" for the mind. Or we can talk of "psychosocial reproduction" to mean the perpetuation of self in the relationships formed while living, and left behind when a person dies. This is a form of perpetuation of the individual. The primary aim of physiologic reproduction is perpetuation of the species.

Now, taking the four dimensions of function and the seven dynamic processes described above, we can construct a Matrix of Integrated Function. This helps to show how all functions are integrated and the possible effects of one dimension on another. It also gives a general guide for organizing information, applications and need for change with regard to health and wellness.

This is the purpose of Figure 1-3. The twenty-eight blocks can be studied one at a time, but always in the context of their

# Matrix of Integrated Function

| DYNAMICS | DIMENSIONS | | | |
|---|---|---|---|---|
| | Physiologic | Mental | Psychosocial | Spiritual |
| Homeostasis | | | | |
| Nutrition | | | | |
| Stress Adaptation | | | | |
| Work | | | | |
| Rest | | | | |
| Growth | | | | |
| Reproduction | | | | |

FIGURE 1-3

relationship one to the other in a dynamic, interdependent system.

Look at this figure again and speculate how any one block may affect or be affected by any other one.

## Health States

When it comes to health, whether of the body or the mind, it seems that we exist in one of three different states. These are:

1. The absence of disease. In this state, we are free from all dysfunction and malfunction.

2. The presence of signs and symptoms. In this state, we are aware that something is not working as it ought. Pain or other unpleasant feeling, and nonspecific loss of function, or hyperfunction tell us something is not right and we should check it out.

3. The presence of definite disease. In this state, whether or not it is fully diagnosed and has a name, we know that something is definitely not working right and needs fixing.

Figure 1-4 is an attempt to relate the health states to each other over any time frame. As you review your life, or the last year or two, you will see a picture of movement among these three health states.

# Wellness and Health States Over Time

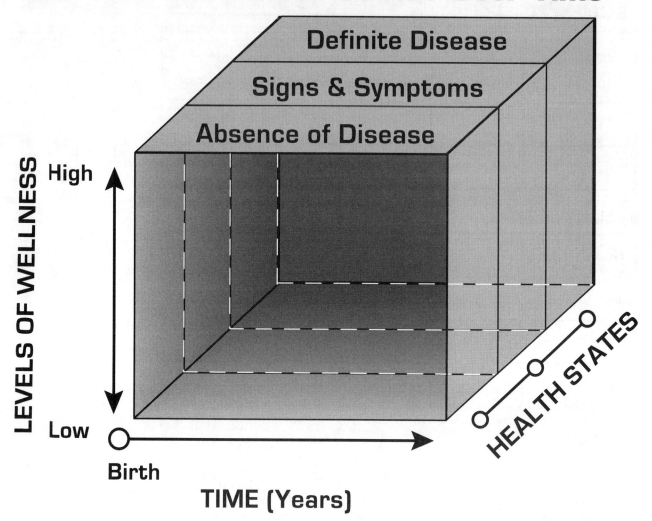

**LEVELS OF WELLNESS**

High

Low

**Definite Disease**

**Signs & Symptoms**

**Absence of Disease**

**HEALTH STATES**

Birth

**TIME (Years)**

FIGURE 1-4

The old concept of health left us only these three states of health. The new concept of "wellness" gives an additional dimension to health. In each state of health, the level of wellness can vary. For example, you may be entirely free of disease, or free of signs and symptoms of disease, but have low level wellness. On the other hand, you may have a definite disease, even a terminal disease, but have a high level of wellness. This is shown on the vertical axis, while the horizontal axis is a time scale.

Use this three-dimensional graph to help focus a general examination of how your level of wellness relates to your health state. Think of wellness as the product (of knowledge, effort, attitudes, emotions and beliefs) that helps us to live the best life possible, regardless of the health or illness state of the body.

Now that we have examined what we mean by self and how it relates to health and wellness, we must define whole-person healing. Understanding the self is the foundation; understanding whole-person healing is the framework.

# Whole-Person Healing

The framework offered for this personal wellness and self-realization approach is a synthesis of the best features of four models of healthcare. These are: the Biomedical Model, the Psychosomatic Model, the Biopsychosocial Model and the Holistic Model.

## The Biomedical Model

The Biomedical Model was defined when the principles of science were applied to understanding how the body works. Use of the scientific method for discovering, testing and using new information led to great developments in understanding normal and diseased states. This contributed greatly to diagnosing and treating physical diseases.

However, a rigid dependence on the scientific approach to healing resulted in a depersonalized system of care, a concentration on drugs and surgery as treatments and an emphasis on dealing with symptoms and single disease states instead of the whole person.

The medical knowledge and understanding gained up to the eighteenth century provide a good perspective to review the dramatic achievements of science and twentieth century medicine.

Figure 1-5 is a summary of the model of health up to the eighteenth century. It reflects the beliefs that:

1. There were four fundamental elements: air, fire, water and earth.
2. There were four fundamental qualities: hot, dry, cold and wet.

3. There were four constituent humors (fluids) of the body: blood, yellow bile, black bile and phlegm, which originated in the heart, liver, spleen and brain, respectively.
4. Human behavior could be grouped according to four temperaments: sanguine, choleric, melancholic and phlegmatic. These temperaments were determined by the dominant body fluid. Thus, a sanguine person (cheerful, talkative, self-centered, undependable) had an excess of blood. A choleric person (optimistic, confident, aggressive and inconsiderate) had an excess of yellow bile. A melancholic person (sensitive, perfectionistic, depressed and moody) had an excess of black bile. A phlegmatic person (calm, efficient, passive and lazy) had an excess of phlegm.

The use of the model to treat disease was simple. If a disease was due to excess blood, bleed the patient. If the disease was accompanied by hot and dry symptoms, treat with compounds or other methods to produce the opposite qualities of cold and wet.

It took the discoveries and theories of chemistry, physics, anatomy, physiology and bacteriology in the eighteenth and nineteenth centuries to make modern medicine possible. The current work in gene therapy, fetal surgery, organ transplant, designer drugs targeted to specific tissues and tremendously complex diagnostic instruments show the remarkable achievements of approximately one hundred and fifty years of science.

The healthcare model that emerged from this scientific foundation is what is called the Biomedical Model. It became

# The Eighteenth Century
# Unified Model of Healthcare

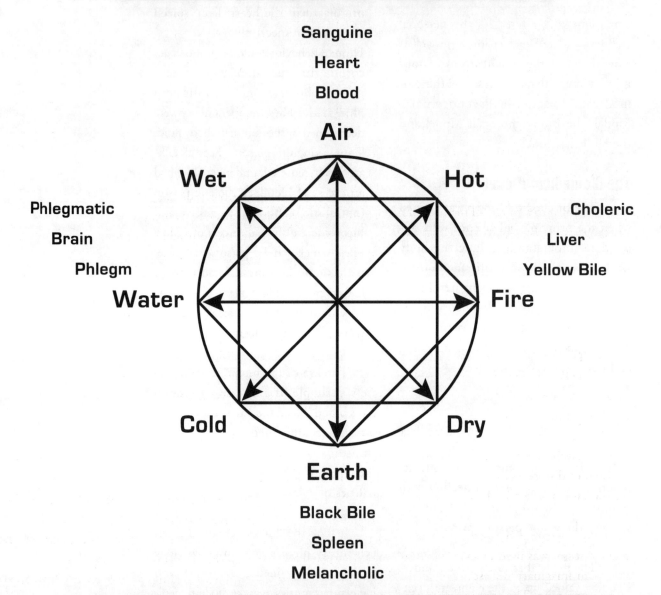

Sanguine
Heart
Blood

Air

Wet · Hot

Phlegmatic · Choleric
Brain · Liver
Phlegm · Yellow Bile

Water · Fire

Cold · Dry

Earth

Black Bile
Spleen
Melancholic

**The unified model of matter, health states and body function
which influenced the practice of medicine in the eighteenth century.
This model was the basis for the first personality type indicator.**

**(Adapted from Ackerknecht, 1982)**

FIGURE 1-5

formalized by the *Flexner Report* on medical education in the United States and Canada published in 1910 by the Carnegie Foundation for the Advancement of Teaching.

The recommendation of the *Flexner Report* was to teach and use only information that could be supported by the scientific method. Facts must be based on experimentation, objectivity and reproducible methods of testing.

This led to a model of medical education based on a reductionistic approach to understanding body function. Mechanisms at the cellular level became more important than how the mind and body affected each other.

## The Psychosomatic Model

The Psychosomatic Model grew out of the medical specialty of psychiatry and emphasized that the mind and body interacted in the disease process and in healing. Thus a "psychosomatic disease" was an expression of disease symptoms in the body with a cause or effect in the mind.

At one time, the term "psychosomatic disease" was used in some circles to mean "an imaginary disease." This is not its true meaning. The term refers instead to the condition that a two-way interaction exists between the body and mind.

The Psychosomatic Model became established in the 1930s as psychiatrists observed that a patient's illness was frequently associated with psychological stress and conflict. It was referred to as an integrational model and held that genetic, experiential, behavioral and environmental factors were involved in the disease pro-

cess. The model lost popularity in the 1950s as the rapid advance in the basic sciences, particularly in pharmacology, provided other ways of treating diseases. And the biomedical model, with the strength of the pharmaceutical industry, continued to dominate healthcare.

## The Biopsychosocial Model

The Biopsychosocial Model was strongly recommended by George Engel in his 1977 paper, "The Need for a New Medical Model: A Challenge for Biomedicine." This model came out of observations that in treating a person's ill-health, the psychology of the person and the social environment must be taken into account in understanding the causes of disease and in prescribing treatments.

The Biopsychosocial Model became the foundation of the medical specialty of family medicine. Several researchers added concepts such as the importance of ethnic and cultural factors.

## The Holistic Model

The Holistic Model became popular at a time when "alternative medicine" was regarded as a challenge to "scientific medicine." The key idea in this model is that any approach to health and healing must consider the object of care as a whole individual with a culture, a set of beliefs and practices, and a set of relationships and needs. Care for the whole person should address prevention, diagnosis, treatment and rehabilitation using any effective means of optimizing human function and healing.

The concept of holism was first introduced by Jan Christian Smuts in his book *Holism and Evolution* in 1926. The

*At one time, the term "psychosomatic disease" was used in some circles to mean "an imaginary disease."*

concept, however, did not become popular until the 1960s and 1970s, and the American Holistic Medical Association was organized in 1978.

Alternative medicine became popular in the 1980s as more consumers sought other means of healing besides drugs, surgery, chemotherapy and radiation therapy. The interest was reflected in such publications as *The Alternative Health Guide* and articles in leading medical journals. *The British Journal of Medicine* and *The New England Journal of Medicine* both published major articles on the subject in 1983.

A gradual increase in articles in mainstream science journals occurred through the decade of the eighties. Alternative medical practices, which may include treatments and therapies from folk medicine to established systems such as acupuncture and naturopathy, were discussed. Aakster, in his 1986 paper, "Concepts in Alternative Medicine," gave a review of the major alternative approaches and included acupuncture, homeopathy, naturopathy and paranormal medicine.

Beyond discussions in journals, the consumer was quietly leading a revolution in healthcare. An explosion of information in alternative therapies occurred in the decade of the nineties. A 1993 study by Harvard researchers, led by David Eisenberg, MD, and published in *The New England Journal of Medicine,* discussed the prevalence of use and the costs for alternative medicine. It showed that approximately one-third of American adults used some form of alternative medicine in 1990, and out-of-pocket spending was about $13 billion.

This information attracted international attention. In 1997, when the same group repeated the study, they showed that approximately 42% of the adult population used some form of alternative therapies with expenditures of approximately $27 billion. When the study appeared in the *Journal of the American Medical Association*, mainstream healthcare woke up.

A more recent survey by Stanford University, American Specialty Health Plans and Health Net revealed that, in 1998, 69% of adults used some form of alternative therapies. The more startling data from this survey was that 55% of these consumers reduced their use of conventional medicine.

The coming of age of alternative medicine research and acceptance of many of the therapies as complementary to conventional medicine can be dated from the fall of 1998. This occurred when the American Medical Association devoted all ten of its medical journals to the subject of alternative therapies.

The emergence of alternative medicine as a major consumer-led force is an outcome of the appeal of the holistic model.

## The Health Promotion Model

Taking the best features of the above models, a more recent model can be defined to summarize what is taking shape after three decades of discussion and slow changes. This model has not been officially or formally named, but the designation is obvious.

We should call it the "Health Promotion Model." The Office of Disease Prevention and Health Promotion within the US Public Health Service has even entrenched the framework of health promotion in its "Healthy People 2000" program.

The Health Promotion Model can be thought of as an approach to health and healing with the following broad outline:

1. The object of care is a whole person with potential for great good and great evil.
2. Disease prevention and optimization of the person's capabilities are of prime importance.
3. Proper diagnosis, treatment of and rehabilitation from disease must follow the scientific method.
4. Other modes of therapies must be established by the scientific method with an openness to incorporate these when they are shown to be effective and safe, even before the scientific mechanisms of action are clearly established.
5. The objective of health and healing is an enjoyable quality of life for as long as possible — promotion of "the pursuit of happiness."

The relationships among the various models of healthcare are shown in Figure 1-6. The Health Promotion Model is the current model. It is a synthesis of the best features of the older models. This is shown by having the principles of scientific medicine, mind/body integration, behavioral medicine and whole person healthcare incorporated into the model. The summarizing concept for all this is the term "wellness."

The next level of evolution of healthcare is being referred to as "Integrative Medicine." This is the leading edge of medicine. Integrative medicine refers to the incorporation of other therapies besides drugs, surgery, chemo and radiation therapy, along with all the goals of health promotion.

Many of the therapies once called alternative are now being used as adjuncts to conventional treatments. The term "complementary therapy," which was popularized by Prince Charles of England, is the term used to refer to those alternative therapies that have been accepted by many mainstream practitioners. These include acupuncture, chiropractic, Chinese herbal medicine, massage therapy, homeopathy and naturopathy. In many cases, the research evidence is incomplete, but the decision to use is made on the basis of two criteria:

1. Is it safe?
2. Is it effective?

The mechanism of action may be incompletely understood, but there is now an openness to consider the possible benefits of therapies once classified as "quackery."

Mind/body medicine is the set of behavioral and spiritual techniques that serve to integrate the functions of body and mind. These are becoming commonly used for stress management and as adjunct techniques in treatment of all diseases. These techniques include relaxation, guided imagery, biofeedback, prayer and faith healing, and meditation.

The establishment of a center to study alternative therapies at the National Institutes of Health is a major step forward in bringing promising complementary therapies into the mainstream. The National Center for Complementary and Alternative Medicine became official in the fall of 1998.

What of the future? We predict that the future model will be a wellness model. This will become entrenched by the year

*The objective of health and healing is an enjoyable quality of life for as long as possible — promotion of "the pursuit of happiness."*

# Evolution of the Healthcare Model

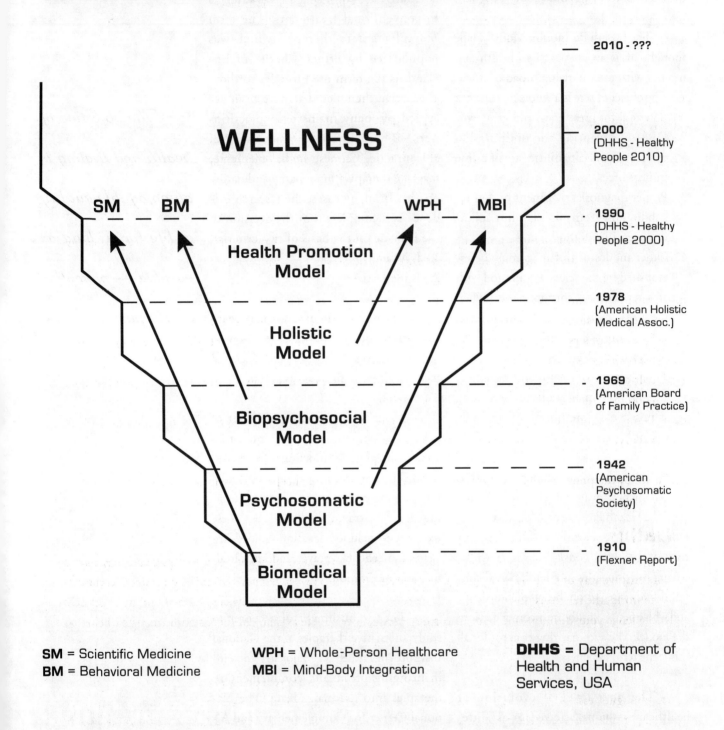

FIGURE 1-6

SM = Scientific Medicine
BM = Behavioral Medicine

WPH = Whole-Person Healthcare
MBI = Mind-Body Integration

**DHHS** = Department of Health and Human Services, USA

2010, the one hundredth anniversary of the *Flexner Report*. "Healthy People 2010" contains the seeds for a revolution in American healthcare because it involves you, the people, like never before. Check out the website (www.health.gov/healthypeople/), and see that your input is invited.

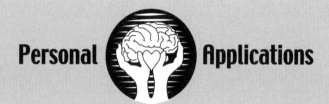

# Personal Applications

So how do the foundation of understanding the self and the framework of whole person healthcare contribute to personal wellness and self-realization? The following principles must be applied.

1. A person is the composite of functional dimensions operating as an integrated whole.
2. The dimensions of human function are physiologic, mental, psychosocial and spiritual.
3. The core of a person's being, which is derived from contributions of all four dimensions of function, is what we have come to call "self."
4. Self-care is the process of taking individual responsibility for prevention, optimization of function and getting good professional help when needed in the healing process.
5. Whole-person healing refers to the use of conventional and complementary modalities of care to involve all four functional dimensions in the healing process.

The following practical applications will help to individualize the concepts dealt with in this chapter.

## Directions:

The greatest benefit from this discussion will be to stimulate your own thoughts. For example, you may have a more creative way of expressing or illustrating the relationships between body and mind, the person and the rest of the world, the relationship among the various models of healthcare or the knowledge base of human functions. To challenge your thinking and make this study personal, complete as many of the assignments listed below as you care to.

As you complete the activities you select, add the pages you write to a notebook binder. If you are so inclined, use your thoughts, essays and the additional materials you collect not only as aids in your personal health promotion, but also as ideas for a book or syllabus of your own creation. There are many avenues to use wellness and health promotion materials. If you are in the wellness business, think of yourself as an educator and seek to develop a curriculum of your own.

In the space after each numbered item below, write the first thoughts and ideas that come to mind.

1. Look at each of the illustrations in Figures 1 through 6 for two to three minutes. After studying each schematic, write down what the illustration is telling you.

   Figure 1-1 (p. 5):

   Figure 1-2 (p. 7):

   Figure 1-3 (p. 9):

   Figure 1-4 (p. 10):

   Figure 1-5 (p. 12):

   Figure 1-6 (p. 16):

2. On Figure 1-4, try to graph the last three years of your life.

3. Write your own definitions for health, wellness, illness, pleasure, pain and happiness. (Don't think about what the experts say or even what the dictionary says. Just write what comes to your mind.)

Health is...

Wellness is...

Illness is...

Pleasure is...

Pain is...

Happiness is...

4. Design and draw a symbol that illustrates your concept of total well-being. Write here your first thoughts about what that symbol might be.

5. Write an essay titled "My Dissatisfaction with the Current Healthcare System, and How I Would Change It If I Had the Power."

6. Discuss the meaning and generalizations of the story at the beginning of the Preface. Write an ending to the story.

7. Tell a story that includes buildings, foundations, storms and survival.

If you take the time to do the above activities, you will find that instead of just getting information and new ideas from this material, you will be taking these thoughts and ideas and creating a synthesis based on your own knowledge and experience. This, to us, is the joy in learning.

# Reflections

One of the sources of enjoyment for us as we teach and lead discussions in health and wellness is to recall stories that add meaning and understanding to the factual material. Here is a story that got expanded over the years.

· · · · ·

A certain farmer sold his property to an urban real estate developer. The new owner intended to destroy everything on the property and build a suburban housing complex.

Walking over the property one day, the developer saw a stone protruding out of the ground at the site that he felt was ideal for his model home. This site would showcase his property and give such a grand view of the surroundings. He centered his whole plan on this selection.

The stone appeared to be small, unimportant and rather unattractive. It was not marble or quartz or any desirable building material — just a common rock, an ugly stone. The developer tried to remove the stone himself, but it was larger than he thought. He gave the assignment to his heavy equipment manager.

The manager thought it would be a small matter to have a bulldozer pry the stone loose and dispose of it when they started moving earth to dig the foundation for the model house. So nothing was done at that time.

Several months later, all the plans were in place and the crew was ready to begin digging the foundation for the $6 million house. The earthmovers started their work. An early task was to clear all the loose rocks and soil. The manager remembered the ugly stone.

"Hey, guys. Just dig it up and dump it somewhere out of the way."

The earthmovers and bulldozers worked all that day but as they moved the earth around the ugly stone, it kept getting bigger and bigger. The developer and the architect were called in. The manager explained, "We can't seem to find where it ends. The more we dig around it the larger it gets. Maybe you have to blast it or use it as part of your foundation."

"No way," the builder said. "That ugly, shapeless mass of good-for-nothing rock has to get out of the way."

The earthmovers worked all week and couldn't get the stone uncovered. Nothing could shake it from its position.

In exasperation, the builder called in the blasting crew. "Blast this ugly thing into kingdom come."

The blasting crew did its job and shattered the uncovered part of the stone into a million pieces. The earthmovers came back to remove the debris and finish uncovering what was left of the ugly stone. But again, they couldn't find the end of the stone. It kept getting larger the more they dug around it.

The builder finally gave in and the architect redrew the plans to incorporate what was left of the ugly stone into the foundation of the model house.

Several years later, a great earthquake shook that part of the country. All the houses in this grand suburban community were destroyed — except for the model home, which had the remains of the ugly stone in its foundation.

• • • • •

As you ponder the above story, some thoughts about the self, programming of the mind and early childhood experiences may come to mind. Some of the questions may be related to other ideas in this chapter. Our discussions on this led to the following questions:

1.  Do we need another model to direct our thinking or organize information about health and wellness?
2.  Is "the pursuit of happiness" really a part of health or does that human desire more properly belong to philosophy and religion?
3.  How do we define health, illness and wellness?
4.  Is it important to understand "self" and "self-realization" in order to be healthy or to pursue personal wellness promotion?

The deluge of health information, the confusion of marketing schemes and the sometimes conflicting claims of research findings leave an individual unsure about what to believe about health. A broad framework and a synthesis of general principles may be useful for personal health promotion.

We have tried to capture factual and symbolic information in each of the illustrations. For example, in Figure 1-6, the shape and position of the various healthcare models convey a sequence, a broadening of ideas and a contribution to the emerging model.

In Figure 1-1, size in the relationship of body to mind, the position of the brain and the broken lines among the functional areas of the mind are intended to convey concepts about how the person works. The mind is "bigger" than the brain. All functions of mind, whether at the conscious or subconscious level, may be fed by the same information processing mechanisms.

Figure 1-2 captures a hierarchical relationship among the four dimensions of function, the knowledge base for each dimension and the emotional components that make up a person. This schematic lays the foundation for the theme of the four dimensions of pleasure and pain.

Figure 1-4 gives time for analysis and personal application. It also exercises the mind to conceptualize in a three-dimensional perspective. This takes more effort for some than others. Moving up or down along the "Levels of Wellness" scale, while moving in and out of the three health states over time, stimulates a personal review of life in general. It is a challenge to push the mind into three-dimensional thinking. But such challenges are part of wellness promotion.

Self-care and whole-person healing involve personal responsibility and a search for optimum function. Fulfillment and satisfaction are goals of health promotion.

"The pursuit of happiness" is not only a part of health, but happiness is the greatest goal of health and health promotion. Therefore, religion and philosophy need to be examined for their contribution to, or obstruction of, health and wellness. Happiness seems to be an outcome instead of a charted goal in life. But conscious decisions, and the attitudes about events over which we have no control, affect our happiness.

Can we define happiness? It may be one of those things you know when you have or don't have, but you can't put it into words. Our attempt at definition is: "happiness is the sense of deep, inner conviction that life is good and worth living." Happiness is the why and how for going the distance.

Throughout these years of discussing Personal Wellness, the following simple definitions of health, illness and wellness seem to be the most useful.

*Health is the presence of proper function in body and mind.*

*Illness is the absence of proper function in body and mind.*

*Wellness is the product of the effort and attitudes we bring to the process of living the best life possible.*

High level wellness is the positive, vibrant, optimistic, productive, realistic, joyful way in which we function in sickness or in health.

As we have discussed and defined the self, we can now look at processes for optimizing the self. This calls for self-examination, self-understanding, self-acceptance, self-management and self-actualization.

Several educational efforts to teach health promotion have used various devices to focus on personal responsibility. These include the University of Wisconsin-Stevens Point SPICES model.

The acronym "SPICES" stands for the six-dimensional view of wellness. These are Societal, Physical, Intellectual, Career/Occupational, Emotional and Spiritual.

Other models that I feel give very instructive views of health and wellness are:

1. The Equilateral Triangle model of Allen and Yarian which arranges the soma, psyche and spirit as the points of a triangle with three equal sides.
2. The Cube Model of Eberst which uses six dimensions of health arranged as the six sides of a Rubik's cube. The six dimensions are physical, emotional, mental, spiritual, social and vocational.
3. The *American Journal of Health Promotion* model in which publisher Michael O'Donnell defines health promotion using the "five dimensions of optimal health." These dimensions are emotional, physical, social, intellectual and spiritual.
4. The *Spirit, Mind and Body Interconnectedness* model described by Hawks *et al*. This model arranges the spirit, mind and body in a spiral with the spirit at the center, the mind as the middle level and the body as the outer ring.

These conceptual models of wellness provide helpful views of the attempts to describe the integration and interdependence of function in an individual. Models are attempts to capture ideas and relate a body of knowledge to real-life applications. It would be extraordinary if no new models appear over the next few years.

However, what is needed is not another conceptual model. What is needed is application and real-life experiments — individual experiments in personal wellness.

*High level wellness is the positive, vibrant, optimistic, productive, realistic, joyful way in which we function in sickness or in health.*

To go the distance, you have to know yourself. Know the speed with which you live and slow down when that is indicated. Challenge yourself to make time for yourself. Read this book in a slow, contemplative mode, not as a speed-reading exercise.

## Carol's Turn

I attended a workshop back in 1990 with our daughter who was in the seventh grade at the time. The theme of the day was that people could be divided into four personality types called Sanguine, Choleric, Phlegmatic and Melancholic. At the end of the day, we came away with, as our daughter put it, "a yuuuccckkkyyy feeling" from wallowing in body fluids.

The workshop, however, gave me an idea. I could hardly wait to discuss it with Al. Suppose we take the four dimensions of function, physiologic, mental, psychosocial and spiritual, and use them as personality types. Would they explain general categories of human behavior?

*When I go the distance, I have to take myself along.*

Many of the people I have known over my forty-something years of living can fit into four groups. There are those who are naturally talented and suited for physical activity and pursuits; people who are naturally gifted for demanding mental and analytical work; people who are naturally caring, helping and supportive; and people who have deep spiritual insights and live inspirational, noble, fulfilled lives, seemingly naturally.

Our discussion led to these conclusions:
1. The four dimensions of human func-

tion are not sufficient to describe temperaments or personality.
2. In the face of all the knowledge we have currently about human physiology and psychology, it seems absurd to classify people according to dominance of a body fluid.
3. It probably would be equally absurd to classify people according to dominant dimension of function, if such a dominance could be determined.

I found that what I needed from this discussion was to apply the principles of self-care and whole-person healing to my life.

I have struggled over many years to control a severe case of obesity, which I believe has a strong genetic factor. I share the related psychosocial factors in Chapter 7. After trying and failing at everybody's diet or weight control program, I came to the conclusion that I had to use my own knowledge of myself, take control of my behaviors and do it for myself. An organized framework has helped me to construct a personal program that is being effective in my own time frame, for my own purposes.

This framework of personal health promotion aims to optimize pleasure and lessen pain in all dimensions of function. It may be an attempt at progressive change from one of "Do's and Don'ts and Can'ts and Ought To's." I feel this gives an optimistic outlook to personal health promotion.

As this new paradigm for healthcare in the twenty-first century takes hold, I believe people will face life and healthcare with more optimism, caring and "wellness promotion." Reform is happening at the theoretical level, the practical level and the personal level. This makes life more enjoyable. Is this part of "the pursuit of happiness?" I believe it is.

When I go the distance, I have to take myself along.

# EXAMINE YOUR CORE BELIEFS AND PERSONAL PHILOSOPHY OF LIFE

*"Wisdom is the principal thing. Therefore, get wisdom; but with your getting, get understanding."*

King Solomon

TWO

*Dedicated to*

*Families who touched our lives in very significant ways:*

**Thomas Uncle and Ellen Auntie (Mr. & Mrs. I.R. Thomas)**

*In appreciation for casting your bread upon the waters. It shall return after many days. But, most of all, thanks for your love and support.*

**Rob and Vimala Abraham**

*Thanks for your friendship that drew us into the Indian community of the Washington, DC, area.*

**Harry and Finnie John**

*Thanks for making us a part of your family celebrations and for a genuine example of unconditional friendship.*

our incidents contributed to the development of the ideas shared in this chapter. The point of these illustrations is to show that we have the potential to constantly adjust and improve the basis upon which we act. This is good when the change represents growth toward greater fulfillment.

As humans, our internal guidance system is programmed by our beliefs. The essence of the knowledge we acquire drives our actions on both conscious and subconscious levels. Our personal philosophy of life is our core beliefs. They guide our course and produce the standards against which we measure our values, our purpose and our meaning in life.

The philosophic framework of this book is this: we are what we believe. Our belief system, what we hold to be true at the very core of our being, is the drive that determines our personal path and our quality of life. We become what we believe we are. Therefore, we need to examine our beliefs and make necessary adjustments.

In the process, a greater harmony between beliefs and reality should develop. This is a personal and mostly private matter. But that is what we are talking about — personal wellness. Therefore, here and throughout this discourse, we cannot and do not want to persuade you to believe what we believe. Our aim is to stimulate your personal examination of your own beliefs and values, and to encourage you to aim for consistency between your beliefs and your behaviors.

The latest biologic evidence from researchers such as Herbert Benson of Harvard University School of Medicine shows a strong connection between our belief system and our biologic function. Psychology and religion have long held beliefs to be central in the understanding of what makes people do what they do. Science is now providing the empirical evidence.

See what incidents in your life may have affected you as the following experiences affected us. As you recall your own memories, write down some ideas for later sharing, discussion or writing.

## The Devil, Dead or Alive?

One of my close friends startled me one day with a remark about the Devil. He said, "I have met the Devil, and I am he." Following through on this thought, we explored our beliefs about the existence and nature of the Devil, also called Satan; how our beliefs and interpretation of what we were taught changed over time; what we believed at this point in our adult lives; whether any or all of that was true; whether any of it can be proved or disproved; how what we believed affected the way we lived; and whether any of what we believed about a Devil really mattered in our lives, for our well-being.

Our discussion spanned the disciplines of religion, psychology and physics. Did God create a Devil? If there is no Devil, can there be a God? The questions from the field of psychology were: Is the capacity of the human mind for evil the real Devil? Are personality disorders the

*Our belief system, what we hold to be true at the very core of our being, is the drive that determines our personal path and our quality of life.*

source of behaviors for which the Devil gets the blame? The question from physics was: How can the Devil enter the human mind? Or, if he cannot physically enter, how does he communicate with humans?

The answers were all personal and unscientific.

## Faith or Presumption: Case of the Manila Cab Driver

This incident took place on the streets of Manila, in the Philippines. I was riding a bus to get from Makati Hospital to the Manila Sanitarium and Hospital. At a red light, the bus stopped and a taxicab pulled up alongside. The driver of the taxi reached into his glove compartment, took out a Bible and read for a few seconds. He suddenly closed the Bible, threw it back into the glove compartment and took off full speed ahead. The bus remained at the intersection because the light was still red.

My thoughts were about why the taxi driver did what he did. Did he think the light was green? Did he feel invulnerable to accidents because of something he just read? Or did he see that the traffic was clear, no cops were around and he could get away with breaking the rules? And that, immediately after reading the Bible! It didn't appear that he surveyed the traffic carefully.

## "To Pee or Not to Pee — Nurse, That Is the Question."

I was ten years old and had to lie in bed for three months with my left leg in traction in the hospital in Kingstown, St. Vincent. A new Matron (equivalent to a Director of Nursing in a US hospital), a recent graduate from a British school of nursing, came to take charge of nursing care at the hospital.

One of the policies our new Matron instituted was to pass bedpans and urinals to the bedridden patients only at set times of the day. The schedule was three times a day, right after meals. If one of us needed the use of these implements at other times, we had to hold it for the next scheduled time of service.

We were on an open ward of about forty beds. The bed next to mine was occupied by a gentleman around fifty-five years of age. Mr. King had broken one leg while working on the docks.

One day, he needed to use a urinal and was told he had to wait for about two hours according to the schedule. He told the nurses that he couldn't wait and if they didn't want a wet floor they would bring him a urinal right then. The nurses felt they had to stick to the rules and denied him the "pee-jug," as it was known on the ward. With one leg in the traction apparatus, Mr. King pulled himself off the side of the bed, unwrapped his pajama bottoms, and proceeded to relieve himself.

Of course, this triggered a rapid response from the nurses. One ran to get a pee-jug, and another hurriedly brought a screen to put around Mr. King's bed. One ran to get a mop, and a fourth kept a lookout for the Matron.

## "We Will Speak Proper English from This Day Onwards."

As a young high school teacher in Richland Park, St. Vincent, I felt that I could make a difference in upgrading our everyday usage of the King's English. I was teaching English grammar in Forms 1 and 2 (equivalent to ninth and tenth grades in the USA). The two languages spoken on the island were labeled as "Good English" and "Bad English." All of us spoke these two languages — one in school and the other as soon as we left the classroom.

One day for English class, I decided that we would tackle the problem of Bad English. Each student would give an example of a sentence in Bad English, then recast it in Good English. For example, "Lay arwe go to de shap an buy a piece ah sahlfish." In Good English this sentence became, "Let us go to the shop and buy a piece of salted fish." The outcome of this exercise was to acknowledge that we knew Good English, to resolve to quit using Bad English from that class period on and to practice Good English for the rest of our lives.

Needless to say, none of us ever made the change that day nor for many years after that. Changes in use of Bad English came only as we got established in different environments. Over thirty years have passed since that creative English grammar class, and when we get together it is amusing and enjoyable to slip into the Bad English dialect. I heard that some of the islands are organizing their version of what used to be called Bad English into a dialect with rules of grammar and pronunciation. Who would have predicted that?

• • • •

When it comes to human behavior, and more specifically to health behavior, why do we do what we do in the way we do it? How do our beliefs about topics like the devil, God, creation, evolution, death, classification of people, etc., affect our lives? How does our treatment of other people affect our feelings of well-being? Why is it so difficult to make desirable changes, but so easy to pick up bad habits?

Part of the Health Promotion Model concept is taking personal responsibility for health. The outdated approach to health is not thinking about health until illness strikes, and then surrendering the body to the experts to be healed by whatever means necessary.

Intuitively, it seems good and useful to examine beliefs and attitudes as a preliminary to advocating changes in thinking and behavior. In one of his graduate courses, Dr. Burt used to give his students the challenge to examine their "presuppositions" about life, health, other people, goodness and badness, etc., before they designed educational and community programs.

A personal examination of beliefs may start with a few definitions. A **fact** is information that is held to be true. **Truth** may be defined as facts or conditions that are proven, established or accepted to hold for all times. (Facts change when new information is gathered or discovered. Does truth change?)

**Beliefs** are distillations of facts and truth that are filtered through individual experience and held with some degree of confidence. (Do beliefs change with experience?) **Perceptions** are the interpretation of facts and events filtered through personal beliefs.

A **theory** is a reasonable explanation supported by the known facts, and can be modified, replaced or expanded as new facts come to light. A **paradigm** is a general world view of a body of knowledge, or a model or belief that influences how knowledge is used.

**Knowledge** may be defined as facts, truths, beliefs, perceptions, theories and paradigms processed in the mind. **Understanding** is the acceptance of the usefulness of knowledge.

**Values** are the standards by which knowledge and understanding guide behavior. **Wisdom** is the conclusion about how knowledge and understanding affect the realities of this world, or any other reality there might be.

The above definitions are what these terms mean to us, given our exposure or lack of exposure to information from experts and ordinary people, as well as the slant of our life's experience. A good exercise at this point is for you to write your own definitions for the above terms. Another good exercise is to research what the classical and modern philosophers have to say about these subjects.

In dealing with knowledge, facts, truth, etc., how do we discover new information? The primary force is the capacity of the human mind to capture, process, store, retrieve and use information. Information enters the mind through observation, reasoning and intuition. Within a belief system where a Supreme Being exists, a case can be made for revelation.

A past period of human history was called the "Age of Reason" because it was believed that through observation and reasoning (cause to effect, deductive and inductive), truth could be discovered. The current "Age of Science" began with observation and reasoning, but with the added dimension of experimentation. A few examples are called for at this point.

The revolution in the field of medicine and healthcare started with Louis Pasteur when he disproved the law of spontaneous generation of life — that maggots automatically came to life from decaying meat, or mice automatically materialized anywhere old rags and corn were left. Pasteur conducted experiments that combined reason and testing of reasonable explanations to establish theories and facts.

Pasteur's greatest contribution was the germ theory of disease, developed between 1857 and 1885. Pasteur's work, and the efforts of Joseph Lister to introduce the use of antisepsis (hand washing, sterilization of instruments and use of disinfectants), were major breakthroughs in science.

In 1867, Lister linked the discovery of bacteria by Pasteur with a theory fruitlessly championed by Semmelweis in 1847.

Semmelweis had observed that many women died being examined by physicians who had not washed their hands following performance of an autopsy. At the clinic next door, run by midwives, the death rate was only about one-third that of the clinic run by physicians and medical students.

Semmelweis pleaded with the physicians to wash their hands before they examined the women, but his efforts were in vain. Frustrated and insane, Semmelweis died in 1865, at the age of forty-seven.

Lister started the practice of hand washing and sterilization of surgical instruments two years later.

Alexander Fleming's discovery of penicillin in 1928 was the next cornerstone in the foundation of scientific medicine. This led to the development of an extensive line of antibiotics and generated a major field of research in chemotherapy — not to mention the pharmaceutical industry.

The scientific method became the best way to discover and establish new information. The principles of the scientific method are:

1. An observation leads to a question.
2. The question leads to a possible explanation called a hypothesis.
3. The hypothesis leads to designing experiments in a way that can be repeated by others.
4. The results of the experiment lead to confirming or modifying the explanation.
5. This leads to generating and testing other possible explanations.
6. Knowledge increases and a theory develops.

The "Age of Science" is being superseded by a "New Era." This New Era is threatening to religion and science because it is feared that the scientific method will be abandoned and a "cult of spiritism" will take over.

What I think is evolving is an "Age of Tolerant Synthesis" where the best of the past is being integrated to make the best future.

Thus, the great philosophies and religions, science and the humanities, music and the arts, the trades and the professions, old-world, New World, Third World and First World, East and West all have something to contribute to the uplifting of the human condition. This is being synthesized in an emerging atmosphere of respect, appreciation and understanding for personal beliefs, cultural differences and personal worth across artificial lines of human stratification.

The competition, distrust, self-interests and concern for the bottom-line are still major factors, but inclusiveness and willingness to listen to other viewpoints are increasing.

This emerging atmosphere of tolerance gives a very hopeful sense of the new revolution in knowledge. As knowledge increases, no human can have it all, understand it all or use it all. (Why do some people act as if they do?)

This revolution brings uneasiness on the personal level in terms of what is truth, what is acceptable, what is right, what is good and what should I do. One way to find direction in a changing sea of information is to examine the personal past. See how personal beliefs have been established

*Values are the standards by which knowledge and understanding guide behavior.*

and modified. Determine what your core beliefs are. Make adjustments where indicated to achieve personal goals. Evaluate what standards or set of rules you have chosen to live by and settle for a level of effort that does not overtax the stress adaptation mechanisms of the body.

Some personal experimentation in living is helpful and enjoyable. There are those who would say that living is the greatest experiment in the universe.

At this point, it may serve a useful purpose to review your ideas, beliefs and personal philosophies on the following topics:
- the origin of life,
- the nature of the universe (from the big bang to the big crunch?),
- the nature of human beings,
- purpose in life,
- destiny in life,
- an after-life,
- a previous existence,
- death,
- good,
- bad,
- right,
- wrong,
- evil,
- suffering,
- stratification among humans, and
- the level of control you have over life's events.

If at all possible, write out *your* thoughts about these subjects — not what others have told you, not what the experts say, not what you believe other people would want you to say, not what you have to say to remain a member of any group, but what you yourself have within yourself.

*"I used to know for certain that the earth and everything in it was created in the year 4004 BC."*

What people believe or perceive about reality affects what they do and how they behave. One young woman expressed it this way:

"I used to know for certain that the earth and everything in it was created in the year 4004 BC. Jesus Christ, a member of the Supreme Godhead who created the earth, became incarnate human two thousand years later and would come back to purify the earth two thousand years after that. This meant that by the year 2000, life as we know it here would end. To be good enough to receive eternal life instead of eternal hell fire, I had to keep all the rules all the time without any mistakes. My life has been no fun."

There is enough knowledge in every dimension of human function, and sufficient methods to use this knowledge, for humans to live enjoyable lives regardless of the events over time. The human need in this New Era is a need for applying knowledge to life's daily hassles and demands in a way that tips the pleasure-pain balance on the side of health-promoting pleasure.

Tipping the balance involves not only an appreciation of the integration and interdependence of functions within a person, but also the integration and interdependence of peoples, cultures, branches of knowledge, different professions and different philosophies. This is happening in the Age of Tolerant Synthesis where "live and let live" and "live and help live optimally" philosophies are struggling towards the forefront. The Health Promotion Model of human interaction may be a good foundation for such progress.

The emerging Wellness Model will focus this effort and bring forces together that will transform the healthcare industry and transform our social condition. It is beginning to happen. Not too long ago, I visited the Prevention and Wellness Director of a large healthcare system. The level of community involvement was intriguing — the public school system, community self-help organizations, government social services and churches of all denominations were in partnership with the health system to affect community health. And the children and youth were the primary focus.

This is how we are going the distance as a community of wellness promoters.

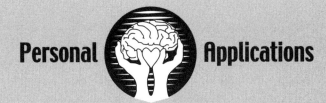

# Personal Applications

## Directions:

The following activities will help make this discussion personally meaningful. Select those that connect with your interests and write your first thoughts in the space provided. Develop the exercises with additional thoughts, ideas and information to add to a journal or notebook.

1. Write a statement titled "My Purpose and Mission in Life."

2. Write an essay on "My Beliefs about the Origin of Life on Earth, the Nature of the Universe, and If and How Life on Earth Will End." (It is reported that about one dozen asteroids approach the earth each year. A large asteroid hit is thought to be responsible for the extinction of the dinosaurs. What do you think of life on earth ending in a "lake of fire" followed by a deep freeze?)

3. a. Write down what you believe about what happens at death.

b.   Compose the eulogy and obituary you would like to have used after your death.

c.   Make a list of ten things you want to do before you die.

4.  Write a letter to a friend describing what your ideas of "the good life" were as far back as you can remember having an opinion, how those ideas changed over time and how the realities of your present life measure up.

5.  Rate your quality of life on the following scales by putting an "x" at the point on the line where your feel you are trying to capture what you really think about the way things are, and not what you wish things to be:

Physical health status:
low_____high

General anxiety level:
low_____high

Financial security:
low_____high

Quality of relationships:
low_____high

Sense of purpose and meaning:
low_____high

Overall happiness:
low_____high

6. Use the following diagram to discuss good and bad, right and wrong. First, define good, bad, right and wrong. Then list examples of things that may fall into each of the four blocks.

Good is...

Bad is...

Right means...

Wrong means...

|  | Good | Bad |
|---|---|---|
| **Right** | | |
| **Wrong** | | |

7. Consider sports. Take basketball, hockey and football. Notice how often players commit fouls and try to deny they did, or how often they break the rules of the game and try to get away with it. In terms of learning right from wrong, what effects do you think these sports have on children?

8. Comment on these reasons for doing things:

a. "Everyone does it."

b. "Do it. If it feels good, it must be good."

9. In the table of "Inventory of Personal Interests" below, check all those you feel are important for you to act on for your personal health status and well-being. Of all the items checked, select the top four and rank them with #1 being the most important.

# Inventory of Personal Interests

| | | | |
|---|---|---|---|
| ☐ | better physical fitness | ☐ | greater self-confidence |
| ☐ | improved nutrition | ☐ | greater intelligence |
| ☐ | stress management and reduction | ☐ | better memory |
| ☐ | disease prevention | ☐ | more willpower |
| ☐ | more or better quality of sleep | ☐ | more control over events |
| ☐ | improved sex life | ☐ | more money |
| ☐ | weight control | ☐ | more creativity |
| ☐ | cure for current illness | ☐ | fewer worries |
| ☐ | greater self-acceptance | ☐ | better communication skills |
| ☐ | improved self-esteem | ☐ | better decision-making skills |
| ☐ | better personality | ☐ | more control over bad habits |
| ☐ | less social anxiety | ☐ | greater satisfaction in life |
| ☐ | more privacy | ☐ | greater joy in living |
| ☐ | less loneliness | ☐ | more feelings of hopefulness |
| ☐ | better relationships | ☐ | greater feeling of purpose |
| ☐ | greater social involvement | ☐ | more meaning in life |
| ☐ | less negative emotions | ☐ | more positive emotions |
| ☐ | better career | ☐ | more inner peace |
| ☐ | less hectic schedule | ☐ | more satisfaction in loving |
| ☐ | more education | ☐ | more opportunities to be loving |

Top four:  1._____  2._____

3._____  4._____

10. Examine Figure 2-1, Personal Responsibility for Wellness. Comment on how to apply it to your life.

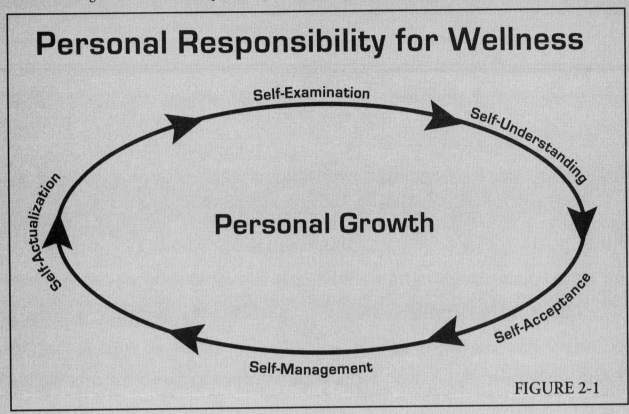

FIGURE 2-1

11. Discuss or write out your personal opinions on the following questions:

a. How important is physical attractiveness to well-being and happiness? Is the body a god or a temple? If a god or a temple, who worships?

b. Besides health and disease, are your dietary habits influenced by beliefs about right and wrong, sin and not sin?

c. When does human life begin?

d. Are there hidden meanings and instructive symbolisms in dreams?

e. Does a creationist or an evolutionist view of life make any difference?

f. Does a "spirit" entity inhabit human minds and physically take leave at death?

g. Has the human race improved over time physically, mentally, psychosocially, spiritually?

h. How does "self-actualization" or "self-realization" relate to selfishness, self-centeredness, selflessness, sacrifice and altruism?

i. Is there intelligent life, other than humans, in the universe?

j. Should the state regulate parenting by establishing licensing requirements?

k.  Is there any life for humans after death?

l.  If you were able to have all you want, what would be your lifestyle?

m.  If you had the power to change one factor that affects well-being for the entire human race, what would you change?

n.  In your observations of society at large, how do you see class structure, and what are some of the reasons for stratification among human beings?

# Reflections

Some of the beliefs, presuppositions, perceptions, knowledge and attitudes that helped to shape this discussion are:

**1.  Physiological function is the substrate and basis of all other functions of human beings. If the life-sustaining mechanisms of the body cease to exist, all other functions are lost.**

This position cannot be scientifically tested. It is a position reasonably assumed given a certain view of knowledge. Consequences of this position include beliefs about communication with the dead; past lives; reincarnation; the existence of God, the devil and angels; and what happens at death.

Personal beliefs on these subjects may not be important to health of the body, but settling or examining them may contribute to health of the mind. Health of the mind influences health of the body, so they may be important after all!

Based on the assumption above, what is the human spirit, and is spirit the same thing as "the soul"?

As a physiologist, I define the human spirit as the functions of the mind that process the larger questions of life such as meaning, purpose, connection to cosmic forces and the drive to find satisfaction in life. But from this perspective, the spirit, the human spirit, does not exist without the physiologic substrate.

Another area of discussion from the above statement is the question of origin of life. Given the complexities of physiologic mechanisms, how do you establish whether life began by design or by accident? How does either position affect the way people live?

2. **Human beings possess a great capacity for good and a great capacity for bad. Evil is bad willfully perpetrated.**

This necessitates a definition for good and bad. "Good is that which promotes the attainment of optimum function in all dimensions, for self and others, for the longest possible time."

"Bad is that which destroys or obstructs the attainment of optimum function for self and others for any length of time."

Sometimes, what appears to be good might turn out to be bad and vice versa. An optimist finds something good in most if not all bad things.

A general purpose of life statement can be "life is for discovering and optimizing our capacity for good, and discovering and controlling our capacity for bad." Final control of bad may be its total elimination. Is that possible? Is that probable? How?

Good and bad may be generally applicable, but right and wrong may need further definition on more personal terms, since specific codes and authorities will come into play.

3. **Quality of life is more important than quantity.**

*"Life is for discovering and optimizing our capacity for good, and discovering and controlling our capacity for bad."*

This can lead into discussions ranging from the use of heroic measures to sustain life, to when does life begin, and why do most humans want to postpone the time of death. Is quality of life purely subjective, or are there any objective measures?

These questions may be important to decisions on establishing a living will, the choice of a method of family planning and care of the elderly.

4. **All dimensions of human function are interdependent and integrated, and the whole is greater than the sum of the parts.**

A division into functional capacities and dynamic processes is convenient for study and examination, but no function occurs in isolation. The expression of function may be more prominent in one dimension or another but the whole person is involved in every action whether or not this is recognized on the level of awareness.

For proper mental function to occur, the nerve cells and transmitter substances in the brain must function in set electrochemical patterns. They must have glucose for energy and amino acids to build the proteins they use.

Likewise, the combination of biologic mechanisms and the environment determine our psychosocial characteristics. The synthesis of biology, environment, principles learned and life experiences together chart the development of the spirit.

5. **Rigid control of behavior according to fixed codes and exercise of willpower may not produce the highest quality of life.**

Observations by experts, such as Ornstein and Sobel who studied healthy people, reveal that living with passion and vitality may involve breaking some of the rules some of the time. Flexibility in following rules and recommendations while holding to non-compromise on some major principles is characteristic of spontaneous living and joyful coexistence.

The analogy I like to use is that of the reflex principle in physiology. A reflex action is one that is coordinated by the nervous system below the level of consciousness and results in quick responses. It occurs according to fixed rules of physiology but is not controlled by the reasoning, thinking, decision-making part of the mind.

Similarly, a mental reflex action is the quick response from the mind for information in answer to a question, or the humorous rejoinder or repartee that generates a laugh in its listeners. It is triggered, not arrived at, through processed reasoning.

A psychosocial reflex is an automatic action of caring and reaching out to people without having to weigh all the implications in terms of risks and benefits.

An example of a spiritual reflex is a spontaneous moment of response to something of beauty or inspiration that lifts the mind above the immediate to conclude, "It is well with my universe and my soul."

Reflex behavior is abundant in children. Here is one example that comes to mind. Check your memories to see what comes to your mind.

•  •  •  •  •

Our children, at the time, were ages five, three and one. Here is the memory:

The usual gang of friends was riding at top speed around the apartment building in Spartan Village at Michigan State University. The group of about ten ranged in age from two to six. Our oldest child was one of the leaders. Our three-year-old always seemed to hang back and bring up the back of the pack.

One day as I returned from classes, I stopped to watch them ride. As they rounded one end of the building, a little girl about three years old fell off her tricycle. Our three year old immediately jumped off his Hot Wheels, threw his mount aside and rushed over to assist the fallen rider. There was no sign of thinking or planning or decision-making about what to do.

I understood more that day about my son's behavior than anything in any class I had ever taken. I decided to not push him to be up there with the leaders of the pack. He seemed to be programmed with strong psychosocial reflexes for caring and watching out for others.

•  •  •  •  •

What I am saying here is that a fulfilled life, a happy life and a life with lasting pleasure may not be one lived with dogged efforts to keep all the rules. I have seen many examples of the neurotic behaviors characteristic of efforts to live legalistically and to exert control over every area of the life of another person. It is not a happy state of affairs for anyone involved.

6. **Control over life's events through planning and conscious choice may not be as real or as extensive as it appears to be.**

*Our three-year-old immediately jumped off his Hot Wheels, threw his mount aside and rushed over to assist the fallen rider.*

It seems that despite our best efforts to plan and chart our lives, many of the major deciding factors and turning points occur outside of our control. We can discuss many sides of the implications of this observation and how it may differ in different belief systems.

Where do coincidence, random chance and the involvement of a Supreme Being meet in the everyday affairs of human beings? The answer is a very personal blend of belief in what a person is taught, what is modeled in the behavior of significant people in the person's life, what is absorbed from authorities and what is learned from experience.

7. **The major quest in life seems to be to find comfortable acceptance in who you are and where you are going, whom you are with and what you are doing.**

This seems to sum up the areas of understanding yourself, accepting the things that can't be changed, changing the things you want to change, and doing it with friends who share a similar general direction in life.

The Prayer of Serenity by St. Francis of Assisi is appropriate here:

"Lord grant me the serenity to accept the things I cannot change, to change the things I can, and the wisdom to know the difference."

8. **Nothing happens before its time, and whenever something happens, its time has come.**

Dealing with time and having a world-view of time affects how we live and how stressed out we become about getting things done and about what things we should get done. Time management has been a major topic in numerous books and workshops. There is much good in learning to manage time.

However, since time is really passive and the same for everybody, maybe a better thing to do is manage yourself in the framework of your understanding of the importance, value and appreciation of the passage of time.

One gentleman in one of our discussion groups expressed his view this way:

"For many years of my life, I used to believe that I had only a short time (a matter of five to ten years) to be on this earth, and that the world on a whole would be destroyed shortly after that. To compound matters, I believed that within that short time to live, there was a cut-off time called the close of probation during which I had to be perfect in every behavior or I would be condemned to burn in hell fire with the devil and the evil angels.

"I always felt that I never had enough time to get all the good things done that I wanted to do. I also became so preoccupied in trying to be good every day in every little thing that I couldn't see or envision the larger goals of life. I used to feel as if I were pushing a large rock up a steep slope, and for every step of upward progress, I slipped nine-tenths a step downwards.

"Now, I find it fun to work through all this to the point of finding peace with my personal efforts to discover the good and bad within and deal with it. I can now plan as if I had a full lifetime to accomplish my life's goals, and at the same time accept that I may only have this moment and no more."

9. **Something good comes out of most bad things, sooner or later.**

This is a belief that seems to function as a protective mechanism when we are confronted with bad things in life. It seems that we have met more people with this outlook than people with the opposite outlook of "something bad is always lurking behind whatever good is happening to me."

10. **Given the opportunity, most human beings will choose to live where they have freedom to pursue self-determined goals, rather than where others control their thoughts and actions.**

This is seen in the history of forms of government where walls and restrictions are erected to keep people in, and forms of government where walls and restrictions have to be erected to keep people out. The changes in the geopolitical world over the past ten years have demonstrated that many people strive for freedom of expression and self-determination. The population's striving is only a collective expression of the individual pursuit of freedom, which is part of the pursuit of happiness.

11. **One of the anchors of satisfaction in life seems to be to have a strong belief that what you spend most of your time and effort on is worthwhile, fits with your world view of life, and contributes in some way to a high quality of life for self and others.**

This not only speaks to career and job satisfaction, but to leisure time as well. Many of us have little choice over what exact job responsibilities we perform, or where we perform them. Much of work and career is spent trying to find satisfying work. The career pattern of the eighties and nineties seems to be to switch careers two or three times before age fifty in an effort to find something more satisfying or more stable.

One of the saddest commentaries on a personal career is to hear someone say:

"I feel trapped in this job for the last twenty years. I do it only because it is a means to a paycheck. I hate the pressure of having to race the clock and fight the traffic to get to work, and when I'm at work I wish I didn't have to be there. Is this all there is to a career?"

12. **Unconditional love may be only a myth when it comes to humans. Maybe God alone is capable of unconditional love.**

Some humans may strive towards unconditional loving. Some, like Mother Teresa, may come closest to demonstrating it. It may be, however, that a lot of unconditional loving goes on in the quiet and unknown of everyday human existence, unnoticed by others but experienced by the lover and the beloved.

Some of the most beautiful human relationships are demonstrations of efforts to love unconditionally — efforts to value and support people without regard for their past mistakes, their present flaws and their future possibilities, good or bad. If humans strive to do this, how does God deal with humans who seem incapable of doing everything right all the time?

*"I hate the pressure of having to race the clock and fight the traffic to get to work, and when I'm at work I wish I didn't have to be there. Is this all there is to a career?"*

Our beliefs are the fuel for living. But it may be that in preparing to go the distance, we forget to plan for fuel.

In January 1996, the heating system in our house did not work on one of the coldest days of the year. The service person came and diagnosed the problem as an empty oil tank. How could the tank be empty when our oil supply was on an automatic schedule with the oil company?

Apparently, I had canceled an old service agreement and told the oil company that I would choose another company or call them to resume delivery. The arrangement was made in the summer and I forgot about it. An emergency delivery solved the problem, and the lesson was not lost.

This discussion on a philosophical framework for personal wellness does not aim to teach anything new, or change your personal beliefs. It is not an automatic supply of "oil" for the furnace of the mind. It is not an emergency delivery of fuel.

Its aim is to remind, to help focus and to encourage personal efforts to ponder the larger questions of existence and to add meaning to efforts to take charge of what is controllable in life.

One of the prominent pieces of information in the health promotion literature is the summary of the factors affecting quality of life. This was first published as a document, *The Ten Leading Causes of Death in the United States*, in 1979, by the Centers for Disease Control in the US Department of Health and Human Services. It included a "Quality of Life" circle showing that, of the factors determining quality of life, 24% was linked to genetics, 12% was attributable to the healthcare system, 16% was environmental, and 48% was connected to lifestyle.

It is currently accepted that over 50% of the factors affecting our quality of life is related to lifestyle. Figure 2-2 presents this in graphic form for impact.

Current life expectancy in the USA is 76 years. The fastest growing segment of the population is those living to be a hundred and more. Current research is showing that it is possible to increase the length of the healthy years of life. But because of the fear of chronic disease and loss of function, sixty-three percent of people responding to a recent survey said they do not want to live to be one hundred. (Survey con-

# Quality of Life Factors

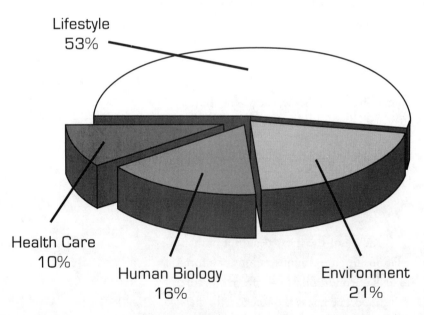

Lifestyle
53%

Health Care
10%

Human Biology
16%

Environment
21%

**(Adapted from Anspaugh, 1994.)**

**FIGURE 2-2**

ducted by the American Association of Retired Persons.)

At some point, the individual settles for a belief about the goodness of quality versus quantity. To go the distance, the belief system sets the clock — allowing for accidents and acts of God, of course.

## Carol's Turn

Al and I grew up in different cultures. However, our belief system and approach to life was shaped by the same subculture. We read mostly the same books, were taught the same religious beliefs, shared similar values and world view, and had similar neurotic behaviors.

I believe that most people have neurotic behaviors, and it is interesting to see examples of it. My understanding of a neurotic behavior is something humans do that is in direct conflict with what they claim to believe. The conflict may lead to a mismatch between what they believe the world should be like, and what reality is. Neurotic behavior ranges from mild conflicts in everyday life to the pathological. So the experts tell me.

Some illustrations of the conflicts in beliefs that we have worked through together over the years come to mind.

When we were at the University of Virginia, Ralph Sampson was the star on the basketball team. There was a Saturday game with the North Carolina Tarheels who had Michael Jordan and James Worthy on their team. This was a game Al really wanted

to see, but since it was a "holy day" for us, he felt he shouldn't.

His solution was to put the kids to bed, go to our bedroom, lock the door and watch the game on TV at low volume. To me, this was a classic expression of neurotic behavior. Al's debate on this issue was not about neurotic behavior but about sin and not sin.

I also recall on one occasion when we went grocery shopping, and we had packages of meat in the shopping cart. He was careful to avoid being seen by our minister who was in the grocery store at the same time. Al must have felt embarrassed to be known as a non-vegetarian by an authority figure who was a vegetarian. To my layperson's understanding of "neurotic," this again was a classic example.

Over the years, we have tried to examine why we do certain things and how we feel about the need for change. The primary need for change was our goal to help our children avoid as many conflicts in living by rigid rules as we had experienced. We were taught to be ultraconservatives, and our children were facing a more liberal environment. How do we adjust without losing our major values and principles?

One of the triggers to review our beliefs started when we were at Andrews University in Berrien Springs, Michigan. The questions finally got resolved about nine years later. They related to very fundamental beliefs, and we review the process here only as an illustration.

Al has always kept me involved in his class work. Not just as a helper but as an active participant in discussing ideas, especially new ideas from his course materials. One day he came home from a class in philosophical biology and was really disturbed.

At that session, a Hebrew language professor had described the account of the creation story of Genesis as the "use of picturesque language common to Hebrew writers that in no way attempted to give a historical account of earth's beginning." We were both fundamental believers in a literal six days of creation events "in the beginning."

*We survive on the conclusion that the good outweighs the bad, and our pleasure has been greater than the sum of all the pain.*

This discussion grew more pleasantly intense at Michigan State University. Some of his fellow graduate students would question his beliefs in stories of the Bible. They would ask questions like, "You mean there was a tree in the garden and Eve ate the apple and gave one to Adam and that was their sin?"

"How about another explanation like, after Adam and Eve discovered that they were of opposite sexes, Eve seduced Adam before they had permission to begin the process of procreation?"

If the original Genesis account was in "picturesque Hebrew," maybe these graduate students had a picturesque point.

Similar questions were asked about stories of the Bible such as Balaam, "You mean that God got frustrated with Balaam and finally told him to go on this journey and then sent an angel to block his way so that a donkey could get in the final word?"

Or how about Jonah? "You mean that God could find only one man to take a message to Nineveh and had to guide a whale to swallow him and vomit him up on the shore of this country after three days of oxygen deprivation?"

After several years of off-and-on discussions about these subjects, Al finally came up with a resolution. He said he had a concept of how his beliefs in creation, his acceptance of the Bible as inspired scholarly literature and his interpretation of the information available in the debate on the age of the universe fit together. By this time he had taken me to see the film "A Brief History of Time" based on the book of that title by Stephen Hawking.

He proceeded to explain a theory he called "A New Theory of Creation." It included explanations for the age of the earth, the origin of the universe, something he said scientists called dark matter and light matter, nothingness and bubbles, and somethingness and wobble, and expansion and contraction, and special creations according to rotational cycles, and life on other planets in other galaxies, and other jumbles of ideas that I don't want to try to comprehend.

My question was, "Does it really matter, anyway?" To me, it didn't. I have a very simple belief system that doesn't get troubled by such ideas. To him, it meant a great deal because a core belief had been challenged, and he had resolved his questions.

One beach incident may illustrate my point. It occurred at Ocean City, Maryland. We were in the water riding the waves when a big wave knocked us down. I was pushed up on the beach. But Al was sucked under the wave and got caught up in the undertow. When he finally surfaced, he started swimming out to sea. Later he explained that he thought he was heading for the beach but was still disoriented by being roughed up by the surf.

We have had fun experimenting with adjusting our beliefs and practices. Our guide has been the authorities we subscribe to and what we believe we have learned from life's experiences. There is a wealth of information available, and our problem has been to limit the sources of information and advice to what we felt were the credible sources for us.

Another of the core beliefs we dealt with is the question of whether life's events are all preprogrammed, directed by God, or simply left to chance and the laws of nature. We had interpreted the events that brought us together as more than mere chance.

Meeting at an odd hour of the night because of our need to work on campus was the first event. About two months after our first date, Al decided that we should not date exclusively because of the social pressures due to our racial difference. However, as a result of my sprained ankle, we ended up spending a lot of time together with him helping me to get to classes. When we finally broke up at the end of the quarter, I thought that was it.

Curiously, he broke his ankle and came back to school on crutches. How would he get around on campus in the dead of the Michigan winter? He had moved to off-campus housing, which was less expensive, and was walking about one-half mile to a 7 o'clock morning class, on crutches.

I had a car on campus so I would get up and take him to class. This time together gave us more opportunities to know and understand each other, and the friendship grew into the romance that is now twenty-nine years old.

As we review these years, interpret what our realities have been, and read the opinions and ideas of the experts, we tend not to place such great importance on co-incidences as we did back then. However, we still maintain that our view of life was right for the time. We take the good and bad of life in stride. We survive on the conclusion that the good outweighs the bad, and our pleasure has been greater than the sum of all the pain.

I think that the book, *The Examined Life* by the Harvard philosopher Robert Nozick, had a lot of impact on Al's ideas as he led discussions in these aspects of wellness and health promotion over the years. Books like that are for him and not for me.

I prefer lighter fare such as *The Peak to Peek Principle* by Robert H. Schuller; *The Road Less Travelled* by M. Scott Peck; *Notes from a Friend: A Quick and Simple Guide to Taking Charge of Your Life* (this was neither quick nor simple but instructive) by Anthony Robbins; *Dare to Win* and *The Aladdin Factor* by Jack Canfield and Mark Victor Hansen; and, of course, the inspirational and motivational articles in the *Reader's Digest*.

When I put together my life experiences, my values and belief system, the social environment I grew up in, the joys and sorrows of mothering three children (and losing a fourth at midterm because of the Dalkon Shield), and the challenges of crossing mid-life in the nineties, my layperson's summary is as follows:

1. Life changes as growth occurs, but "where there is life, there is hope."
2. As humans, we tend to be our harshest critics, our most unforgiving creditors and our worst taskmasters.
3. Self-acceptance precedes other people's acceptance.
4. Thank heavens for true friends both young and old.
5. When the clouds part and the sunshine breaks through, you know deep down that life is worthwhile even though clouds may again cross your sky.
6. Socrates is supposed to have said, "The only life worth living is the self-examined life." These days everybody wants you to examine everything (or they offer to examine it for you for a fee, of course). Maybe the over-examined life isn't worth living either.
7. Experiencing pain makes pleasure more meaningful.

I believe that people everywhere, regardless of how much or how little formal education they have, know their personal systems of beliefs. Examining this belief system, with input from reading other people's ideas and insights, can contribute to approaching life at any stage with more confidence and healthy pleasure.

Two other stories come to mind as I close this chapter. One, I wonder how different our lives would have been if we had not moved to the Washington, DC, area in 1981. Al had been offered a full-tuition scholarship from the University of North Carolina at Chapel Hill to do a master's degree in public health in cardiovascular epidemiology. He turned it down. It is interesting to review the beliefs and decision-making process that led to that turning point in our lives, and to

be at peace with it.

The other is our decision in 1974 not to be part of the lawsuit that sent the A. H. Robbins company, the makers of the Dalkon Shield, into bankruptcy. We had a good case but accepted the token payment. What were our beliefs and the decision-making process that led us to pass up a chance at around one million dollars as awarded to others? Probably neurotic behaviors! That was a turning point in our lives that caused some adjustments in beliefs. We have come to acceptance and peace with that also.

Beliefs, more than facts and figures, are the game-masters of the circus of our lives. Each person is different. Each belief system is to be respected. We grow as our beliefs bring harmony, peace and comfort with acceptance of ourselves, and acceptance of others as they are.

To go the distance, I must know what I believe, even when the belief is that it is not important to examine my beliefs.

# UNDERSTAND THE BASICS OF PERSONALITY THEORY

*"To love and to give,*

*these are the supreme virtues."*

Rabindranath Tagore

Three

*Dedicated to*

**Al's six brothers, three sisters and their families**

*We want to do our part to take the "func" in dysfunctional and just shorten it to "fun."*

*and to*

**Carol's brother, sister and their families**

*We wish we could see you all more often.*

*P*art of the discipline of higher education is the absorption in one area of study and research to the exclusion of others. It is a matter of time, energy and interest. In the fourth year of a doctoral program in human physiology, I had no appreciation for what was happening in the field of psychology. My only course in psychology was an introductory course in college where the emphasis was on learning dates, terminology and names to regurgitate on tests to get a good grade.

However, personal life events stimulated the interest that led me to search for a layperson's overview of personality theory. Here's the story:

• • • • •

The second of our three children had episodes of temper tantrums that ended with him passing out, turning blue at the lips and having mild convulsions.

My area of concentration in research was cardiovascular physiology, and the first explanation I thought of was "blue baby syndrome"—a structural problem with the heart and major blood vessels. But the doctors could find nothing wrong with either his heart or the electrical patterns of his brain. One physician mentioned something about ego and super-ego conflicts, middle child syndrome and possible need for psychoanalysis.

Our health insurance (pure illness insurance in those days) didn't cover such needs, and I decided that I should learn about those things myself. (Our son outgrew those episodes and today, at twenty-four, is one of the gentlest and most thoughtful young adults I know, if you'll pardon a biased father.)

• • • • •

What came out of that personal study, and what I have used in the classroom over the past fifteen years in one form or another, I call "A Layperson's Summary of Personality Theory."

"In the beginning, there was Freud." That's what many of us took away from our college psychology class back in the 1960s. However, before Freud proposed his psychoanalytic theory of personality in 1905, the discipline of psychology had to be established as a science.

## Historical Perspective

A brief review of the history of Psychology sets the perspective for modern personality theory. This information is gathered at the textbook level from works such as Wayne Weiten's, *Psychology: Themes and Variations*; Baughman & Welsh's, *Personality: A Behavioral Science*; H. J. Eysenck's, *Fact and Fiction in Psychology*; Morton Hunt's, *The Story of Psychology*; C.S. Hall's, et al., *Introduction to Theories of Personality*; Nathan Brody's, *Personality in Search of Individuality*; J. Hettema and I. J. Deary's (eds.), *Foundations of Personality*; Raymond Barglow's, *The Crisis of the Self in the Age of Information — Computers, Dolphins and Dreams*; L. A. Pervin's (ed.), *Handbook of Personality — Theory and Research*; and K. Craik, R. Hogan and R. Wolfe's (eds.), *Fifty Years of Personality Psychology*. There are many other excellent textbooks of psychology, but I mention here only those from which I gleaned information for this summary.

Important early influences on the development of psychology before Freud include the ideas of Hippocrates (fourth century BC) who:

- used philosophical methods based on the nature of matter which was thought to be composed of four elements — earth, fire, air and water;

- taught that human function was based on four body "humors" — blood (corresponding to fire), black bile (corresponding to earth), yellow bile (corresponding to air) and phlegm (corresponding to water). These humors, working together, fueled the machinery of life; and

- classified people into two groups based on physique: thick, muscular, strong — subject to strokes; and thin, delicate, weak — subject to tuberculosis.

The disciples of Hippocrates described behavioral temperaments based on the theory of a predominant body humor. Thus, excess blood produced a sanguine temperament, excess yellow bile a choleric, excess black bile a melancholic, and excess phlegm a phlegmatic.

Galen, in the second century AD, revived and popularized the humoral classification of Hippocrates.

In the eighteenth and nineteenth centuries:

- Gall and Spurzheim developed phrenology, which associated bumps and indentations of the skull with personality.

- Kretchmer classified manic-depressive psychosis and schizophrenia and related

them to three basic types of physique: asthenic (frail/thin); athletic (muscular/vigorous); and pyknic (plump).

- Wilhelm Wundt, the "father of psychology," combined philosophy from Hippocrates with techniques of the scientific method then being applied in the field of physiology. Wundt established a laboratory for research in psychology at the University of Leipzig in 1879.

- G. Stanley Hall founded the first American research laboratory for psychology at Johns Hopkins University in 1883.

Sigmund Freud, a neurologist by training, was the first to introduce the idea of a prominent role for the unconscious. His method of study, called "psychoanalysis," grew out of treating patients with mental disorders, and probing his own personal anxieties, conflicts and desires.

Carl Jung and Alfred Adler were early disciples of Freud who developed their own theories within psychoanalysis.

In 1913, John B. Watson proposed that the study of the conscious or unconscious be abandoned because they could not be studied by the scientific method. He advocated the study of behavior, which could be observed directly, and study results could be subjected to verification by others.

In the 1940s, Hans Eysenck, merging Carl Jung's typology of extraversion and introversion with his own typology of neurotic states (stable and unstable), came up with a cluster of factors distributed around the four temperaments of sanguine, choleric, melancholic and phlegmatic. In a chapter titled "Personality and Eysenck's Demon", in his book, *Fact and Fiction in Psychology*, he presented a merged version of personality factors. He suggested getting away from the old terminology by using the trait names which are "the results of a considerable amount of empirical research."

In the 1940s, William Sheldon proposed another classification of styles of human behavior based on a biological premise. This was probably inspired by the classification of physique by Hippocrates. Sheldon had conducted what he thought were well-designed experiments to match body type to personality traits and came up with the endomorph, mesomorph and ectomorph classification scheme.

Later researchers abandoned this classification because its premise was suspect and its methods were flawed by experimenter bias. However, Sheldon's work was important because it connected genetics to body type and to behavior.

The next major school of thought, the humanistic movement, began with Carl Rogers and Abraham Maslow in the early 1950s. Around this time, B. F. Skinner published his work *Science and Human Behavior* which proposed theories similar to Watson's, but in an even stronger tone.

The work of these researchers led to the establishment of three major views of personality (and therapy) referred to as Psychodynamics (the first force), Behaviorism (the second force) and Humanism (the third force). The theories and other areas of research which do not fall into these three schools of thought are called the Factor and Typological theories, and the Field theory. These latter theories emphasize personality traits and are based more on biological rather than mind processes.

The contributions of Gestalt psychology, dealing with learning and perception in a "whole-person view," may be grouped with Humanism. Also, Existentialism, which rejects the concept of the unconscious and relies on studies of immediate experience, can be placed in the humanistic school of personality psychology.

For purposes of this lay summary, the groupings of Psychodynamic, Behavioristic, Humanistic and Biological (Trait/Factor/Typological Theories) will be used.

A brief overview of the major contributors to the various personality theories may be helpful for an appreciation of the complexities of explaining human behavior. This may serve as a stimulus for more in-depth study on the subject for enjoyment and personal applications. But first, a definition of personality:

"Personality is the individual's unique set of behavioral dynamics, generally consistent over time." This is a composite definition from the sources I reviewed for this summary.

A definition I memorized in grade school went like this: "Character is the sum of the qualities of a man's mind, of his soul and of his body. Personality is the sum of those qualities which other men see or feel." (When this was written, "man" was used to mean all humankind.)

# The Psychodynamic Theorists and Their Theories

This school of thought held that personality developed from the conflicts between the conscious and subconscious. The major points are listed here as a barebones outline.

## Classical Psychoanalysis

### Sigmund Freud

- Behavior is the outcome of the interplay of three structures of personality:
  1. the id — the primitive, instinctual drives of biology, which operate on the pleasure principle and demand immediate gratification;
  2. the ego — the rational, decision-making component of the mind which operates on the reality principle; and
  3. the superego — the moral component of personality blending knowledge of social standards and the conscience.

- Personality resulted from the interaction and conflict among these three structures acting across three levels of mind function: the conscious, preconscious and unconscious.

- Other concepts contributed by Freud include instinctual drives, libido, defense mechanisms, five stages of psychosexual development, penis envy, fixation, the Oedipal complex, dream analysis and free association.

## Individual Psychology

### Alfred Adler

- an early associate of Freud

- developed an "individual psychology" that differed from Freud's

- contributed concepts on the effects of birth order and child-rearing practices, the development of inferiority or superiority complexes and the results of efforts to compensate for these.

## Analytical Psychology

### Carl Jung

- a contemporary of Freud who disagreed with Freud's emphasis on sexuality

- blended religious views into a theory describing a personal and a collective unconscious

- promoted the concept of archetypes and the introvert-extrovert personality types

- described four psychological functions: thinking, feeling, sensing and intuiting

## Interpersonal, Social and Ego Psychology

Several theorists, without discarding the Freudian doctrines, developed their own systems of psychoanalysis based on their extensions of the major principles. These "neo-Freudians" took parts of the psychoanalytic foundation and extended them by accounting for the influence of personal, cultural and social factors.

**Karen Horney**

- first female personality theorist

- emphasized interpersonal relationships and the growth principle

- described a healthy personality as "a balance among tendencies to move towards people, move away from people, and move against people;" imbalance produced neurotic behavior

**Heinz Hartman** and **Anna Freud**

- dealt more with the ego and conscious processes than with the id and unconscious processes

**Erik Erikson**

- proposed the first model of personality development and change across the lifespan

- held that ego and social interaction were more important than biological factors in determining personality

- believed that development continues throughout life and proceeds through eight stages:
    1. trust versus mistrust (one year old)
    2. autonomy versus doubt (two to three years old)
    3. initiative versus guilt (four to six years old)
    4. industry versus inferiority (six to puberty)
    5. identity versus confusion (adolescence)
    6. intimacy versus isolation (early adulthood)
    7. generativity versus self-absorption (middle adulthood)
    8. integrity versus despair (the aging years)

**Eric Fromm**

- emphasized that personality development was strongly influenced by social factors

- offered the principles of "the existential dilemma" to describe the inherent conflict between our connection to nature as other animals and "our uniquely human possibilities"

- attempted to merge Freud's views with the social theories and philosophy of Karl Marx

- proposed character types or orientations (productiveness and non-productiveness) based on differences in social interaction

**Harry S. Sullivan**

- first American personality theorist

- developed the "interpersonal theory of personality"

- explained three modes of experience: prototaxic (undifferentiated or momentary states of the newborn), parataxic (associational or connecting events in early childhood) and syntaxic (the logical mode of connecting things and events to reality)

- other concepts include personification (good-mother/bad-mother, good-me/bad-me, me/not-me), the self-system (a complex arrangement of factors relating anxiety and interaction with others) and seven stages of development similar to Erikson's eight stages

## Transactional Analysis
**Eric Berne and Thomas Harris**
- popularized a form of psychotherapy called transactional analysis based on the concept of three ego states, the child (largely emotional and remaining embedded in each person); the parent (the precepts and beliefs, "shoulds" and "should-nots" internalized from the childhood perceptions of parents); and the adult (the mature, rational, cognitive self)

- the ego states are involved in each transaction or unit of social behavior

- transactions between people can be complementary or crossed, and therapy involves helping people to see what "games" they play in inappropriate roles

# The Behavioral and Cognitive Theorists and Their Theories

The basis of this view of personality is that personality develops as behaviors are learned. This learning is simple or complex, and the process is open to empirical study.

## Classical Conditioning
**Edward Thorndike**
- established stimulus-response relationships, reward-and-punishment and trial-and-error learning

**Ivan Pavlov**
- worked with dogs and described the conditioned reflex

## The Birth of Behaviorism
**John B. Watson**
- launched the era of behaviorism in psychology

- incorporated the principles of conditioning as explained by Thorndike and Pavlov

## Operant Conditioning
During the 1920s to the 1960s, behaviorism became the dominant branch of psychology and efforts were made to establish it as a natural science equivalent to Newtonian physics.

**B.F. Skinner**
- famous for using the "Skinner Box" to gather objective data on the acquisition and extinction of behavior

- developed theory of "operant conditioning" of rewarding small changes in behavior to produce more complex learned behaviors

- trained animals to perform unusual feats and applied the results of his research to human learning

## Stimulus-Response Learning
**John Dollard and Neal Miller**
- emphasized the role of habits, conditioning and reflexes in behavioral development
- defined a drive as a stimulus for any action, and a cue as the stimulus for a specific action

## Social Learning

This view held that learning of behavior occurs more by absorption than by conscious effort, and that the social context is crucial to understanding behavior.

### Albert Bandura

- called his theory "reciprocal determinism," meaning that the behavior and the environment interact and affect the person according to the person's interpretation and beliefs

- described a "self-system," which provides a reference for the behavior-environment interaction

- defined "self-efficacy," which is the self-perception of how well one can function in a given situation

- taught that behavior is guided mainly by self-approval or self-criticism, and the key to change is to build strong efficacy expectations and realistic outcome expectations; these lead to persistence and hard work

### Walter Mischel

- studied factors that would predict behavior and found that the situation may be more important than the personality traits

- researched "the delay of gratification" (the ability to forgo immediate gain for future reward) as an important part of the cognitive model of influencing child development

### Julian Rotter

- concluded that people develop "generalized expectancies" when certain acts are rewarded or not rewarded

- researched "locus of control" which may be internal (control with much self-direction and self-management), or external (control with environmental and higher authorities having a big influence)

### Martin Seligman

- described "learned helplessness" and its relationship to stress and depression

- proposed an "explanatory style" as the basis of the personality traits of "overall optimism" and "general pessimism"

### George Kelley

- developed the idea of "personal constructs" to show that conscious attitudes and ideas are part of what shape personality traits and behavior

# The Humanistic Theorists and Their Theories

The general view of personality in this school of thought is that the normal healthy personality develops from an interaction between the person and the environment. The person acts as a whole entity and experiences the world consciously and with purpose.

## Holistic Humanism

The rise of the concept of a human being as an integrated whole with inherent potential for positive growth was a reaction to the pessimistic view of psychoanalytic thinking and to the robot-like stimulus-response development of behaviorism.

**Abraham Maslow**

- held the basic assumptions that: (1) human beings have genetically built-in needs, capacities and tendencies which are basically good or neutral, not evil; (2) healthy development involves fulfilling the potentials of these basic capacities; and (3) psychopathology results from denial and frustration of the essential nature

- described a hierarchy of needs with four basic needs — physiological, safety, belongingness and love/esteem — beyond which is self-actualization, the highest need to be addressed when the basic needs are met; self-actualization consists of pursuit of metaneeds or being-values such as truth, justice, beauty, simplicity, fairness, etc.

## Person–Centered Psychotherapy

**Carl Rogers**

- defined a "self-structure" (the self as it is) and the "ideal self" (what a person would like to be)

- proposed that the combined self seeks "congruence" with the composite physical-psychological being (the organism)

- congruence exists when self as it is and the ideal self match reality

- the single motivating force is the self-actualizing drive, and the goal in life is to become self-actualized

## Gestalt Psychotherapy

Gestalt psychology is based on the concept that a set of sensations are perceived as a meaningful whole, with the whole being greater than the sum of the parts. This deals mainly with mental perception, learning and problem solving.

**Kurt Lewin**

- described "life space" as the total set of factors affecting a person's behavior at any given time

- proposed a theory of personality, motivation and social behavior called the "field theory"

## Existential Psychology and Personality

The basic theory of existentialism is that there are no cause-and-effect relationships. There are only sequences of actions and experiences. A human being is a whole, not a composite of body and mind. There is no unconscious mind. To understand human experience requires openness without preconceived theories. Humans should not be managed, controlled or exploited.

The philosophers **Martin Buber** and **Martin Heidegger** strongly influenced this branch of psychology, the main points of which are:

- "being-in-the-world" is the whole of human existence
- there is no separation of person and environment

- existence can be in three primary world-regions: the Umwelt (the physical surroundings), the Mitwelt (the human environment), and the Eigenwelt (the psychological and physical self)

- the equivalent to self-actualization is called authenticity — to fulfill one's potentials is to live the authentic life

- development throughout life is a constant "becoming"

## Personology

**Henry Murray**

- named this branch of psychology "personology," to apply to the study of "human lives and the factors that influence their course"

- saw each individual as unique, and each interaction between two people as unique

- advocated that brain function was the basis of psychological processes and that the past, present and anticipated future play a role in individual events of life

- known for his Thematic Apperception Test

## Biological Theorists and Their Theories

The foundation to this view of personality is that people have certain stable, enduring characteristics or traits that determine their behavior.

## Traits of Personality

**Gordon Allport**

- believed that conscious thoughts and wishes, not unconscious needs and impulses, were responsible for how people behave

- authored the first textbook on personality in 1937

- proposed that personality was composed of a constant and a variable portion, the constant portion made up of traits expressed consistently

- described the relationship among traits, attitudes and habits: a trait is general and expresses itself in several habits; the attitude is more general than the habit but more specific than the trait

- developed measures of personality called "A Study of Values," and the "Ascendance-Submission Scale"

- his study of terms that described human behavior led to the definition of the "Five Factor Model" of personality, which describes the five independent traits of personality as extroversion, agreeableness, conscientiousness, emotional stability and culture

## Factor Analysis

**Raymond Cattell**

- applied the statistical technique of factor analysis to the trait descriptions of Gordon Allport

- derived a "Sixteen Personality Factors Questionnaire" which describes an individual by sixteen paired characteristics

**Hans Eysenck**

- believed that personality traits are mostly inherited but that behavior is learned

- described four personality types: extraverts/introverts, normal/neurotic, normal/psychotic, high intelligence/low intelligence

• • • • •

The above superficial review of personality theory may bring to the mind of readers two stories that seem to make the academic rounds. One is of a group of blind men describing an elephant to one another. Each description depended on the part of the elephant the individual was holding.

The other story goes like this:

A college freshman asked his teacher on the first day of classes, "Professor, what is science?"

The professor answered, "Science is looking for a black cat in a dark room."

The student came back the next day and asked, "Professor, what is philosophy?"

"Philosophy," the professor explained, "is looking for a black cat in a dark room where there is no black cat."

The next day, after his psychology class, the student came back with a third question. "Professor, what is psychoanalysis?"

"Psychoanalysis," the professor patiently explained after some thought, "is looking for a black cat in a dark room where there is no black cat, and finding one anyway."

• • • • •

The following are my personal conclusions about psychology based on my understanding of personality theory as a layperson.

1. Some basic traits that determine how we behave are inherited. The influence of these traits is on the neurophysiologic level of receptors and transmitter substances in the brain, and also at effector systems that control function.

2. The social environment, the learning mechanism and the information absorbed from the environment are important factors in unfolding and shaping behavior. It seems that a child is born with a basic package of behavioral tendencies, and the environment unfolds and molds the personality in a two-way interaction.

3. The codes of behavior, values and standards of conduct taught or expected help to shape specific behaviors.

4. The experiences of life (both unplanned and unanticipated, and the results of conscious choices) affect personality and behavior throughout the life-span.

5. Development and growth are always possible as long as the capacity for understanding and decision-making is functional.

6. If the mind is exposed to knowledge of how personality is shaped, it can use this understanding to initiate movement into desirable pathways. This may occur consciously and subconsciously.

7. From Freud to Bandura and current researchers, each theorist has contributed valuable insights based on their work, their life experiences and their own personalities. However, older theories based on false premises should be abandoned.

8. Application of personality theory and therapy seem to be moving away from categorizing and labeling people to applying general principles on which people can make adjustments to meet the challenges of present circumstances. A life-span perspective seems to be more widely used.

9. Laypeople are capable of constructively applying psychological concepts to problems of everyday life. Summary materials, self-help groups and knowledge of available professional therapy can assist this application.

10. Personal health promotion should include an effort to understand the basis of one's behavior, to accept the things that cannot be changed and to try to change the things that can be changed.

# Personal 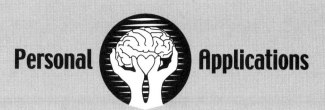 Applications

## Directions:

To apply the broad concepts of personality theory to an understanding of self, use the outline in section A below to review your personal history. Then rate yourself on the behavioral scales in section B.

A. Major Influences and Determinants of My Personality and Behavior
As you read each item, write down the first thoughts about yourself that come to mind.

### The Physiologic Factors

1. General, physical (ethnic, athletic, strong, weak, etc.)

2. Specific physical factors (right- or left-handedness, body size, etc.)

3. Sensory systems and organ function (sight, hearing, touch, etc.)

4. Sudden and extreme reactions ("hot-tempered" or "freezing-up")

### The Mental Information Processing Factors

1. Capacity to deal with information, memory

2. Early interests (in creative writing, speaking and performing, etc.)

3. Drive for formal education (self-driven or parent-driven)

4. Type of schools attended through high school (one-room, no science curriculum, etc.)

5. Type of work enjoyed (outdoors, agricultural, office, factory, etc.)

6. Career interests

**The Psychosocial Factors**

1. Birth order and position among siblings

2. Social group and how regarded by other groups

3. Personal characteristics (shyness, boldness, etc.)

4. Child-rearing philosophy of your parents

5. The religious climate of your home and society

6. Emphasis on getting an education

7. Social values (helping others, improving their living conditions, etc.)

8. The dominant atmosphere in your home (accepting and encouraging, critical and lots of "put-downs," etc.)

## The Spiritual Factors

1. Distinction between religion and spirituality

2. Beliefs relating to experiencing joy, and happiness with obeying detailed rules

3. Sense of goodness or sinfulness, and approval or disapproval by higher powers

4. Belief about the purpose of life

5. Belief about the noblest avocation

6. Belief about the hardships, pain and suffering in this life

7. Belief about other people's interests, comforts and advantages in relation to your own

8. Belief about the reason for being good all the time

9. Belief about the love and accumulation of money

10. Belief about an after-life

B. With the above summary in mind, describe your characteristics and behavior on the following scales. Keep in mind that all pairs of behavioral characteristics are a range of possibilities along a continuum, and the interplay produces individuality and uniqueness. Place an "X" on the line to show where you think YOU are at this point in life. Try to think of things as they are, not what you would like them to be.

(These scales are only qualitative and subjective adaptations of the major personality traits as discussed previously. They are to be used only for personal introspective study, not to assess other people. After each rating, itemize some of the major behavioral characteristics that you see as related to the trait.)

1. introvert _____extrovert
   (Under what circumstances do you feel self-conscious and shy, or expressive and uninhibited? Have you always felt this way?)

2. neurotic_____normal
   (If neurotic behavior is maladaptive behaviors based on conflicts between beliefs and reality, can you identify any such conflicts in your background?)

3. psychotic_____normal
   (If psychotic behavior is a tendency to harm yourself or others out of a sense of distorted reality, have you ever actually done so, felt driven or had an impulse to do so?)

4. intelligence:
   low_____high
   (Do you think that your capacity to learn, understand and manipulate information was inherited or cultivated?)

5. unpleasant_____agreeable
   (How do you think other people would rate you on this scale?)

6. unscrupulous_____conscientious
   (Under what circumstances do you feel inclined to bend the rules?)

7. closed-minded_____open-minded
   (How open do you feel about new experiences and people different from you?)

8. emotional_____stable
   (How do you make decisions — on gut instincts after gathering the facts, or in combination — and how do you respond to upsetting situations and people?)

9. humble_____assertive
   (What is true and false humility, or effective assertiveness?)

10. suspicious_____trusting
    (In dealing with other people, are you too trusting, or too suspicious?)

11. practical_____imaginative
    (Does being imaginative and experimental with life lead to risk-taking?)

12. tense_____relaxed
    (In which situations do you feel uptight and pressured, or free and relaxed?)

13. locus of control:
    internal_____external
    (What beliefs seem to correlate with external — outside factors control your life more — or internal — personal decisions and abilities — locus of control?)

14. low efficacy_____high efficacy
    (If efficacy is your personal sense of how successful you can be in producing desired outcomes, how do you see efficacy in relation to locus of control and religious beliefs?)

15. optimism_____pessimism

(How would the people closest to you rate you in terms of optimism and pessimism?)

(If you have access to the Internet, you may want to look up some personality scales as comparisons to this application. One is currently found at http://keirsey.com. The Myers-Briggs Type Indicator can be taken at www.personalogic.com. Select "Life Decisions," then "Careers," then "Choose the Career for You." The Myers-Briggs Type Indicator is a twenty-question assessment which is immediately scored.)

C. Write an essay titled: "Why I Like or Dislike my Name and/or Body (Size and Shape of the Whole or Parts).

# Reflections

This examination of personality and behavior for personal application is neither suitable for research nor clinical diagnosis. But I believe it is useful for health promotion in the normal, healthy population, which is the context in which it is used. It should give a sense that personality is not static; that change occurs over time; that desirable changes, within certain limits, can be planned; and that drastic changes, such as seen in religious conversion and cultism, are possible.

Some professionals would argue that it may not serve any good purpose to have laypeople play with personality theories. In fact, it might make professional work more difficult if someone has prior knowledge of personality theory when they have to take personality tests or other psychological diagnostics. Prior knowledge may influence their answers, and a false picture may result.

At one time, it was thought best (especially in psychoanalysis) that the patient be unaware of the aims and methods of therapy. The mystery of the process and the extraordinary abilities of the professional were considered necessary to successful therapy.

Carl Rogers attacked that attitude with his introduction of client-centered therapy. I believe there is more to be gained from the public's understanding of psychological theories than the risk of inaccurate answers to either research or diagnostic questions on tests.

When I do the above evaluation on myself, several incidents, episodes and experiences come to mind that illustrate the influences that shaped my personality and behavior, and some of the changes over time. Some of the major influences relate to physiologic factors such as left-handedness, having a nasty temper from childhood and being "cross-eyed."

Other factors include mental factors such as a sharp memory from early grade school and enjoyment of performing before large crowds but being very shy on a person-to-person level. The psychosocial factors, as I see them, are being a middle child (number five out of eleven) and growing up as an ethnic minority in a predominantly black culture. The spiritual factors are trying to harmonize religious beliefs with everyday life and belief in an after-life.

A few illustrations from my background would serve to show some of the factors that I see as operational in making me who I am. I recommend such a look backwards not in the sense of psychoanalysis, but in a sense of review of personal history. As you read this, think about incidents in your life that may illustrate some of the major influences on your personality.

1. **Influences on my shyness and self-consciousness**

I recall the derogatory remarks of children, which were not as hard to endure as those from adults. They described my crossed eyes and ethnic make-up in very creative and picturesque language. I can still see those people now, and hear them say the words that stung so deeply then, but now the bitterness, hurt and resentment are gone.

The worst one was "You coolie boy, your eyes look like a dog just farted in them." Imagine what we do to children when adults make observations like that on the basis of a physical imbalance.

## 2. Near disasters with a hot temper

In several fits of uncontrollable rage, I came close to stabbing one brother in his chest with a butcher knife and did end up scarring him with a double-edged razor blade. It was only after we were in our late thirties that this brother and I could talk freely about this eight-inch scar on his thigh and wonder together why things like that happen, how we survived without some permanent damage and how our parents survived raising us!

Nowadays, I see myself as a great pacifist, extremely patient, very forgiving and accepting of other people, and shy and outgoing according to the situation. The difference over time has been the influence of the people I came to have close association with; the hopes, prayers and expectations of my parents; education and a modified understanding and practice of religion; and my close inner circle of wife and children.

Even so, I sometimes wonder what monster lurks beneath the surface and what events might trigger an eruption. Suppose someone breaks into my home and attacks my wife and daughter. What rage and murderous instincts might that bring to the surface? Or is that capacity eradicated? Is there a monster inside being held at bay?

## 3. On being left-handed in a right-handed world

During my early grade school years, the prevailing theory of dealing with left-handedness was to change it into right-handedness by the teacher hitting you on the left hand with a wooden ruler every time you were caught using the left hand.

My grade school buddy, Leroy Morgan, and I devised a routine to get through my in-class penmanship exercises. He had a beautiful handwriting and could quickly produce his work, then do mine in a disguised version of his while I held his and pretended to be writing it myself. It worked well, and I continued to write with my left hand for the homework.

As an eight-year-old, I felt a great sense of anger and dislike for this teacher. I was greatly relieved and felt rescued when she had to leave the school.

I sometimes think about what might have happened if that teacher had stayed at that school throughout my grade school years. Could my anger and hot temper have led to a violent confrontation? Would I have grown up into a life of deceit and criminal activities? Quite possibly. The teacher who succeeded her was, for me, the greatest grade school teacher that ever lived, Edward Macarno

## 4. Temptation to tell a lie in church

One of the strict practices of the religious group we were part of was to have a prescribed lesson to be studied every day of the week. In the group meeting at church, each child had to raise a hand when the attendance record was taken and say aloud if you had studied the lesson all seven days or not.

Imagine the conflict in confessing before your peers and adults to not studying the lesson. Or to saying you studied when you knew you hadn't and thus committing a sin in an attempt to look good! So you try hard all week, but you forget one or two times, and everybody else seems to be perfect at it every week. So you endure confessing being less perfect than the others, or telling a lie in church! I was glad to see the record keeping of daily study discontinued and my children saved from those conflicts.

But on the other hand, is it not the facing of conflicts like this and making the right choice that strengthens character? Maybe I should hope then that our children have more of these conflicts and make the wise choice! In this case, to be comfortable and accepting with having others know what they are, or what they are not, without the need to cover up.

Health psychology across the life-span is a developing field. Some major studies are under way in this and related disciplines. Studies such as the Baltimore Longitudinal Study of Aging conducted by the National Institute on Aging show that extraverts are happier than introverts in mid-life. Low scorers on the neurotic scale adapt better to change than do high scorers.

Other studies show that pessimists get sick more frequently than optimists. Type A personalities (competitive, hostile and driven) are more likely to develop heart disease.

Many studies are being conducted to see whether people can change behaviors. The results so far are very encouraging. With the use of a combination of interventions such as meditation, positive affirmations, stress management, exercise, nutrition and relaxation, Type A personalities are making changes that relate positively to fewer second heart attacks in people with heart disease.

There seem to be a causal relationship. Some people refer to "cancer-prone personalities," for example. On the other hand, the relationship may be more basic. The presence of certain personality/behavioral traits may be part of a make-up where the physiological functions are concomitantly more at risk. Whatever the basis, there seems to be a strong connection between personality, behavior and health.

Some people may have a stronger, hardier or more resilient style of behavior. These characteristics may be accompanied by a stronger resistance to diseases and greater vitality, vim and vigor. There seems to be some connection. But again, is it cause and effect, or is it part of the same basic make-up? Future studies may clarify this.

The point of this chapter, however, is not whether you can change personality or behavior and change health and wellness. The point is that understanding how you became who you are and who you are capable of becoming brings certain confidence to the pursuit of personal growth and enhancement of well-being. Getting to this understanding is, in itself, growth and wellness producing. This enhances performance. Performance is what counts on the outside, and personal satisfaction is what counts on the inside.

To go the distance, we have to understand how we became who we are.

*Performance is what counts on the outside, and personal satisfaction is what counts on the inside.*

# Carol's Turn

In college in the late sixties, I had one very confusing course in general psychology. I was turned off from the social sciences and wanted to pursue art instead.

I was hoping that Al wouldn't get into the private applications of these concepts. He loves to tell stories about his childhood; about fights and conflicts among his seven brothers; about growing out of these conflicts to mutual respect and understanding; about the adventurous life of growing up as a left-handed, cross-eyed, ethnic minority on a Caribbean Island; and about being left-handed in a right-handed world during medical technology training.

He is comfortable with this type of illustration. I was not. I have been more private and reserved, and maybe that's my prominent personality trait. I am comfortable with that. However, I see myself changing in this regard as I have spent more time in these discussions. It's not so bad to share your life with others, but there is a limit.

I think one of the major factors in personality development is the method of parenting under which we are raised along with the biologic inheritance. I may have discounted the importance of this when I consciously decided to have no contact with my biological parents who gave me up to be raised by relatives.

I have chosen to keep fully absorbed in my life and let them have the life they chose. I wonder if one of these days I would feel it important enough to my comfort or to theirs to find out what has happened to my biological parents. This discussion on personality is stimulating traces of interest, but, presently, I feel no great need one way or the other.

Wouldn't it be interesting for some therapist to read into my attitude some form of denial? Right now I really don't care, because I am too busy struggling with trying to get to a level of physical fitness that I never had the time, energy and resources to pursue.

Al thinks that maybe some subconscious need to find out if my mother is alive or dead may be holding me back from doing the things I need to do, the things I am capable of doing to make a greater contribution. With this in mind, I spent a weekend with Iyanla Vanzant, author of *The Value in the Valley: A Woman's Guide Through Life's Dilemmas* and *In the Meantime: Finding Yourself and the Love You Want*. This "Wonder Woman Weekend" was inspiring and revealing. The probing techniques for understanding the self were intriguing. But I came away with the same conclusion. I don't need to reconnect with my biological parents. I have enough to concentrate on with three adult children and a three-year-old granddaughter!

For going the distance, I have to put the past behind me and move ahead with an optimistic view of the second half of life.

# EXAMINE YOUR PLEASURE, PAIN AND ADDICTIVE BEHAVIOR

"*Pleasure is frail like a dewdrop, while it laughs it dies.*"

Rabindranath Tagore

"*Do not put off till tomorrow what can be enjoyed today.*"

Josh Billings

Four

*Dedicated to*


**Eric and Sue Khandagle, and Sureka**

*In appreciation for the many pleasures we shared, and the pain we have endured together.*

Imagine babies born without the ability to feel pain. As these children begin to explore their surroundings, they can throw themselves into anything from any height, break bones, smash fingers, cut themselves deeply and burn themselves severely without feeling anything. Nothing in the environment gives feedback of injury or danger. Imagine the degree of concern and watchfulness required in caring for such children.

The *Southern Medical Journal*, in its August 1995 issue, reported on the case of two brothers born with this condition. The scientific term for the condition is "congenital insensitivity to pain" or "hereditary sensory and autonomic neuropathy."

Imagine losing the ability to experience pleasure. This happens in cases of severe depression and in some patients with Parkinson's disease. These conditions have helped to shed light on the brain chemistry of pleasure and pain.

It is easy to talk about pleasure and pain but a little more difficult to define and understand the human ability to experience pleasure and pain, and the role pleasure and pain play in all human interactions. In this chapter, we will examine some basic ideas about pleasure and pain, and their functions in human behavior.

These topics became a core part of this material after I did a seminar on addictions. One individual in the group felt free to share her experiences and viewpoints about personal addictive behavior.

One of the rules of self-disclosure that we follow in all our discussion sessions is that we should give careful consideration before revealing private information or personal behavior to see if it would make us or our listeners uncomfortable. In this case, the individual started by saying that her weekend had been "one magnificent pleasure high." She had had one male lover visit one day, and a female lover the next. At that point, the group stopped her from giving further details.

However, she had some interesting insights which she wanted to share, and she asked to talk to me privately. She gave permission to use her story. Here is the story, reconstructed and paraphrased with details changed to protect privacy, but essentially factual as told. I had no reason to think that it was a concocted story, and no reason to verify it. I accepted it as truth. See what you think.

• • • • •

"It seems that in my adult life I have developed a stronger and stronger addiction to sex. In my mid-thirties, I feel driven to make love as often as I have the opportunity — two, three and even five times a day. In the process, I have had several lovers of both sexes, with some relationships lasting from a few months to several years, and more than one at the same time.

"I have tried to analyze the situation from a viewpoint of what is right or wrong, what is healthy or unhealthy, what is normal or abnormal, and whether I have a desire to change and why. At this point, I can manage my life, which consists of work, school and social activities. I feel that I have control of my circumstances, and have no reason to change. I accept the health risks of having multiple lovers and enjoy my life as it is.

"In trying to understand how I became this way, I look back to my family circumstances and my childhood. My father was an alcoholic and spent little time at home. I grew up in a medium-sized town where outward behavior was supposed to be prim and proper, but everyone had hidden lives doing what they could get away with.

"At about seven years of age, I became the youngest member of a group of teens and pre-teens who ran around together and did fun things. One of the fun things the older boys did was to introduce the girls to sex. I was introduced at eight years of age. By the time I was eleven, sex was a regular part of our gang activities, and I was beginning to enjoy it. From then on, it seemed that sex was the subject that occupied most of my thoughts. I feel lucky that I didn't get pregnant or contract sexually transmitted diseases. Maybe I can't get pregnant. I have never tried to, but I am beginning to think that it would be nice to have a baby before I am forty.

"I think that the tendency to become addicted to something is inherited, and the environment determines what we become addicted to. I feel addicted to sex, but I really don't have any good reason to want to break this addiction. Am I looking at this realistically, or is there another way of looking at this from a wellness perspective which I should consider?"

• • • • •

How do you respond to such questions? My first reaction was to point out that I am not a psychologist, trained counselor or therapist. My opinions were opinions and beliefs from the viewpoint of health promotion and wellness. I ended by referring this person to a counselor and giving information about self-help groups on addictions.

Again, this subject can be the topic of an entire book or a full course by itself. In this chapter, we will share a perspective in the hope of contributing to self-understanding.

## Definition of Pleasure

Pleasure is the perception of pleasant and enjoyable stimuli. This may vary in degree from the state of existing without pain, the baseline, to euphoric states of climactic ecstasy that may overwhelm the consciousness and cause fainting.

In human experience, pleasure may be immediate, short-term, long-term or delayed. Gratification is often used as a synonym for pleasure, but it carries an additional meaning of self-centered pleasure. Pleasure, as a mode of human experience, can be examined without evaluation based on beliefs and religious teachings. The final integration of pleasure in personal experience, however, must be considered within the context of beliefs and values.

Immediate pleasures produce pleasant feelings described by such terms as thrilling, surge of joy, climactic, euphoric or ecstatic, occurring over a short time frame — from an instant to a few hours. "Immediate" refers to the time between the stimulus and the response.

Short-term pleasures produce the same feelings over a few days to weeks. The time frame between stimulus and response is longer than immediate. The mechanism is the same, but the intensity of the response may not be as high as immediate.

Long-term pleasures are those derived from planning and creative devising where an anticipated reward is achieved through postponement of the immediate and short-term pleasures, or through unexpected positive results from working at otherwise unexciting tasks. This happens in doing work that has to be done to achieve certain goals, while putting aside activities that might be pleasurable but not directly contributory to the goal.

# The Dimensions of Pleasure

Pleasure can be described in the four dimensions of functions discussed in the model introduced previously. Thus physiologic pleasure is the perception of pleasant feelings originating in the physiology of the body. For example, a roller coaster ride (for those who can endure such things) produces pleasure because of the effects of changes in motion and gravity on the body. The adrenaline rush is part of the chemistry of the experience.

The physical arousal that is part of the sex act is also physiologic, based on nervous and hormonal mechanisms.

Mental pleasure is the pleasure originating in the ability of the mind to process information. This involves gaining knowledge and the ability to deal with information, pleasant memories, feelings of accomplishment and creativity. The excitement of synthesizing information or having new ideas and creative inspirations are pleasures originating in the mind's ability to receive, process, store, retrieve and use information both on the conscious and subconscious levels.

Psychosocial pleasure is the pleasure originating from our feelings about ourselves, and the interaction with other people, things and processes in the environment. This includes being comfortable with who we are, being confident, caring, having positive self-regard and earning the gratitude and positive evaluation of others. Knowing the joy of being a friend and having friends, contributing to the welfare of a group and sharing enjoyable activities, are examples of psychosocial pleasures.

Spiritual pleasure is pleasure originating from our sense of purpose and meaning in life, our sense of the "rightness" in what we do and how we live, our feeling of connectedness to the human family and our felt needs to be connected to some Power or Person of cosmic dimensions. This sense of transcendence over the human condition can be a source of pleasure that can only be described as spiritual.

Categorizing pleasure in this dimensional scheme does not mean that these pleasure dimensions act independently. Pleasure is experienced as a whole-person phenomenon. It is likely that the same biochemical mechanisms are involved. The observation here is that pleasure may originate in any of the four dimensions of function. An understanding of this may contribute to a better understanding of ourselves as pleasure-seeking organisms, with the ability to balance pleasure toward more health promoting pleasures.

It is not necessary, thankfully, to examine pleasure in order to experience pleasure. An understanding may lead to a better appreciation of often-overlooked pleasure. For example, in the normal functioning of the body when pain is absent, there is no specific pleasure stimulus, but the absence of pain and the smooth functioning of a healthy body are pleasurable — just the consciousness of it. Many other everyday occurrences are pleasurable not by producing pleasure stimuli in the body, but in the psyche and in the spirit.

## Definition of Pain

Pain is the perception of unpleasant, hurtful feelings sometimes called "noxious stimuli." The word "noxious," used in the scientific and medical description of pain, means harmful or hurtful. This is mostly used in reference to physical pain, but the same meaning is useful for pain in the other dimensions as well.

Pain is often described as acute, chronic or referred. Acute pain is immediate or short term, while chronic pain remains over a long period of time. Referred pain means the sensation of pain comes from one location but the cause of the pain is in another location in the body.

In terms of quality, pain is described as sharp, dull, throbbing, crushing and excruciating. Pain may be so severe as to overwhelm the consciousness and produce fainting.

## The Dimensions of Pain

Pain in the physiologic dimension is always a signal of something abnormal, but it serves a useful purpose. It serves as a warning of potential or actual tissue damage, abnormal pressure or spasm in organs, or actual death of tissue. This pain is the easiest to understand because it is a protective mechanism for the physical body. Unless you have hereditary insensitivity to pain or damaged nerves, you have felt physiologic pain and understand its function.

Mental pain originates in the mind's ability to handle information. Hurt may derive from the personal perception and interpretation of information received from others, or from personal memories of past hurts, guilt, regrets and self-blame. The knowledge and awareness of mistakes, missed opportunities, wrong decisions, loss, and misuse or lack of information can produce pain that is as real as physical pain. The sensation or quality of the pain is different because it does not originate in tissue damage. It originates in the mind's capacity to process and interpret information.

Psychosocial pain has to do with the negative valuation of self and self-perception in relation to others. Thus shyness and self-consciousness; low self-esteem; lack of confidence; devaluating treatment from others; feelings of embarrassment, shame and disgrace may produce pain as real and with similar effects as if tissue or organ damage did occur.

The origin of this pain is in the mind's capacity to define and know the true self and make judgments in comparison with other people. The quality of the pain is different from physical pain but the effects on the person are just as real; and, as we shall see later, these psychological effects have real biological consequences.

Spiritual pain has to do with the lack of purpose and meaning, feelings of hopelessness and despair in terms of everyday challenges, as well as the transcendent questions of life. The origin of this pain is in the mind's capacity to define and seek meaning, purpose and satisfaction in life.

## Addictions

After a review of many of the current theories of addictive behaviors, I am led to the conclusion that anything that generates pleasure or soothes pain in any dimension of function has the potential to establish an addiction.

Let us define an addiction as a behavior that has the following components. This is a summary of the literature reviewed on this subject.

1. There is a craving, drive or compulsion (weak or strong) for the object, whether the object is a substance or an activity.
2. The craving, drive or compulsion is temporarily satisfied when the object is obtained.
3. After some time, the satisfaction wears off, the craving returns and the object is again sought to satisfy the drive. The "dosage" of the object may have to be increased over time to give the same level of effect in pleasure production or pain alleviation.
4. The substance or the behavior occupies a disproportionate amount of thoughts, energy and resources compared to its usefulness in promoting positive growth in the person.
5. The time, energy and resources spent on the object delay or sabotage the achievement of other more worthwhile goals for health, standard of living and contribution to the common good. This may produce guilt feelings.
6. The addicted individual generally has thoughts about the negative effects of the substance or behavior and thinks about or makes some efforts to escape.
7. Addictions may be mild or severe, negative or positive, and to single or multiple substances or behaviors at the same time.
8. An attempt to break the addiction is accompanied by some withdrawal symptoms, which can range from mild to severe.
9. The pleasure and pain effects are more immediate and short term. The long-term consequences may be negative or positive. Risk is part of the excitement and attraction to engage in the activity.
10. When the individual is not engaged in the addictive behavior, or is removed from the environment that is conducive to the activity, there is a feeling of ability to control the behavior. However, availability and the environment weaken that sense of control.
11. A positive addiction promotes health, personal productivity and better relationships, is moral and ethical, is recognized and is kept within limits that reduce possible long-term damage. Examples are addiction to physical activity such as running or racquetball and mental activity such as reading or daydreaming. The positive addiction may

be controlled to avoid damage to body or mind.

12. A negative addiction destroys health, personal productivity and relationships; is immoral and unethical (or leads to immoral or unethical behaviors); may provide an escape from reality; may or may not be recognized; and gets out of control with long-term negative consequences. Examples are addiction to smoking, alcohol, mood altering drugs, watching TV and spectator sports, or uncontrollable spending. Negative addictions may be more difficult to control.

13. An addiction may be focused in the physiologic, mental, psychosocial or spiritual dimension, but the effect is on the whole person.

## The Mechanisms of Pleasure and Pain

Pleasure and pain are coordinated in the limbic system of the brain. For physical pleasure and pain, nerve endings serve as receptors for the stimuli. The nerve impulses generated then travel along particular nerve pathways to channel the impulses into the brain. They release neurotransmitter substances, such as norepinephrine and dopamine, and trigger electrical circuits in the emotional centers of the brain. The results are projected to the cortex where the sensations are perceived.

For pleasure and pain originating in the mind, for example, psychosocial or spiritual, there is no nerve input from the body. However, our understanding is that the same mechanisms may be involved. The same neurotransmitters, electrical circuits and brain centers project the results to our

level of consciousness. The difference in quality of the sensation may be that the brain has no physical pain or pleasure receptors of its own (none as yet identified by our scientific techniques). It seems to be only a coordinating center. However, thoughts originating in the mind generate pleasure and pain.

The experience of pleasure and pain triggered from what is seen and heard is different from direct stimulation of physical pleasure and pain. Beauty or ugliness, pleasant or discordant sounds trigger pleasure or pain sensations as part of information processing and relate to previous knowledge and experiences. This also illustrates the integration of these experiences. Different people have different perceptions and appreciation of beauty. To some it may be more mental, while to others it is a more spiritual experience.

In the drawing of the brain found in the color section, note which areas of the brain are referred to as the limbic system. This area of the brain integrates the emotions and gives us the ability to experience pleasure and pain (Figure 5-16, p. 143).

Keep in mind that:

1. Pleasure and pain are whole-person phenomena. The perception occurs in the conscious part of the brain (the cerebral cortex). The coordination of the inputs, whether they arise from the physiologic, mental, psychosocial or spiritual mechanisms, occurs in the limbic system.

2. Particular neurotransmitters are involved. Norepinephrine, adrenaline, dopamine and endorphins seem to be part of the brain chemistry that modulates these experiences. Researchers have

identified dopamine depletion from nerve terminals as the mechanism that is responsible for the experience of unpleasant effects of long-term use of cocaine. This is probably why it takes larger doses to produce the same high with most drugs.

3.  The emotional response to pleasure and pain is triggered before the conscious control centers. More will be said on this in Chapter 10 on emotions and motivation.

# The Highest Pleasures, Greatest Pains and Strongest Addictions

As I surveyed the literature, discussed these topics in a classroom setting and reflected on human experience over the years, I concluded that we can identify the pleasures and pains that are the most profound in human experience. Since personal perception and belief play a role in the experience and interpretation of sensations, there will be individual differences. However, some general observations can be made, based on our understanding of the nature and mechanisms of the human experience of pleasure and pain. See what you think.

In the physiologic dimension, pleasure stimuli include things that are comfortable in terms of temperature and texture (a warm bath), things that are relaxing in terms of reducing muscle tension (a total body massage), things that produce sudden changes in the effects of gravity or velocity on the body (roller coaster rides) or things that generate a coordinated nervous system

discharge (the sexual climax). Of these, the sexual climax seems to be the most intense pleasure experience of which the system is capable without artificial interference with brain chemistry.

The most intense physiologic pain is associated with the death of tissue. Judged by patients' reactions and the amount of painkillers necessary to reduce pain, physicians estimate that the pain of bone cancer may be the most excruciating pain humans experience. The source of the pain is death of tissue and the release of chemicals that stimulate pain receptors. The pain receptors generate a huge number of nerve impulses that travel into the pain centers of the brain.

Mental pleasure comes from understanding information and using information to solve problems, generate new ideas, recall pleasant experiences through memory and have creative insights. Of these, creativity (the conception, development, birth and maturation of products of the mind) may give the greatest pleasure. (The product does not have to be life changing or exotic. Everybody is capable of creative insights to one degree or another. That's the way the system works.)

The greatest mental pain may be the experience of anxiety, loss, guilt and regret. All these seem to be connected and integrated with psychosocial and spiritual functions. Severe depression, which has a basis in brain chemistry, may be one of the greatest pains experienced in this dimension. There may be precipitating factors of loss, guilt and regret associated with some forms of depression.

In the psychosocial dimension, our experience of pleasure and pain is in the evaluation of the inner self. Self-confidence, balanced with the positive valuation of others, is pleasure producing. Extreme social shyness and self-consciousness, low self-esteem, feelings of shame and disgrace, and lack of self-confidence are painful.

The highest pleasure may be the experience of realistic, positive regard for self, while valuing someone else to the point of being willing to give up self for the other. The greatest pain may be loss of this positive self-regard accompanied by feelings of shame and utter disgrace.

The highest spiritual pleasure may be coming to the point of having resolved the question of a purpose in life and an acceptance of human mortality. This resolution involves coming to terms with human limitations and finding a basis for redemption. Redemption here is used in the generic sense to mean a condition that compensates for or negates the frailties and weaknesses of humanity. This answers the search for meaning, the questions about immortality, connection to the rest of the cosmos, and the unknown of life after death. Religion helps or should help in this area.

The greatest spiritual pain may be purposelessness and meaninglessness in life.

This involves lack of resolution of the question of connection to other parts of the universe, while struggling against our mortality. This is being spiritually lost.

The generic process of redemption is the process by which our greatest pains are turned into pleasures. For example, when the intense physical pain of a disease process is relieved by complete healing and the pain comes to an end, this is physiologic redemption.

When a mind, trapped in ignorance and frustration of its capacities to develop, is cultivated through learning techniques of handling information (reading, writing, reasoning), this is mental redemption. Teach an illiterate adult to read, and see redemption in action.

When someone in despair about their personal worth is befriended and brought to feel value and caring from another human being without having to pay back the friend, this is psychosocial redemption.

When a sense of purposelessness, meaninglessness and hopelessness is changed into strong purpose, meaning and hope for this life and for any other life there is, that is spiritual redemption. Redemption is part of wellness.

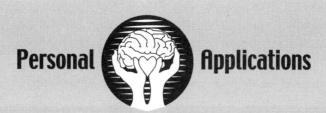

# Personal Applications

## Directions:

Check your agreement or disagreement with the following summary statements in section A, and then fill in the summary tables of personal pleasure and pain in sections B and C. Work with the suggestions in sections D, E, F, G and H only if you feel comfortable with the recall exercises.

A. Seven summary statements present the main principles from the discussion above and lay the foundation for the personal applications to understanding self from a pleasure and pain perspective. These are:

1. The brain is the biologic base, and the mind is the functional coordinating instrument that gives humans the capacity to experience pleasure and pain.

   [  ] agree       [  ] disagree       [  ] unsure

2. Our pleasure and pain drives seem to be the foundation for the rest of the drives that regulate human behavior and experience.

   [  ] agree       [  ] disagree       [  ] unsure

3. Even though we can examine pleasure and pain in a dimensional format to aid in understanding ourselves, all pleasure and pain are experienced as a whole person, and each dimension affects the others to some extent. The physiologic dimension is the lowest, and the spiritual dimension is the highest level in the hierarchy. It matters more to have found meaning and purpose around which life can be focused than how many T-bone steaks are consumed or how many times a week you make love.

   [  ] agree       [  ] disagree       [  ] unsure

4. The highest pleasures and the greatest pains in life deal with the greatest questions of life, over the long haul.

   [  ] agree       [  ] disagree       [  ] unsure

5.  It seems to be a human tendency to want to be in pleasure, to feel good, all the time. This is not possible. The system may not be able to tolerate or grow on continuous pleasure experiences. It may be that pain is a necessary balance to increase the human ability to find satisfaction in pleasure.

[  ] agree        [  ] disagree        [  ] unsure

6.  It is abnormal to seek or desire pain and suffering.

[  ] agree        [  ] disagree        [  ] unsure

7.  No pain, at the time it is experienced, seems desirable or beneficial. But some good seems to come from most pain. The sum of life experiences seems to be to have the pleasure outweigh the pain in the long haul.

[  ] agree        [  ] disagree        [  ] unsure

B.  In the table below, write a word or phrase in each cell to describe a pain experience. For example, in the cell Mental/Stress Adaptation, "guilt" may be one pain experience. In the cell, Psychosocial/Rest, "loneliness" may be a pain experience. There are no right or wrong answers.

## Human Pain Experiences

| Dynamics | Dimensions | | | |
|---|---|---|---|---|
|  | Physiologic | Mental | Psychosocial | Spiritual |
| Homeostasis |  |  |  |  |
| Nutrition |  |  |  |  |
| Stress Adaptation |  |  |  |  |
| Work |  |  |  |  |
| Rest |  |  |  |  |
| Growth |  |  |  |  |
| Reproduction |  |  |  |  |

C. In the table below, write a word or phrase in each cell to describe a pleasure experience. For example, in the cell Mental/Stress Adaptation, "getting rid of guilt" may be one pleasure experience. In the cell Psychosocial/Rest, "solitude" may be a pleasure experience. There are no right or wrong answers.

## Human Pleasure Experiences

| Dynamics | Dimensions | | | |
|---|---|---|---|---|
| | Physiologic | Mental | Psychosocial | Spiritual |
| Homeostasis | | | | |
| Nutrition | | | | |
| Stress Adaptation | | | | |
| Work | | | | |
| Rest | | | | |
| Growth | | | | |
| Reproduction | | | | |

For sections D and E, you may want to write your thoughts in a private journal, or just think about them without writing anything down.

D. As you review your life, what are some of your most pleasant memories?

E. As you review your life, what are some of your most painful memories?

F. What are some of the most beautiful scenes you have witnessed?

G. What kind of music do you enjoy?

H. What is co-dependency?

# Reflections

Integrated pleasure and pain give the final evaluation of the quality of life. This is where happiness, fulfillment or satisfaction in life is truly defined. This is what success means — when the integration of the pleasures and pains of life comes out on the positive side for healthy pleasures. This is what humans seek and need.

The teaching that pleasure is sinful may have led many to live in frustration. I recall that in a strict religious environment, the term pleasure was often associated with sin, wrong, bad and severe punishment. Because of this, it seemed that there was always a question of "what sin am I committing now" associated with even the innocent pleasures such as playing in a volleyball tournament — competition was regarded as not just bad but sinful.

The review of human pleasure and pain in the personal applications above may lead to raising our level of wellness through decision-making to increase healthy pleasures, deal with inevitable pain and control addictive behavior.

The exercise above may take you into some unfamiliar ways of looking at life and may risk getting intensely personal. Take a few cells at a time and see what thoughts and ideas are stimulated. Here are some examples of what I mean. See what ideas come to your mind. You don't have to agree with anything I say. There are no right or wrong answers.

## 1. Physiologic Homeostasis

When all body parts and functions are operating normally, we tend to overlook the pleasure of a healthy body — the existence of the most marvelous, miraculous, living machinery we know. We take our biochemistry for granted because there is no intense feeling in this baseline condition. If we consciously appreciate the marvels of a body with all its potential, instead of only being aware of it when pain and illness occur, we may increase our pleasure. We may increase our awareness of healthy pleasure and our capacity to experience pleasure.

The body is so susceptible to pain and malfunction that it is a marvel that most of us function well most of the time. It is a miracle that we heal and recover so well, so frequently. It is inevitable that we experience pain, malfunction or loss of function. What can we do to enhance function, postpone loss of function and recover function when lost?

The potential for addiction lies in the biochemistry of the brain. Chemical addiction (substance abuse) is the prime example of how this works. Chemical addiction may occur to anything that produces pleasure or soothes pain.

## 2. Physiologic Nutrition

The pleasure of the process of eating and the pleasure stimulation from the foods we eat dominate our feeding behavior (at least in the countries where food is in relative abundance). Many of us eat what we eat because of the enjoyment of eating. The foundation for this is laid in customs and habits developed in childhood, rather than in the nutrient content of the foods we eat.

Pleasure we should have, but there are foods that give short-term pleasure with long-term pain consequences. It seems that part of the decision-making of what and how much we eat should take into consideration the pleasure functions of food and the pain consequences of ill health. This can help in making choices that enhance health, reduce the odds for certain diseases and optimize our biochemical functions.

I believe some foods are addictive for people with the susceptibility for addictions. The physiologic part of this mechanism, based in the biochemistry of the cells, may be only one part of the condition. The mental part of the equation includes knowledge and discipline. The psychosocial part includes the social functions of food and the self-assertiveness (or lack thereof) of the individual. The spiritual part of this is the meaning and significance of food in the belief system of the individual. Food addiction is one example of the integrated nature of all human behavior and the pleasure-pain interaction of all dimensions.

If we were to examine each block of the matrix in a manner similar to 1 and 2 above, it would make this a very long chapter — possibly a book by itself. Therefore, I will go through each of the remaining blocks in a list fashion giving my thoughts on the pleasure, pain and potential for addiction related to the particular human capacity. See what ideas come to you as you consider the following points.

3. **Physiologic Stress** — pleasure stimulated by adrenaline rush; pain generated in organ malfunction (ulcers, spastic colon); potential for addiction to adrenaline highs, leading to risk-taking and extreme physical stimulation.

4. **Physiologic Work** — pleasure in physical exertion, in activities such as gardening or playing racquetball or manual labor by choice; pain in damage of muscle, joints or bones; potential for addiction to adrenaline and endorphins (runner's high).

5. **Physiologic Rest** — pleasure in the relaxation of tired muscles and deep, restful sleep; pain in tense muscles, tension headaches and chronic insomnia; potential for addiction to lethargy and excess sleep.

6. **Physiologic Growth** — pleasure in the normal maturing process from infant to aged adult; pain in the adjustment to various stages and in losing function as the upper limits of life are approached; no potential for addictive behavior.

7. **Physiologic Reproduction** — pleasure in the mating act and nurturing a fetus; pain in the process of childbirth; potential for addiction to sex.

8. **Mental Homeostasis** — pleasure in knowing, having the capacity to know, and feeling in balance between lack of information and information overload; pain in the awareness of lack of knowledge (when you know you don't know), or in information overload; potential for addiction to certain sources or modes of information such as TV or reading (especially exciting novels).

9. **Mental Nutrition** — pleasure (short term and long term) in feeding the mind with good, nourishing, creativity-stimulating, growth promoting information; pain on reception of bad news, human tragedies; potential for addiction to sources of junk food for the mind (trashy information, pornography, TV news recap of all the murders of the day, music videos, etc.)

10. **Mental Stress** — pleasure of the chemical rush during stress — increase in productivity under stress; pain in the process of distress and increase in guilt and doubt; potential for addiction to the adrenaline rush of stress (may be one reason for procrastination of tasks with a massive, stressful effort just before deadline).

11. **Mental Work** — pleasure of accomplishments; pain in failures and frustrations; potential for addiction to work that is enjoyable (workaholics).

12. **Mental Rest** — pleasure in variety, mental relaxation and periodically "emptying" the mind; pain in monotony of exertion and feelings of burden from having too much to pay attention to (this is probably a good definition of anxiety); potential for addiction to the medium which produces variety or relaxation.

13. **Mental Growth** — pleasure in the discovery of new information as mental capacity matures and as wisdom accumulates; pain in awareness of ignorance and waste of mental capacity; no potential for addiction.

14. **Mental Reproduction** — pleasure in creativity; pain in frustration of creative abilities; potential for addiction to some aspects of the creative process such as daydreaming and fantasizing.

15. **Psychosocial Homeostasis** — pleasure in a balanced self and keeping relationships in balance; pain in disharmony within self and in relationships with others; potential of addiction to some of the social aspects of relationships (dependence on companionship).

16. **Psychosocial Nutrition** — pleasure in processes and things that feed and build up the self and positive relationships; pain in processes and things that tear down the self and destroy healthy relationships; potential for addiction to social processes that enhance this pleasure, or to social processes that soothe this pain, for example, team sports or dependence on a social support system.

17. **Psychosocial Stress** — pleasure in fulfilling social roles that earn positive self-regard and the regard of others; pain in social ineptitude and loss of positive self-regard; potential for addiction may be to dependency on social role for positive self-value.

18. **Psychosocial Work** — pleasure in building ego strength and self-defense mechanisms; pain in weak ego and overexertion such as for caregivers of chronically ill dependents; addictive potential seems unclear.

19. **Psychosocial Rest** — pleasure of voluntary solitude; pain of constant interaction with people or pain of loneliness; potential for addiction to group activities as a means of avoiding loneliness.

20. **Psychosocial Growth** — pleasure of maturing socially; pain of social immaturity; no potential for addiction.

21. **Psychosocial Reproduction** — pleasure of perpetuating self through relationships; pain of unsuccessful or broken relationships; addiction potential? Not clear if there can be an addiction to certain personalities or temperaments?

22. **Spiritual Homeostasis** — pleasure of spiritual balance in positive and negative emotions, settled beliefs and values; pain in imbalance and lack of a core set of values and beliefs; potential for addiction to processes that promote or promise spiritual certainties, for example, group meetings and exciting speeches.

23. **Spiritual Nutrition** — pleasure in activities that feed or strengthen the spirit and uplift the soul; pain in experiences that dampen the spirit and beat down the soul; potential for addiction to things that produce pleasure or that soothe pain, e.g., religious services and rituals?

24. **Spiritual Stress** — pleasure in maintaining optimistic, positive attitudes and transcendental experiences; pain in struggling against pessimistic, negative attitudes like hopelessness; potential for addiction to whatever produces pleasure and soothes pain.

25. **Spiritual Work** — pleasure in searching for meaning, truth, beauty, goodness and purpose; pain in frustration of this search; potential for addiction to what produces pleasure or soothes pain.

26. **Spiritual Rest** — pleasure in personal peace and inner security; pain in personal disharmony and inner insecurities; potential for addiction to whatever produces peace or soothes pain of inner discord and disharmony.

27. **Spiritual Growth** — pleasure in developing positive, mature faith, hope and trust in transcendent values; pain in accumulation of doubt in core belief system; no potential for addiction.

28. **Spiritual Reproduction** — pleasure in connecting to an infinite source of being for an infinite period of time; pain in losing connection to an infinite source of being; potential for addiction to whatever produces the pleasure and soothes the pain.

The above reduction of pleasure and pain may seem redundant and in some cases nonspecific. Human nature is so complex that any attempt to dissect whole-person processes such as pleasure and pain may seem futile — similar to our attempts to fully describe personality. However, the above breakdown leads to discussion and insight on a personal level that makes it useful. Each person puts an individual meaning to the aspects that are of interest. Some of the ideas above may be wrong. We have thrown them out for discussion and stimulation of your personal thoughts, not to feed you what is proven right or wrong.

The thoughts and ideas above are for triggering your own ideas. For example, I said that in the spiritual dimension, the pleasure that is analogous to physiologic pleasure in the dynamic of reproduction is the pleasure of "connecting to an infinite source of being." This means ensuring perpetuation of the self for all times, similar to how physiologic reproduction perpetuates the self for a lifetime.

To a religious person, this may make a lot of sense. There is pleasure in a feeling of closeness in constant connection to a personal, all-powerful God (or there should be, if the nature of that God is accepted as loving and caring). People talk about being "born again," and demonstrate great and effusive joy and rejoicing. To an non-religious person, this may be utter nonsense.

Here are some other questions to help in the personal application of understanding pleasure and pain:

1. Can the absence or end of pain be pleasurable? Can the absence of pleasure, or loss of the ability to experience pleasure, be painful?
2. What personal differences may influence how we relate to pleasure and pain?
3. Why has sexual activity been part of some religious rituals throughout history?
4. If, in the process of this personal application, you identify any negative addictive behaviors, are you willing to go to the next level of wellness by seeking to change such behaviors?
5. How can you optimize pleasure? (Physiologic pleasure, mental pleasure, psychosocial pleasure and spiritual pleasure.) What is the balance to be achieved?
6. What role does a sense of humor play in dealing with pleasure and pain? What factors seem to contribute to cultivation of a healthy sense of humor?
7. What is hedonic pleasure? What are your beliefs about pleasure and sin and punishment?

• • • • •

An experience from childhood comes to mind. This may trigger similar memories for you:

Our neighbors had a bird-pepper tree close to our property. We were taught that using pepper was wrong — even sinful. But our neighbors used pepper and they seemed to enjoy it. The peppers were very tiny and bright red when ripe. But, as I found out, they may be the hottest peppers in the world!

One day, I decided to try one. I sneaked off into the garden next to the pepper tree, plucked a few peppers and stuck them into my pocket. Hurrying back to our kitchen, it felt exciting to be on the verge of a new experience.

I took a loaf of penny-bread, put the usual butter and brown sugar onto it and added pepper. My first bite of pepper! Oh, what a feeling! Burning pain from hell! It felt as if my tongue was swollen and raw. My eyes watered and I rubbed them with my hands. Now the pepper was in my eyes. What misery!

It was a long time before I tried pepper again.

# Dealing with Addiction

One way to recognize an addiction is to try to give up the behavior. The "whole-person" reaction to the absence of the behavior (addiction to a substance or a process) will give an indication as to whether the addiction is weak or strong, positive or negative, and whether change is necessary.

Of course, a positive addiction may only need to be kept from getting extreme. A weak negative addiction may be changeable through personal efforts, but a strong negative addiction may require outside help.

Stanton Peele, in his book *The Meaning of Addiction: Compulsive Experience and Its Interpretation*, defines an addiction as "an unhealthy or pathological involvement with physical, emotional or environmental factors." Biological, cultural, social, situational, ritualistic, developmental, personality and cognitive factors influence this physical and psychic dependence.

This is what we have been calling a negative addiction. The addict, Peele says, "disregards health, personal well-being and social propriety in order to continue the behavior."

Peele defines a normal self, an ideal self and an addicted self, and believes that an addiction is more related to the individual make-up and adjustment to the environment than to properties of the addictive substance or process. He proposes the following susceptibility factors in the establishment of an addictive behavior:
1. social class (any class can be affected but there is more in lower social classes);
2. parents, peers and the social environment;
3. ethnicity, beliefs and culture;
4. stress situations;
5. inadequate social support and intimacy;
6. lack of positive rewards in life;
7. lack of values toward moderation, self-restraint and health;
8. antisocial attitudes, aggression, alienation and lack of achievement;
9. fear of failure, intolerance of uncertainty and belief in luck or magic; and
10. low self-esteem, lack of self-efficacy and external locus of control.

Along with the above analysis, Peele offers a cure: "Since addiction short-circuits achievement of real-world rewards, find some meaningful activity around which you can wrap your life." The question is what and how. That is the personal pursuit.

Francis Seeburger, in his book *Addiction and Responsibility: An Inquiry into the Addictive Mind*, observes that an addiction is "the state of having given over control to a behavior or habit," "an enslavement," "a way of being in surrender of self to a substance or process." The addiction is tempting, tranquilizing, disburdening and self-perpetuating.

That may apply to both positive and negative addictions. In a negative addiction, the additional components are: harmful to health (physiologic), indicates moral failing, entangling time and resources (mental), leads to alienation and broken relationships (psychosocial), and reflects a lack of real meaning in life (spiritual). Thus, the whole person is involved in a destructive pattern of living, which risks security and offers up self as a sacrifice to an object of worship. The reward is to receive pleasure or decrease pain.

Seeburger proposes that the causes of addiction lie not in the substance or process but in the person and the environment. He believes there is a genetic and psychological predisposition to become addicted; that availability, opportunity and access contribute to the establishment of addictions; that social and societal factors such as permissiveness and consumerism help to push use and consumption; and that direct or symbolic mood or sensation modification help to perpetuate the addiction.

He also thinks that it is possible to reach the ultimate goal of freedom from any addiction where there is "detachment in which there is no obsession with having or avoiding" a substance or process. Thus, an alcoholic may get to the point of non-addictive use of alcohol.

To get to this state of controlled response to pleasure producing or pain relieving behavior, Seeburger gives the following advice:

1. Make the right effort — know the rules and steps to build strength to resist temptations not merely to avoid vice.
2. Cultivate positive traits, retain good ones and seek to expunge bad ones.
3. Replace addictions with healthy pleasures, and seek pleasure options with positive, long-term rewards.
4. Cultivate resistance.
5. Change negative abstinence into positive embrace of self-restraint.
6. Adjust to belief changes — liberation and freedom may only come after bottoming out.
7. Seek activities with greater satisfaction in life.

The above list presents ideal things to do but not how to do them. Many people find practical help through programs such as the "Twelve Step" process (and the many variations and adaptations) first established by Alcoholics Anonymous. The National Directory of Self-Help Organizations provides a list of self-help groups with the services they offer and phone numbers.

Professional help can be obtained through referral or recommendation to licensed practitioners. University-based addiction programs and counselors are a good source of help and generally less expensive than private practitioners.

As an exercise in applications, develop a plan to help a close friend break a pattern of negative addiction to anything of your choice.

One of the aims of this chapter is to produce introspective analysis of the role of pleasure, pain and addictive behavior in overall living. In light of the topics covered here and the knowledge processed over several years, reflections on my life experiences indicate some general, shareable thoughts. In considering my parents, their peers and social environment; my life and social changes in adapting to the American culture; and my children's lives and adjustments to adulthood, I make the following observations:

1. I believe that the propensity for addiction is inherited, and that there are different degrees of expression of the addictive drive.
2. Moral standards, religious dogmas, and general value systems need to be balanced approaches. Extreme rigidity or extreme permissiveness may help to establish addictive behaviors.
3. When good humor, optimism and enjoyable recreational activities outweigh frustration, discouragement and inactivity, there is more enjoyment of life and better handling of inevitable pain.
4. There seems to be nothing as effective as pain and suffering to purify the mind, stimulate creative thoughts, clarify the beliefs and generate spiritual growth.
5. An "amusement park" existence, where you move from one thrill ride to the next for the physiologic excitement, can be fun for a day or two; but if you want a full experience of the park, examine how the rides work, get to know the caretakers, visualize how things can be made better and

work towards doing so. That will provide lasting, integrated pleasure.

6. It may be that everyone is addicted to something. Addiction may be good or bad. It depends on the overall effects on life and everyday function.

7. Happiness is integrated pleasure and pain over the long haul. Both pain and pleasure seem to be necessary for lasting happiness.

## Carol's Turn

Without revealing uncomfortable details of my personal life, I want to share some thoughts on childhood pain, adult pleasures and chronic physiologic pain.

I have shared before about the pain of rejection on the basis of gender. The pleasure of finding love and acceptance is the sweetest experience in life. The joys of intimacy, caring, support and sharing make life worthwhile.

The pain of a constant battle with obesity has given me opportunity to reflect on how humans value one another. I read somewhere that obesity is the fourth leading cause of discrimination behind race, religion and gender. It is painful to experience devaluing treatment by many people when their attitude is based on body size.

It is said that you can control your feelings and determine how other people's attitudes make you feel. Maybe I have not established that level of control. People's negative attitudes and comments hurt, and more so, when it is from relatives or people you know should know better. It is plea-surable to be accepted by true friends for what and who you are.

In Chapter five, I will share my method of dealing with obesity by taking control. I used to depend on other people and the methods of the experts. But gaining the knowledge to proceed with self-directed treatment, even when my primary care physician advised differently, is a pleasurable experience. There is special pleasure in achieving realistic goals.

The core of my belief about a fulfilled life was to devote myself to raising a family and being a happy homemaker. The economic realities of the last twenty years have dictated that that dream be modified. However, the greatest fulfillment and pleasure in my life has been to anchor a Christian home for a devoted husband and to see three children grow to responsible adulthood, give or take a mistake or two. This has given purpose and meaning to my life. The careers I had to acquire along the way were secondary and were for contributing to the primary goal.

After twenty-nine years of marriage, I can summarize by saying that I have lived a satisfied life. I have had my share of inevitable pain. But all in all, life is worthwhile.

To go the distance, the pleasure must outweigh the pain.

# UNDERSTAND HOW
# THE BODY WORKS:
# THE PHYSIOLOGIC DIMENSION

*"...there is no ready-made success formula which would suit everybody. We are all different. The only thing we have in common is our obedience to certain fundamental biologic laws..."*

Hans Selye

Five

# Dedicated to

## Dr. Jerry B. Scott
*Al's major professor at Michigan State University*

*I wish you were still here! You changed my life immeasurably.*

*(Jerry passed away at the tender age of fifty-one, at the peak of his career of bringing in multi-million dollar research projects to Michigan State University. I was one of the last two graduates he sponsored for membership into the American Physiological Society.)*

*and to*

## Francis J. Haddy, MD, PhD
*Former Chairman and Professor Emeritus, Department of Physiology, Uniformed Services University of the Health Sciences*

*I admire you in your retirement as you paint and still keep your hands in physiology research. Thanks for assigning me to work under Jerry's mentorship at Michigan State University twenty-five years ago.*

*M*y task in this chapter is to summarize the major concepts of human function in as simple and straightforward an approach as possible. The seven dynamics from the Matrix of Integrated Function in Chapter 1 will serve as a coherent way to structure this summary. I hope to get the basics of human physiology across to an audience interested in wellness and health promotion.

The anatomy drawings in the color section illustrate the information and supplement this summary. Among all the textbooks I have used over the years, John W. Hole's *Human Anatomy and Physiology* has been my favorite for illustrations and concise summaries. The seventh edition of Hole's book is a revision done by three authors who keep Dr. Hole's legacy available for students of anatomy and physiology. If you want to read more in-depth anatomy and physiology in relation to health or for college course-work, this is the text I recommend.

My purpose is to give an abbreviated review of the major concepts in human physiology. In doing this, there will be major gaps in the information. I hope an overall picture will emerge that will reinforce the great complexities of human function and give a basic understanding of how all the organ systems work together to maintain life.

Life, as we know it, is only possible from the physical point of view because certain conditions exist that allow biochemical processes to continue to "keep the fires burning." The term "homeostasis" was first used by the Harvard physiologist Walter B. Cannon to mean the mainte-nance of internal balance in the conditions that support life.

For example, the body must maintain its state of balance between acid and alkaline conditions. There must be a supply of oxygen and an excretion of carbon dioxide. Water and nutrients must be supplied. Cell function must produce certain molecules and break down others to extract energy and form building blocks for complex molecules needed to perform certain functions. Our discussion has to begin with homeostasis.

# Homeostasis at the Cellular Level

Homeostasis is the state of constancy and balance that exists among the mechanisms that support and maintain the conditions for life. The mechanisms have to be examined on the cellular level first of all.

## The Cell

The cell is the unit of structure and function in the human body. Within the cell, the chemical reaction is the unit of function. Chemical reactions make and break chemical bonds. This is the basis of all of life's chemistry. While some physical processes, such as movement of particles from areas of high to low concentration, assist in some cell functions, the basis of how the body does what it does is chemistry. (I have found that biochemistry textbooks are very fast-acting sleeping aids!)

The basis of chemistry is the structure and properties of the atom, the smallest interacting particle of matter, which has the characteristics of the specific element. The active part of the atom is the electron orbital, which forms and breaks bonds, trapping or releasing energy. The number of protons in an atom determines the qualities of the atom.

Atoms bonding together make up molecules. The structure of an atom and a portion of DNA, one of the most complex molecules in the body, are shown in Figure 5-1.

The atoms most prominently involved in body chemistry are oxygen, carbon, hydrogen, nitrogen, calcium and phosphorus, in descending order as percent body weight. These make up about 98.8% of the body weight. The other elements such as sodium, potassium and chloride, and the trace elements such as copper, zinc, selenium and iodine, make up the other 1.2%.

It was once calculated that all the elements that make up a human could be purchased for less than $10. But all the molecules the body synthesizes from these elements would cost several million dollars! Talk about $6 million person!

All human cells have a membrane, which regulates transport into and out of the cell; a cytoplasm, where many chemical reactions take place; and a nucleus (except mature red blood cells), where the genetic material is stored. A composite cell is illustrated in Figure 5-2.

Cells are three-dimensional physical structures and are adapted to perform specific functions. In the illustration, the various structures shown are common to most cells. Let us look at the major features of the subcellular structures. These are referred to as organelles or "little organs."

## The Nucleus

The nucleus of the cell is the headquarters of operations since it contains the chromosomes which carry the genetic code.

The body is made up of about 100 trillion cells, give or take a few trillion! Each cell contains all forty-six chromosomes (except mature egg and sperm cells which have twenty-three). The function of a given cell is determined by which genes are turned on or off at a given point in its life.

The nucleus of each cell contains all the chromosomes, which have copies of all the genes. The forty-six chromosomes have about 100,000 genes. Genes carry the instructions to make specific proteins, which then carry out their special functions such as transporting oxygen (hemoglobin), giving color to the skin (melanin), speeding up chemical reactions (enzymes) and protecting against infections (immunoglobulins).

Genes are made up of DNA (double-helical strands of deoxyribonucleic acid). The DNA can unwind at specific spots to create copies of the code on the genes. These copies, called messenger RNA, then go out into the cytoplasm to make proteins.

A protein is made by assembling a set number of amino acids in a set order and structure. The genes tell how many of which amino acids, how many strands of simple proteins, and how these strands twist and coil on one another to make a complex protein.

The Human Genome Project, the US government's $3 billion research plan to identify all the genes on the forty-six human chromosomes, should be completed by the year 2003. About six thousand genes have been identified so far.

## The Mitochondria

The mitochondria take in molecules from the digestion of food to produce energy. The energy is obtained when chemical bonds in the food molecule (mainly the carbon-hydrogen bonds) are broken. The energy released is captured and stored as ATP (adenosine triphosphate). The mitochondria are sometimes called "the powerhouse of the cell." The cell gets energy from ATP to power chemical reactions.

## The Ribosomes

The ribosomes are sites of production of protein, for which the commands come from the genes in the nucleus. This process is one of the most fascinating in cell function.

## The Cell Membrane

The cell membrane controls what goes in and out of the cell. This is done by passive transport through open channels, or by special transport molecules in the membrane. In nerve, muscle and some special receptor cells, the electrical charge across the membrane can be temporarily discharged, giving rise to an electrical spike.

What an organ can do is based on what the cells of that organ do. A brief review of organ function will help us capture the basic concepts of homeostasis. Each organ system plays a specific role in maintenance of the delicate balance necessary to support life.

# Homeostasis at the Organ Level

## The Skin

The skin is the largest organ of the body. It is made up of several layers of tissue, each with its own cell type. The illustration (Figure 5-3) shows a section of skin with blood vessels, sweat glands and nerve endings.

The skin functions as a protective covering; as a water, body temperature and salt regulator; and as a sense organ for changes in temperature and pressure. Pain and pleasure receptors abound in skin.

## Muscle

Muscle tissue is composed of cells called myofibers. These are elongated cells which contain proteins organized into myofilaments. Skeletal muscle and heart muscle are more organized than the smooth muscle which lines the internal organs and blood vessels.

In skeletal muscle and cardiac muscle, the thick and thin proteins are arranged in units called sarcomeres. It is the shortening and lengthening of these sarcomeres that cause a muscle to contract to develop force. When many sarcomeres shorten, the myofibrils shorten, then the muscle cell shortens. Many muscle cells shortening together cause the whole muscle to shorten with force.

Thus, the skeletal muscles can produce movement and do work. The heart can pump. The blood vessels can change size to control blood flow. All this depends on the proteins, arranged in a specific order and sliding across each other. In fact,

*The Human Genome Project, the US government's $3 billion research plan to identify all the genes on the forty-six human chromosomes, should be completed by the year 2003.*

this is called the sliding filament theory of muscle contraction. Calcium plays a central role in this process.

The junction between nerve and muscle is the key connection enabling us to control muscle movement. Figure 5-4 illustrates the structure and function of skeletal and cardiac muscle.

## Bone

Bone is living tissue. The bone cell, the osteocyte, and its cousins, the osteoblast and osteoclast, are the central players in controlling bone composition. Bone is active tissue with constant turnover between breakdown and formation. Calcium and phosphate salts are responsible for the hardness of bone. Vitamin D plays an important role in bone health.

Bone functions as protection, to allow movement and locomotion, and to produce blood cells in the marrow. Figure 5-5 illustrates the structure of bone.

## Blood

In contrast to bone, the hardest tissue in the body, blood is the softest. It is composed of a variety of cells suspended in a fluid-protein matrix called plasma.

Plasma is water with proteins and salts. Plasma makes up about 55% of the volume of blood. The other 45% (referred to as the hematocrit) is mainly red blood cells, with a smaller volume of white blood cells and platelets. The blood cells and platelets are produced in the marrow of the bones.

Red blood cells (RBCs) transport oxygen to all tissues and carbon dioxide to the lungs to be excreted. Most of the oxygen and carbon dioxide are transported bound by hemoglobin, a protein in the RBCs. RBCs also carry other proteins which determine our blood types (A, B, AB, O). RBCs live for about 120 days.

White blood cells (WBCs) can move from the blood vessels and travel throughout all tissues where they carry out functions of the immune system. One type of WBC, the granulocyte, eats foreign cells and particles. They live for about twelve hours.

Another type of WBC, monocytes, live for several weeks and patrol the tissues as macrophages. A third type, the lymphocytes, are the main players in the immune system and live for several months to years.

Platelets are not whole cells. They are like fragments of cells, which function to plug injuries in blood vessels and help blood clot. Platelets live for about eight to twelve days. Blood cells are illustrated in Figure 5-6.

An average adult has about five liters (ten pints) of blood. The water in blood is in constant exchange with the water between cells in the tissues, including bone. The volume of this interstitial (between cells) water is about eight to ten liters, including the water in the fluids in joints, the spinal fluid, the fluid in the eyes and around the heart.

The water between cells is in constant exchange with the water within the cells. The volume of intracellular (within the cells) water is about twenty-five liters.

The total volume of water in an average adult is about forty liters. This accounts for about 63% of the body weight in men, and about 52% of the body weight of women. Obese people of both sexes have less water than lean people.

The need for and importance of water for health cannot be overemphasized.

Blood functions to transport cells, oxygen and nutrients to all tissues, to maintain water and electrolyte balance, to carry cellular waste and to provide a proper environment for chemical reactions to occur.

## The Heart and Blood Vessels

The heart and blood vessels keep blood circulating throughout the body. The heart is a mechanical pump (really two pumps side by side), and the blood vessels are the plumbing that conducts blood to all tissues. (Are cardiovascular surgeons and urologists, then, the plumbers of the body human?)

One fascinating aspect of heart function is that the heart can beat without any nerve connections. It generates its own electrical stimulus which triggers the contraction of the heart muscle. A record of this electrical activity is called the electrocardiogram (ECG or EKG). This electrical pulse occurs about seventy-two times each minute in an adult at rest. Each heartbeat starts as an electrical impulse in the node of tissue called the sino-atrial node.

Among the blood vessels, the arterioles are the major points of control of the pressure and flow within the system. The capillaries, the smallest of the blood vessels, are the sites of exchange between the blood stream and all other tissues. The lymphatic vessels collect excess water from between cells and dump it back into the blood stream. Figure 5-7 illustrates the structure and relationships of the heart and circulation.

## The Kidney and Urinary System

The plasma volume and the dissolved salts in the blood are regulated by the action of the skin (sweat), lungs (moisture in the air exhaled), intestines (water in the feces) and chiefly, the kidneys (urine). The entire plasma volume flows through the kidneys approximately once every twenty-four minutes.

The nephron (about one million in each kidney) is the unit of structure and function in the kidneys for filtering the plasma, getting rid of waste and returning the good stuff back to the blood stream. The tubules from all the nephrons join the ureters, which conduct the urine to the bladder.

When the bladder reaches a certain degree of stretch, the urination reflex (the exotic term is micturition reflex) is triggered and the urine is expelled through the urethra.

The bladder of an average adult holds about six hundred milliliters of urine. However, the urination reflex is triggered at about 150 milliliters. Urine output needs to be balanced each day by adequate intake of water. Figure 5-8 illustrates the urinary system.

The urinary system is the main system that regulates water and salt balance. The average adult output of urine per twenty-four hours ranges between one and two liters. This output must be balanced by water intake to maintain the proper internal environment for chemical reactions. This is the reason for the advice to drink about six to eight eight-ounce glasses of water per day. One liter is approximately equal to thirty-two ounces, which is four eight-ounce glasses.

## The Digestive System

The digestive system, also referred to as the gastrointestinal (GI) tract, processes the food we eat by breaking down complex molecules into simpler ones. Proteins are broken down to amino acids and very small proteins called peptides.

Carbohydrates are broken down into simple sugars, chiefly glucose. Fats are broken down into fatty acids and glycerol. Nucleic acids are broken down into nucleotides. These smaller products of digestion can be absorbed into the blood stream for distribution to the cells throughout the body.

The digestive process begins in the mouth with the saliva. The stomach adds its juices which are highly acidic. The small intestine, pancreas and liver add their juices, which are alkaline.

Most of the absorption of food occurs in the small intestine. The large intestine completes the absorption of water, electrolytes and some vitamins.

The action of normal bacteria is essential for the completion of the process, especially to break down fiber. These bacteria also make small amounts of some vitamins such as K and B12.

Fecal waste is expelled when the defecation reflex is triggered due to bulk accumulation in the rectum, the terminal end of the GI tract. The anal canal conducts the feces out at the anus under voluntary control. Figure 5-9 shows the organs making up the digestive system.

All the absorbed nutrients from the GI tract go first to the liver, then to all other tissues of the body for use in production of energy and as building blocks for complex molecules.

## The Respiratory System

In order to produce energy from the food we eat, oxygen must be present in the cells. The respiratory system is designed to bring a fresh supply of oxygen into the body and expel excess carbon dioxide, which is produced during metabolism.

The lungs are richly supplied with blood capillaries. The capillaries lie close to the smallest air sacs, the alveoli. Oxygen moves from the air in the air sacs, across the capillary membrane and attaches to the hemoglobin in the red blood cells. Oxygen is transported to all tissues by the red blood cells. Some oxygen is dissolved in the plasma, but most of it is bound to hemoglobin.

At the tissue level, oxygen moves from the capillaries, across the cell membrane into the cytoplasm and into the mitochondria. The major work of producing energy, mainly from glucose and fatty acids, occurs inside the mitochondria.

Oxygen is the acceptor of free electrons and free hydrogen ions, which are captured to form water. The other product of this metabolic process is carbon dioxide. Carbon dioxide is transported back to the lungs to be exhaled.

Cells cannot survive long without oxygen. If oxygen is missing, or if the energy production cycle in the mitochondria is blocked (by cyanide, for example), the energy producing reactions in the cell stop. The chemical reactions inside the cell cannot go on. Cells die. Then tissues die. Then the organs die. And then, the organism, the person, dies. This is the common pathway for all causes of death — cells are deprived of oxygen and nutrients by some means. Figure 5-10 shows the structure of the respiratory system.

## The Endocrine System

One of the ways all the above systems are made to work and develop together is by the action of hormones. Hormones are chemicals produced in small amounts by specialized tissue. They are dumped directly into the blood stream and stimulate specific actions in other tissues. The responsive tissues have receptors for the particular hormone.

All the glands that produce these hormones make up the endocrine system. The endocrine glands and their major functions are shown in Figure 5-11.

Hormones exert their actions by binding to receptors on cell membranes or inside the cell, and triggering chemical reactions, including gene activity. The response by the cell is to make active molecules such as proteins that carry out the action intended by the hormone. Figure 5-11 illustrates the location of the endocrine glands.

## The Immune System

The other system helping to integrate and balance all body functions is the immune system. The major function of this system is to preserve and protect the entire body from external and internal threats of destruction.

The white blood cells erform the major immune functions. Neutrophils and monocytes are phagocytic — they eat foreign particles. They leave the blood stream and patrol all tissues. They congregate at the sites of infection and inflammation. Monocytes give rise to macrophages which become attached to various tissues.

The major immune functions are carried out by lymphocytes, which are produced mainly in the bone marrow, some in the lymph nodes. A portion of them goes to the thymus where they mature into T-cells. The rest mature in the bone marrow or elsewhere and become B-cells. Both types circulate in the blood, lymphatic system, lymph nodes, bone marrow and secretory glands. They live for several months to several years.

T-cells and B-cells react differently to abnormal and disease causing agents outside or inside the body. T-cells directly attack the foreign particle or secrete a substance that attacks and destroys the foreign particle. This is called cell-mediated immunity. (The AIDS virus destroys one line of T-cells, the T4 line, and greatly reduces cell-mediated immunity.)

B-cells respond to a foreign particle by becoming plasma cells that secrete antibodies. These antibodies are a class of proteins called immunoglobulins which bind to antigens on the foreign particle.

B-cells and T-cells work together in many cases. Some lymphocytes do not become B-cells or T-cells. They are called null cells. Some of these null cells have the ability to destroy tumor cells, virus-infected cells and cells coated with antibodies. Such null cells are called "natural killer cells."

*This is the common pathway for all causes of death — cells are deprived of oxygen and nutrients by some means.*

The immune system gives protection against and enables recovery from many diseases. These responses are also the basis of allergic reactions and tissue transplant rejection. Figure 5-12 shows the cell types of the immune system in relation to the other blood cells and the origin of B-cells and T-cells.

## The Nervous System

The nervous system is the most rapid and most extensive system for coordinating and controlling body functions. From simple sensations to the higher functions of the mind, the activity of nerve cells is the foundation.

The nerve cell or neuron can generate an electrical impulse. This is possible because the arrangement of positive and negative charges across the cell membrane can be briefly disturbed and reestablished. The neuron is said to be "irritable." Figure 5-13 illustrates the structure of a neuron and the events occurring at a synapse.

A stimulus discharges the voltage across the cell membrane by causing sodium ions to move into the cell and potassium ions to move out. The electrical spike created is called an action potential.

The action potential, or electrical spike, is conducted along the length of the axon of the cell to the terminals. The axon terminals have many tiny vesicles, filled with neurotransmitter substances. The action potential breaks the vesicles and the neurotransmitter substance flows out of the terminal into the junction with another neuron. This junction, the synapse, is the point of contact with other neurons to form an electrical circuit.

*Signals about how much of what is acting where must be given in order to have proper conditions to maintain life.*

The functions of neurons and receptors at nerve endings are to deliver electrical impulses into and out of the brain and spinal cord. The brain and spinal cord, the central nervous system (CNS), process the information brought in by the nerves. The stronger the stimulus, the more action potentials flow into the brain.

The receptor cells of the sense organs (eyes, ears, nose, tongue, skin) are specialized to respond to a specific stimulus. They capture the stimulus and conduct the information as action potentials. Each type of stimulus (light, sound, chemical, pressure, pain, pleasure, temperature) travels along specific paths to specific areas of the brain. The stronger the stimulus, the more action potentials — electrical spikes — generated and sent to the spinal cord and brain.

In the eyes, the receptor cells that respond to light are called rods and cones. The receptor cells in the ears are called hair cells which respond to the frequency of vibration (sound) conducted in the air.

For smell, the receptor cells are called olfactory cells which respond to chemicals. The tongue has taste buds with taste cells which detect chemicals.

Perception, storage and recall; interpretation; and responding to and using this information are "higher functions" of the brain. This is where mind comes in. Examine Figure 5-16 to see the relationship of the funcational area of the brain.

The above summary has been an attempt to paint a picture of the vast numbers of mechanisms and events that must be coordinated for the body to function.

This is homeostasis — a second-to-second act of balance and integration.

The systems all depend on one another and interact with one another. Signals about how much of what is acting where must be given in order to have proper conditions to maintain life.

The signals, which indicate changes in the various systems, are called feedback signals. For example, if body temperature falls, the change is sensed in the hypothalamus of the brain. The drop in temperature is registered, and action is taken to bring the temperature up.

Blood vessels of the skin constrict to push blood away from the skin to the deeper tissues (cold bumps appear on skin and hairs stand up). Muscles begin to contract to produce a shiver. These mechanisms help to create heat to raise the temperature. This is an example of negative feedback — a response to bring a set value back to a set point after a change has been detected.

Positive feedback occurs to push a process to a desired limit. A good example of this is the process of childbirth. Small uterine contractions stimulate bigger contractions until the infant is expelled from the birth canal.

Diseases are disturbances and disruptions in the homeostatic mechanisms. The body fights to recover from any of these assaults. From diseases caused by bacteria and viruses to diseases influenced by lifestyle and environment, the cause of the malfunction is a disruption of one or more of the homeostatic mechanisms discussed above.

The magnificent healing power of the body is built into these homeostatic mechanisms. Our self-care and medicines only help to promote the conditions for these mechanisms to work.

We can now move on to exploring the other dynamics of human function.

# Nutrition

Plants can use water, sunlight and inorganic chemicals from the soil to make all their food. Humans cannot. To provide the chemicals needed for energy production and for building the complex molecules required for homeostasis, humans must get a regular supply directly from plants or from animals.

## Nutrients

Nutrients come in the form of organic compounds and inorganic molecules. Carbohydrates, proteins, fats and vitamins are "organic," meaning that the molecules are built upon a backbone of carbon atoms. "Inorganic" means other than carbon-based molecules. (Organically grown produce means grown in soil that has not been fertilized by inorganic, manufactured fertilizers, but enriched by plant and animal matter.)

The inorganic substances are minerals such as sodium, potassium and calcium; and trace elements such as copper, zinc, selenium and chromium.

Proteins must provide all amino acids of which eight are termed "essential" because they cannot be made from other amino acids. The eight essential amino ac-

*The magnificent healing power of the body is built into these homeostatic mechanisms.*

ids are isoleucine, leucine, lysine, methionine, phenylalanine, threonine, tryptophan and valine.

Carbohydrates, or starches, are broken down to simple sugars, which are all eventually converted to glucose in the body. Glucose is the most immediate energy source for the cells. The storage form of glucose is a body starch called glycogen.

Fats are used in the body as fatty acids and glycerol which are energy sources. Fat storage is for longer term energy supply.

Vitamins are organic substances required in small amounts to speed up important metabolic reactions. Several trace elements act as cofactors with vitamins to control metabolic reactions.

Minerals are inorganic molecules needed for important chemical reactions and bioelectricity. Minerals such as sodium, potassium and chloride dissolved in the blood are referred to as electrolytes.

The trace elements such as selenium, chromium and zinc are needed in very small amounts. Much research is currently focused on understanding the role of trace elements in metabolic reactions.

Another interesting function of vitamins and trace elements is their role as antioxidants. Antioxidants are compounds that neutralize free radicals.

Free radicals are generated in the chemical reactions where oxygen is used within cells. The resulting compounds contain oxygen with an unpaired electron. This makes the molecule highly reactive and unstable.

Free radicals such as hydrogen peroxide and the hydroxyl ion can damage cell membranes and DNA. This may lead to cancer, degenerative disease, faster aging and the initial damage to blood vessels that starts the accumulation of plaque.

The body contains natural chemical systems to neutralize free radicals. However, because of the composition of the average diet, especially in developed countries, these systems can be overwhelmed. Extra antioxidants in the diet are recommended if the diet includes animal proteins, fats, fried food, high dairy and low plant products.

Antioxidants include beta-carotene; vitamins A, C, E, B1 and B6; lecithin; indoles (from cabbage and broccoli); and chlorophyll (the green coloring pigment in leaves).

## Nutrition Behavior

An adequate diet is balanced in terms of supplying all the required nutrients. Minimum daily requirements were first established to provide levels that would keep people from developing deficiency diseases. Currently, the major questions at the consumer level with regard to nutrition include:

1. Are important nutrients lacking from our diets because of deficiencies in the soil?
2. What level of supplementation is safe or necessary?
3. Can longevity, degenerative diseases, and mental abilities be influenced by nutrition?
4. Why is eating behavior so difficult to change for better health?

There is now no question that in many places the soil is deficient in important nutrients. The history of iodine deficiency as told in the Oxford University Press publication (1989), *The Story of Iodine Deficiency: An International Challenge in Nutrition*, shows how widespread is iodine deficiency in soil.

Western countries have solved the problem of iodine deficiency and practically wiped out goiter and cretinism (characterized by dwarfism, mental retardation and deaf mutism) by adding iodine to table salt. But there are many countries where dietary iodine deficiency due to iodine deficiency in the soil is still a major problem.

Estimates are that about one billion people are at risk for iodine deficiency worldwide. In the People's Republic of China, about one-third of the population lives in areas with iodine deficiency in the soil.

With our modern methods of cultivation and commercial fertilizers, we cannot be sure that we are getting all our essential nutrients from food sources. A prudent course is to supplement with multivitamins, antioxidants and trace elements. A moderate use is the best advice currently.

High doses of some vitamins have been shown to be toxic. For example, high doses of vitamin A produce liver toxicity. Considerations of how much of certain formulations are absorbed enter into this decision.

There are laboratory tests that can determine what levels of some vitamins and minerals are actually available to the internal function of white blood cells. These tests may become more commonly used to determine how much supplementation is necessary.

Because of the role nutrients play in nerve activity, hormone production and function, and immune system function, it is thought that diet and nutrition may be second only to the genes in influencing aging; many chronic, degenerative diseases; and general well-being. The direct influence on mental abilities and function is not as definitely established. There are claims for tyrosine and choline improving memory and mental alertness.

The research studies to link specific vitamins and minerals to either preventive or health enhancing functions take years to complete. For example, it has been known for about fifteen years that some types of birth defects are related to the lack of specific nutrients in the mother's diet.

It has now been shown definitely that folic acid deficiency during pregnancy is the chief cause of spina bifida. The FDA sanctioned the addition of folic acid (folate) to food such as grains and bread in 1997.

How long should an individual wait for research in order to act on using nutrient supplementation to prevent disease and promote health? The individual decision is a matter of what a person believes and how much trust a person puts in the advice of physicians or other authorities on the subject.

The claims and counterclaims about new and old supplements, and the introduction of myriad herbal therapies, leave many of us confused. In the personal applications section below, I will discuss what course I follow, and how I came to that decision.

*Because of the role nutrients play in nerve activity, hormone production and function and immune system function, it is thought that diet and nutrition may be second only to the genes in influencing aging; many chronic, degenerative diseases; and general well-being.*

The effect of nutrition on longevity is obvious from the statistics on risk of heart disease and cancer. People on diets of high animal protein and fats have more heart disease and colon cancer than those whose diets are based more on plant source. Diet is a major lifestyle factor associated with leading causes of death and disability.

Eating habits are difficult to change because we get programmed with certain tastes, and eating takes on more than biologic meaning in our lives. Genetic and environmental factors set a pattern that is difficult to change with knowledge, decision and discipline.

Several levels of nervous and hormonal input influence the hunger and satiety centers in the brain. Early programming, the social and spiritual significance of food, and marketing appeal set the appetite for food.

The major nutritional disorders in developed and developing countries are malnutrition, obesity, anorexia and bulimia.

In the USA, one in three adults and one in five teenagers are overweight. These numbers are included in the *Healthy People 2000 — Midcourse Review and 1995 Revisions* published in 1995. They show an increase from ten years ago.

According to recent data gathered by the US Department of Agriculture in the survey "What We Eat in America," some improvements in dietary habits have been made. However, when the survey showed that, as a group, adult females failed to meet the recommended dietary allowance for six nutrients (iron, zinc, vitamin B-6, calcium, magnesium and vitamin E), it highlighted major room for improvement. The problem is not a lack of information and knowledge. It is the difficulty of changing eating habits.

# Stress and Stress Adaptation

Hans Selye, famous Canadian scientist, devoted his life to the study of human stress. His research laid the foundation for the medical, psychological and philosophical application of stress physiology to everyday life.

The following points highlight what we understand about stress and stress adaptation:

1. Stress is any demand on human function that pushes homeostatic mechanisms to increased function. This causes excess wear and tear on the whole person.

2. Good stress (positive life events) and bad stress (negative life events) trigger the same mechanisms. The difference seems to be the perception and meaning in terms of pleasure and pain.

3. Good stress may trigger other mechanisms such as endorphins and enkephalins which may strengthen the immune system. Bad stress may also trigger as yet unknown mechanisms that have negative effects.

4. The nervous system and the immune system have a close interconnection in response to stress. The new science of psychoneuroimmunology has shed considerable light on this subject. Good stress, up to certain levels, strengthens this positive connection; bad stress weakens this interaction.

5. Stress is a normal part of life. Our reaction and personal adaptation to the stress response can be moderated and controlled through understanding and use of some practical stress management techniques.

Stressors are the events or conditions that trigger the stress response. The stress response includes increased nervous drive, increased hormone production and general arousal described as "the flight or fight response." The physiology of this response is illustrated in Figure 5-14.

Physiologic stressors include excessive noise (also prolonged sound isolation), extreme temperatures, radiation, pollutants and toxins, carcinogens, extreme physical activity (or inactivity), hunger, thirst and malnutrition.

Other stressors such as anxiety, guilt, low self-esteem and hopelessness will be discussed in the appropriate chapters. The key point here is that the stress response is to push homeostatic mechanisms to a state of imbalance.

The sum of all stressors increases the wear and tear on the body resulting in physiologic malfunctions. In most individuals, a vulnerable system would be affected. If the cardiovascular system is the vulnerable system, hypertension and heart disease may occur.

If the GI system is the vulnerable system, ulcers or spastic colon may result. Similarly, headaches — both tension and migraines — nervousness and depression, arthritis and other symptoms may result from stress.

These physiological changes are the consequences of overdrive of the nervous (sympathetic and parasympathetic drives) and the endocrine systems, coupled with a reduced effectiveness of the immune system.

Stress management includes removal of stressors, escaping from the stressful environment, adapting to conditions that cannot be changed or buffering the effects of inevitable stress through learning techniques to control the stress response. Medications to relieve painful symptoms of stress are helpful, but they do not resolve the problem or provide long-term coping strategies. In Chapter 6, we will review some practical stress management techniques.

# Work

Work is the expenditure of energy to generate force that acts on the environment. Physiologic work by humans involves chemical work and physical activity.

The energy to do work ultimately comes from the sun. It is trapped by plants in the process of photosynthesis. The energy in the chemical bonds (mainly the carbon-hydrogen and carbon-carbon bonds) in food molecules from plants is transformed into high-energy phosphate bonds in adenosine triphosphate. ATP is referred to as "the energy currency of the cell."

The body uses ATP to produce more ATP from carbohydrates, fats and proteins. To maintain the normal body functions at rest requires about twelve hundred calories per day. This is the reason for recommendations that weight reduction diets should not supply less than a thousand calories per day. If the supply of calories falls below what is needed to maintain the basal metabolic rate, metabolism slows down.

For chemical reactions to go on, for mechanical work such as the beating of the heart or moving food through the gut and for body movements such as playing a game of racquetball, ATP is the energy supply.

Physical work leading to physical fitness is essential for maintaining and promoting healthy function of the body. Physical fitness provides better muscle tone, strength and flexibility; increased bone density and resistance to osteoporosis; a strengthened immune system; increased cardiopulmonary fitness and reduction of the risks of heart disease; and an increased overall sense of well-being.

People who keep physically fit enjoy more years of healthy function than people who do not. The consequences of inactivity and a sedentary lifestyle include obesity, increased risk of osteoporosis, hypertension, diabetes, heart disease and cancer.

Balance, moderation and enjoyment are important factors in the pursuit of physical fitness.

## Rest

Physiologic rest refers to physical relaxation of muscle tension and deep, restful sleep. The demands of everyday life produce tense muscles which can be the cause of muscular pain and headaches. Several techniques in deep muscle relaxation and massage can be very helpful.

The human organism needs sleep for the reduction of the level of work it does, for a period of shutdown from input stimulation and for the brain to process all the information captured during the waking period of the day.

Six to eight hours of sleep fill the need for most humans. Individual requirements may range from as little as four to as much as nine or ten.

The circadian rhythm of the sleep-wake cycle is approximately twenty-four hours. The phases of sleep show different electrical patterns as the brain moves from an awake-alert state into deep sleep.

The predominant brain wave form in an awake, aroused state is called beta waves. As relaxation and drowsiness take over, the electrical pattern changes to alpha waves when the eyes close. The first period of sleep is "slow wave sleep" or "non-REM" sleep. This consists of four stages which represent increasing depth of sleep. The four stages of slow wave sleep are:

1. Stage 1 — theta wave stage where slower waves appear among the alpha waves.
2. Stage 2 — sleep spindles, bursts of fast waves, appear as the theta waves change to even slower waves.
3. Stage 3 — slower delta waves appear with fewer sleep spindles.
4. Stage 4 — this is also called delta wave sleep. Delta waves are the slowest brain wave and represent the deepest sleep.

In slow wave sleep, the muscles relax, heart rate and blood pressure decrease, and the GI tract speeds up to push digestive products through. The stages of slow wave sleep follow a reverse order to return to the awake state. On ascending from the

*The phases of sleep show different electrical patterns as the brain moves from an awake-alert state into deep sleep.*

depth of delta wave sleep, rapid eye movement (REM) sleep occurs.

The change from slow wave sleep to REM sleep occurs about every 90 minutes. In REM sleep, the brain's electrical activity is similar to what it is in the awake state, but it is difficult to arouse the sleeper. This is why this phase of sleep is also called paradoxical sleep. This is the stage of sleep when dreaming takes place. The eyes move as if following motion, and other muscles contract to produce erratic body movements. Dreams occur as if real events are taking place. (People who experience bed-wetting report that, in their dream, they were actually urinating at an appropriate time in an appropriate place.)

Our understanding of the mechanism and function of sleep is incomplete. It seems to be an active process with a built-in cycle. New research shows high activity of the emotional areas of the brain during sleep and dreaming.

One possible purpose of sleep is to shut down incoming stimuli to give the brain time to process, sort, file and fit in new information. In the process, many bits and pieces of related and unrelated information from knowledge and experience flow together, creating dreams.

Newborns spend about half their time in REM sleep. This decreases to the point that in the elderly, there is little time spent in REM sleep, and less sleep is needed.

The most common major sleep disorder is insomnia — difficulty falling asleep or difficulty staying asleep. It is believed that the neurotransmitter serotonin plays an active role in sleep. A deficiency in serotonin may be one of the causes of insomnia.

Other causes of insomnia are stress, lack of physical activity, use of stimulants and obstruction of breathing during sleep. Obstruction of breathing, or sleep apnea, may be related to mechanical problems in the airways. It causes frequent interruption of sleep. This condition is more common in men than women.

It is estimated that sleep disorders cost the US economy about $50 billion each year for treatment and loss of productivity.

Sleep disorder medicine is one of the latest specializations in medical science. Sleep laboratories are set up to help diagnose and treat patients for insomnia and other conditions such as narcolepsy (excessive sleepiness and loss of control of muscles even in the awake state). REM behavior disorder, where the person acts out dreams and may cause injury to self, sleep partner or the immediate environment, is also seen.

*It is estimated that sleep disorders cost the US economy about $50 billion each year for treatment and loss of productivity.*

# Growth and Development

The human life cycle begins with the union of the sperm cell (the male gamete) and the egg cell (the female gamete). This merger of the genetic material from each parent is called fertilization.

The product of fertilization is a zygote, a single cell with forty-six chromosomes, twenty-three from each parent. Cell division and travel to the uterus begins, and in approximately one week a hollow ball of cells (the blastocyst) implants in the uterus.

Implantation marks the beginning of the embryonic period of development. The offspring develops from pre-embryo (two weeks old) to embryo (up to the end of eight weeks) to fetus (up to the time of birth).

The odds against an egg becoming a newborn infant are tremendous. It is estimated that a female human is born with about two million eggs. These degenerate until there are only about 600,000 at puberty. During the reproductive years, only four to five hundred will mature to produce fertilizable eggs. On average, approximately 38% of fertilized eggs produce live births.

The prenatal period is divided into three stages: the period of cleavage, the embryonic stage and the fetal stage. The postnatal period begins at birth and ends with death.

The postnatal period is divided into the neonatal period (up to four weeks old), infancy (one month to one year), childhood (one year to puberty), adolescence (puberty to the age of majority), adulthood and senescence.

The control of growth, maturity and aging involves the program of the genetic code, the biochemical environment of the cells, the state of nutrition and the physical and social environment.

Normal growth with an optimal environment seems to allow for a lifespan of 115 to 120 years. The average life expectancy in the USA for infants born in 1996 is approaching eighty years — always a little lower for males and a little higher for females.

*It is estimated that by the year 2020, one-third of the US population will be over sixty-five years of age.*

Death is the inevitable end of life. The major causes of death in adults are heart disease, cancer and stroke. Cancer is on the increase, while heart disease has been declining over the last ten years. Cancer may soon be the leading cause of death.

It is estimated that by the year 2020, one-third of the US population will be over sixty-five years of age. Disease patterns may change as heart disease and cancer are better controlled through a combination of scientific and lifestyle efforts. If current trends continue, it is conjectured that Alzheimer's disease may be the leading cause of death by the year 2020.

## Reproduction

I have dealt with the introductory facts of reproduction above. The bare essentials of the early events in the biology of human reproduction are illustrated in Figure 5-15. This figure illustrates formation of the sperm cells in the testes and the process of fertilization and implantation.

The biochemical purpose in life, the physiologic reason for the functioning of all the systems described so far, and the single biologic goal of existence is the perpetuation of the species.

However, human sexuality serves the species for higher functions as well. The physiologic component of pair bonding is the pleasure generated in the brain when the nervous mechanism of the sexual climax is triggered. The brain registers this surge of euphoria and confers value and worth to the partners involved in producing this highest experience of physiologic pleasure.

Pair bonds promote the formation of the social dynamics that provide for the nurturing of the next generation mentally, socially and spiritually, as well as physically and biologically.

Human sexuality and the sociology of family life are beyond the scope of this book. It must suffice at this point to say that human sexuality is the aspect of physiology that has the potential to be a major force for pleasure and pain, good and bad, and satisfaction and dissatisfaction in life.

# The Major Physiologic Health Problems

Diseases of the cardiovascular system are currently the leading cause of death and disability for adults in developed countries. This group of diseases includes coronary heart disease, in which the arteries that bring oxygen and nutrients to the heart muscle are clogged by plaque. Cerebrovascular disease, which results in strokes caused by blockage or rupture of arteries in the brain, is currently the third leading cause of death in the USA.

In the 45-64 age group in the USA, cancer has overtaken heart disease as the leading cause of death.

The 1999 statistics from the US Public Health Service (*National Vital Statistics Reports*, Vol. 47, No. 9) list the ten leading causes of death among adults of all age groups and all races as:

1. heart disease
2. cancer
3. cerebrovascular disease
4. chronic obstructive pulmonary disease
5. unintentional injuries
6. pneumonia and influenza
7. diabetes mellitus
8. HIV infection
9. suicide
10. homicide

Lifestyle factors are thought to be responsible for roughly 50% of the causes of the top four diseases listed above.

The latest statistics as summarized in *Healthy People 2000 — Midcourse Review and 1995 Revisions* from the US Public Health Service show the following:

1. Approximately 2.1 million people die each year.
2. About 400,000 of these deaths can be directly attributed to cigarette smoking as the primary cause of the disease (heart and lung disease, cancer and stroke) that ended life.
3. Obesity is a major contributor to disease and disability. It is estimated that as much as one-third of the American population is overweight. This is an increase of about 10% over 1980 (National Center for Health Statistics, www.cdc.gov/nchswww/fastats/ overwt.htm).
4. Underage drinking and excess alcohol consumption were responsible for nearly 100,000 deaths.
5. Life expectancy has increased to about seventy-six years, but the health-related quality of life may be declining.

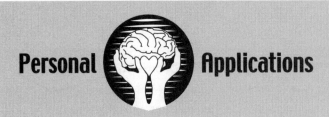

# Personal Applications

## Directions:

Read the following statements in section A and check whether you agree, disagree or are unsure. Complete the other sections only if you have a personal interest in some lifestyle adjustments for promotion of healthy pleasures.

**A.**

1. Some people think that since we all have to die of something anyway, why be so concerned about preventing disease, promoting health and postponing death? The main response is that life is more than a choice of staying alive biologically until death. It is more of an experience to enjoy, to contribute for good and to fulfill a personal purpose.

   [ ] agree      [ ] disagree      [ ] unsure

2. Physical health contributes to the overall experience of living a worthwhile life. Good health is generally prized above wealth and material possessions.

   [ ] agree      [ ] disagree      [ ] unsure

3. The main goals of this chapter are to encourage, stimulate and push people to take action to live healthier lives, with more pleasure and less pain, both in the short-term and the long-term. Increasing the years of healthy function, and striving for a high quality of life in all stages, is a desirable goal.

   [ ] agree      [ ] disagree      [ ] unsure

4. Some common lifestyle choices influence several diseases. Smoking, diet, obesity, physical inactivity and stress are some of the common primary causes of heart disease, stroke, cancer, diabetes and other degenerative diseases.

   [ ] agree      [ ] disagree      [ ] unsure

5. Making lifestyle changes is difficult. The whole person is involved in any change — the biology, the mental discipline, the psyche and the spirit are part of the process.

   [ ] agree      [ ] disagree      [ ] unsure

6. Increasing healthy pleasure and avoiding pain is one perspective that may promote change.

   [  ] agree       [  ] disagree       [  ] unsure

7. Most of the actions needed to make positive changes are the responsibility of the individual. Without adequate pressure or attractive incentives, most individuals are not prepared for the personal responsibility to change.

   [  ] agree       [  ] disagree       [  ] unsure

8. Some people can handle only small changes scheduled over a planned time frame. Others can do better with drastic changes. Many of us get forced into change when some unexpected negative health consequence precipitates action to regain health. For example, a heart attack stimulates action to prevent a second one.

   [  ] agree       [  ] disagree       [  ] unsure

9. A partnership between the individual, the worksite and the healthcare system is helpful in creating the support system that can be most effective to promote health, prevent disease and increase the quality of life. A similar partnership and integration among health practitioners may also contribute to helping individuals live healthier lives.

   [  ] agree       [  ] disagree       [  ] unsure

10. The scientific foundation of healthcare is important, but the knowledge and input of the consumer, and alternative and complementary therapies should be incorporated in the decision making process. It will take some time for all this to achieve a solid foundation for the new atmosphere of cooperation in healthcare. Economic factors seem to be the leading dynamics in the whole arena.

    [  ] agree       [  ] disagree       [  ] unsure

11. There was a time when people considered themselves healthy if they had no obvious disease. This has changed. Health now is defined in terms of not just the absence of disease, but the optimization of function, the prevention of disease, early diagnosis and thereby early treatment, the best scientific therapies and the most effective rehabilitation.

    [  ] agree       [  ] disagree       [  ] unsure

12. It is said that very few humans have died from natural aging — the body reaching its programmed limits of function. Most deaths are from interruption of the homeostatic mechanisms when one system fails due to premature dysfunction.

[ ] agree        [ ] disagree        [ ] unsure

B. Self-Examination I — The Physiologic Dimension
Check the most appropriate answer. Note that for each item your answer will be somewhere on the line between "T" for mostly true or "F" for mostly false. If you don't know the answer, check the "Don't Know" box. Check the "Don't Care" box if you believe that an item is not important to your personal health. Give the answers that you honestly think apply — not what you would like to be true.

## Physiologic Health Factors

| | True or False | Don't Know | Don't Care |
|---|---|---|---|
| 1. My general feeling of well-being is good. | T———F | | |
| 2. I have no known major illness or disease. | T———F | | |
| 3. I get an adequate balanced diet. | T———F | | |
| 4. I do not overeat. | T———F | | |
| 5. I use foods that seem to protect against cancer. | T———F | | |
| 6. My cholesterol level is low-risk. | T———F | | |
| 7. My hemoglobin level is normal. | T———F | | |
| 8. My blood pressure is normal. | T———F | | |
| 9. My blood sugar level is normal. | T———F | | |
| 10. My daily body functions are normal. | T———F | | |
| 11. I have no nagging, chronic pain. | T———F | | |
| 12. I get regular, competent medical checkups. | T———F | | |
| 13. I do not smoke. | T———F | | |
| 14. I use alcohol moderately or not at all. | T———F | | |
| 15. I know basic first aid and CPR. | T———F | | |
| 16. I get sufficient, enjoyable physical activity. | T———F | | |

| | | | | |
|---|---|---|---|---|
| 17. I get adequate, restful sleep. | T——F | | |
| 18. I am satisfied with my sex life. | T——F | | |
| 19. I am careful about my personal safety. | T——F | | |
| 20. I do not use illegal or overuse legal drugs. | T——F | | |
| 21. I have adequate health insurance. | T——F | | |
| 22. I experience physiologic pleasure. | T——F | | |
| 23. I have experienced major physiologic pain. | T——F | | |
| 24. I have no stress-related symptoms. | T——F | | |
| 25. All in all, my pleasures outweigh my pain. | T——F | | |

From the twenty-five items in the table above, list in order (number 1 being the most important and number 4 the least important), four items you feel you need to improve for better physical health.

1.

2.

3.

4.

C.

1. What do you think may eventually be your cause of death? (If you find this subject uncomfortable for you, disregard the question.)

2. The lifestyle strategies to optimize physiologic health and prevent preventable disease are:
   a. Eat a balanced diet high in complex carbohydrates such as grains, cereal, beans, fruits and vegetables; and low in meats, dairy, oils and refined carbohydrates. The Food Guide Pyramid summarizes this recommendation. See Figure 5-16.
   b. Drink about 6-8 eight-ounce glasses of water per day.
   c. Engage in some form of enjoyable physical activity for 30-40 minutes at least three to four times per week.

d. If you smoke, quit. If you don't smoke, don't start.

e. If you drink alcohol, do so in moderation and never to the point of losing mental control.

f. Get adequate, restful sleep.

g. Learn some practical techniques for stress reduction and control.

h. Wash hands with soap and water periodically throughout the day, especially after using the bathroom. This simple action can decrease the rate of spread of infectious disease. (Infectious diseases are on the rise again. It is thought that resistance to antibiotics and lack of hand-washing among the general public, healthcare workers and food handlers are factors contributing to this. Recent surveys have shown that only 61% of men and 74% of women wash their hands after using the bathroom. Other surveys show a reduction in emphasis on hand-washing among nurses and doctors.)

How do you evaluate yourself on the prevention strategies above?

[ ] excellent     [ ] good     [ ] fair     [ ] poor

3. What do you understand by "self-care?" What self-care strategies do you practice?

4. What alternative therapies are you acquainted with?

5. Do you discuss alternative therapies with your physician?

6. Write short summaries of what you know and what you believe about the following:

a. acupuncture

b. aromatherapy

c. Chinese herbal medicine

d. chiropractic

e. homeopathy

f. hypnotherapy

g. massage therapy

h. music therapy

i. naturopathy

j. osteopathy

k. reflexology

## Reflections

It is easy to say "do this, that or the other thing" for improved health and fitness. Making the change when the habit is not part of the lifestyle is more difficult. Most people know what they should do, but they never take the action until they are forced to do so. Sometimes, this is at a point when the choice is to take action or to give in to chronic ailments.

Many times, a small step can trigger long-term action. In other cases, it takes a radical change to produce sustained effort. In Chapter 10, we will discuss some specific steps in motivation, goal setting and other techniques to make changes effective.

Two questions frequently arise in discussions on lifestyle change:

1. How much personal experimentation is advisable? Or, is there a protocol to follow, and whose approval do I have to get before launching on the path of lifestyle improvement?

2. If I lose the enjoyment of my favorite foods, smoking, drinking and "couch potatoing," what will life be worth without them? You have to die of something, so why not enjoy life while you can?

With respect to question one, here are our thoughts:

*However, the ultimate responsibility for health promotion and disease prevention is your own.*

In this "New Era" of personal responsibility, in this culture of high-pressure marketing, an individual has to find credible sources of information. Your physician should be such a source. Unfortunately, the system of medical education coupled with the business side of healthcare has left many physicians unprepared to deal with the issues of lifestyle change.

The current advice, however, is to involve your physician, especially when starting on a new exercise program. Sudden, drastic changes may precipitate damage to the heart or other body system. This should be evaluated before making the change.

On the other hand, don't postpone simple changes that may improve overall health, such as beginning a walking program.

Or take, for example, the issue of appetite control. One simple experiment to illustrate that plant food can be an effective appetite suppressant is to try eating your salad without dressing. It turns off the desire for food! Low salt food is not very appetizing to someone accustomed to high salt and lots of seasoning. We can achieve appetite control through our own manipulation of the refined food content, the salt and seasoning, the animal fat and animal protein content of our food.

The alternative medicine industry is approaching a $50 billion industry. It shows that people are making decisions on their own to try other therapies that may offer help in health promotion, therapy and prevention. Some HMOs have even begun paying for alternative therapies such as acupuncture, massage, therapeutic touch, etc. Many others are planning to follow the lead.

Many anecdotes abound about the effects of various therapies, diets, and healing techniques. Caution, a moderate approach, knowledge and information and inclusion of your current healthcare provider in your decisions are recommended. However, the ultimate responsibility for health promotion and disease prevention is your own.

One personal experiment that yielded positive results for me was the experience that led me to a dietary supplement with all the essential amino acids, vitamins, minerals and trace elements which, I now believe, are a necessary part of my "health insurance." Here is the story:

• • • • •

I was developing pain and discomfort in my wrist and knuckles. To me, these were early signs of arthritis. I would take aspirin to control the pain and "heat" I could feel in the joints. My physician sent me for x-rays and advised that I stay with the aspirin as long as that controlled the symptoms.

One of my great fears is that something would interfere with my racquetball game! I was open to looking at other ways of handling this increasing threat and not merely taking care of the symptoms with painkillers and anti-inflammatories.

In the early summer of 1996, I came across some information citing a study done at the Veterans Hospital associated with Harvard University Medical School. I searched the literature from Med-Line and at the library at the Veterans Administration Medical Center in Washington, DC, and found no such study.

The gist of the study, according to the source on tape, was that a group of arthritic patients for whom all treatments had failed, leaving joint replacement as the only choice, had dramatic relief of their arthritis when they were given Knox Drinking Gelatin every day for a month.

Knox Drinking Gelatin is sold in the grocery store and has been on the market for many years, used by women to strengthen their nails. I saw this as a safe experiment. I purchased the stuff from the grocery store and drank it every day. In two weeks, the pain and heat in my wrists had disappeared, and I didn't need any aspirin. The symptoms of what I believed were the beginning of carpal tunnel syndrome (pain and tingling in the band of tissue in the hand above the wrist after a long session at the keyboard in typing this manuscript) had also disappeared.

I called Nabisco, the makers of Knox, to see what was in their product. They sent me a printout of the composition. The significant content was the eight essential amino acids, plus eleven non-essentials. My reasoning went like this: "If my symptoms were developing because of the lack of at least one of the essential amino acids, some other source of the essential amino acids would have the same effect. Knox is made from beef and pork cartilage, and I try to avoid all pork products in my diet. Also, my diet must be lacking in at least one essential amino acid."

I stopped using Knox for a week and my symptoms returned. I found another supplement, powdered Spirulina (a blue-green aquatic algae with the highest protein content among plants or animals), known to contain all the amino acids, es-sential and non-essential. I couldn't stand the taste of this powder mixed in water, so I went back to Knox.

My search then led to a source of liquid Spirulina flavored with a fruit taste. This I could quickly mix in my skim milk and have a pleasant tasting breakfast drink.

In two weeks, all pain, heat in the joint, discomfort over the carpal bones and tingling sensations were gone. I no longer took aspirin. Racquetball was again pain free. I could type for several hours without discomfort.

Needless to say, I keep drinking liquid Spirulina. Further information gathering led to assurance that the source of the Spirulina was not contaminated but grown under highly controlled, "laboratory clean" conditions. I obtained printouts of the analysis of the composition of this Spirulina and was satisfied that there was nothing that I felt posed a known health risk.

But I was still cautious. I called the US Department of Agriculture Human Nutrition Research Center and learned that Spirulina is being researched as a "designer food" that may solve the world need for alternative sources of protein. Spirulina is about 60% protein — a plant source of protein.

If I stop using Spirulina for more than five days, my wrist pains and heat in the wrist joint reappear. I don't know the exact mechanism of action of this nutritional supplement, but I cannot wait for the research to be done. I believe if I wait, I will end up dependent on some strong anti-inflammatory to control the symptoms.

• • • • •

Stories such as this abound in the information about many products and therapies outside of conventional healthcare. But anecdotes are not scientific evidence. It takes years of carefully designed studies to prove cause and effect and to discover possible negative side effects of any new food sources, drugs or therapeutic measures.

In my case, I feel comfortable experimenting with a dietary supplement that may be addressing my problem directly, instead of just treating the symptoms. With just drug treatment, I may have to go to stronger drugs and eventually have surgery. If I can avoid those options by using a dietary supplement, I will do that as long as it controls the symptoms.

It is a consumer decision to wait for the evidence or to "experiment" within the bounds of available information, checking out questionable recommendations with cautions about unsupported claims.

*There are many claims made for many new herbal products available on the open market. Some are safe, some do neither harm nor good and some are harmful.*

There are many claims made for many new herbal products available on the open market. Some are safe, some do neither harm nor good and some are harmful. There have been reports on ephedra, or mahuang, of having caused about seventeen deaths. The FDA has issued warnings and banned the marketing of this product.

My recommendation is to check things out, gather as much information as possible and proceed with caution. A salesperson is probably not the best source of information on the product being sold. Physicians are becoming more knowledgeable and more comfortable discussing these issues and should be consulted or informed of patients' use of alternatives.

Some of the safe areas for personal experimentation with lifestyle factors may include:

1. Try to cut back on the oil or sugar used in cooking and still prepare tasteful meals. Some ethnic recipes, which call for cups of oil, are just as tasty and more healthful with half the oil. When we bake from scratch, we have found that one-quarter to one-third the amount of sugar called for in the recipe usually is sufficient.

2. Work into your daily schedule a ten-minute stretching and toning routine either in the morning or evening. This may help ease stress and strain, backaches and headaches as muscles and joints maintain their flexibility and tone. If you can't find a suitable place to walk, run or play your favorite sport, run in place at home. Do jumping jacks. Something. Get moving.

3. Try various sources of dietary supplements before settling on one regular source. Not too long ago, many of us used to believe that taking dietary supplements was only "to produce expensive urine." Then we progressed to the point of believing that a multivitamin, multi-mineral supplement was helpful and the synthetic formula was just as effective as the naturally occurring compounds. Now, we are presented with evidence about absorbability and function that indicate that plant derived compounds as close to their natural state as possible may be more beneficial than synthetic compounds.

4. If insomnia is a problem, experiment with physical activity, environmental changes such as lighting, changes in work schedule if possible, reading, getting out of bed and working at something boring until sleepiness comes on

before becoming dependent on pre-scription pills.

Regarding the question of loss of enjoyment of the unhealthy lifestyle:

Find substitute pleasures. Look for enjoyable activities for physical fitness. Find healthy foods that may retrain the tastes to experience pleasure without the risks. The capacity for pleasure and the depth of meaning of pleasure for the whole person increases as health, vitality and zest for life increases. The beginning of change may be uncomfortable because it is new and dif-ferent and may be accompanied by fear of failure. The short-term pain and discom-fort will yield the long-term pleasure of more healthy years, with a higher quality of life.

If you can't always have or do the things that provide pleasure, find pleasure in the things you have or do.

The ideal of good physical health through sound nutrition, enjoyable physi-cal activity, restful sleep and a fulfilling sex life is attainable. It is health promoting and disease preventing for the whole person. The realities of life are that for many people, much of the time, through no fault of their own, the ideal seems far out of reach.

There are people who get sick and die despite their best efforts at living healthy lifestyles and practicing many preventive measures. There are people whose efforts have to be greater and for a longer period of time to achieve the same level of health other people achieve with little effort. Ge-netics, metabolism, personality, inner drive and social environment differ.

A fulfilling, high quality of life is built on the foundation of physiologic health and well-being. However, ultimate satisfaction in life does not depend on a fully intact, optimally functioning body. The whole person may rise above physical incapacities, limitations, diseases and even terminal ill-ness to experience high level wellness. But a healthy body sure helps.

There are two organizations you should contact for further information, questions or materials on promoting good health. They are:

1. National Health Information Center
   Office of Disease Prevention
   and Health Promotion
   330 C Street, SW
   Switzer Building, Room 2132
   Washington, DC 20201
   http://nhic-nt.health.org

2. C. Everett Koop Institute at Dartmouth
   HB 7025 Strasenburgh Hall
   Hanover, NH 03755-3862
   http://koop.dartmouth.edu and
   www.drkoop.com

Write to these organizations for in-formation and booklets on weight control, physical fitness, medical education and con-sumer health, etc.

To go the distance, you have to take care of the machinery that is tak-ing you there.

There are three things I want to comment on from my layperson's perspective. These are: how individual differences affect health, the health information deluge and my understanding of obesity from first-hand experience.

## 1. Individual Differences

During all his years of study of human physiology, Al used to point out that the "normal values" of almost everything were based on or adjusted to "the seventy kilogram male."

It is good to see female physiology being recognized in the past two decades. Last year, Al brought home a book *New Dimensions in Women's Health*. One of the authors, retired Colonel Linda Alexander, RN, PhD, was one of his colleagues in the Department of Health Education at the University of Maryland. Books such as this are giving long overdue emphasis to the subject of women's physiology and women's health.

It is now recognized that along with gender, racial and geographic differences affect individual function. Part of our personal responsibility in health promotion is to know our individual differences and work with them.

Genetics, metabolic rate, resistance to disease and reaction to drugs or other treatments make for uniqueness.

*The fact I need to reinforce to myself is that over 50% of the causes of disease today are lifestyle factors.*

## 2. The Rapid Increase of Information about Health and Medicine

News and information about health and medicine are everywhere. Each day, newspapers, magazines, radio, television and the tabloids carry news about health, disease, new discoveries and reviews of how the body works. It is impossible to keep up with it all.

I have on my desk a copy of the fall 1996 issue of *Time* magazine titled, "The Frontiers of Medicine." The topics range from cancer and gene therapy to aging, AIDS and alternative medicine. The "Modern Milestones" list includes the 1928 discovery of penicillin and the 1995 successful heart transplant from one species of animal to another.

In the face of all this technology, it is easy to think that science and technology can solve all our health problems. The fact I need to reinforce to myself is that over 50% of the causes of disease today are lifestyle factors.

It took me a long time to accept personal responsibility for my health. My background in X-ray technology did not help to reinforce this. I grew up in a healthcare environment and social climate where you ate what tasted good and thought about health only when you got sick.

Now I read a summary of the health effects of obesity (diabetes, hypertension, coronary heart disease, cancer, gallbladder disease, osteoarthritis and gout) and wonder why I couldn't take control of this disease years ago.

### 3. How I Finally Took Control of a Chronic Case of Obesity

As I write this section, I have in front of me a copy of the September 23, 1996, issue of *Time*. The cover picture is a thigh-to-chin photo of a woman in an aqua swimsuit. Her abdomen is flat and well toned. She has good muscle definition and looks the ideal picture of health and fitness.

The caption beside this swimsuit-clad beauty reads: "The Hot New Diet Pill." Below that is a picture of a drug capsule with the word "Redux." Under that, these words: "Redux really seems to work. But is it too good to be true?"

Redux was then the newest fad in weight control. My endocrinologist had said I qualified for the Fen/Phen regimen: the combination appetite suppressant which came before Redux. I reviewed the information on the possible side effects and was too scared to accept the offer. The way my health had been, I felt that if a severe side effect were possible, it would happen to me. So when I learned that primary pulmonary hypertension was already diagnosed in about seventy-five people using Fen/Phen, I made the choice to struggle with other ways of taking control of my obesity. My choice was obviously a good one, since both Redux and Fen/Phen were later banned from the market.

I asked a physician why he prescribes appetite suppressants, and he said that patients ask for them. People are looking for a quick, painless fix, instead of undertaking the difficult work of lifestyle change.

What I have learned about obesity came from firsthand experience and from reviewing literature on the subject with Al. Three of the sources we read that brought us up-to-date on the subject are *Obesity: Pathophysiology, Psychology and Treatment* and two papers from the *International Journal of Obesity*: "Long-Term Intervention Strategies in Obesity Treatment" by S. Rossner, and "Psychosocial Factors and Quality of Life in Obesity" by Stunkard *et al.*

What I understood from all this can be summarized as follows:

a. There are two types of obesity. Simple obesity, which results when genetically normal people overeat and are inactive; and genetic obesity, where there is a defect in the genes that regulate body composition.

The genetic type is less common, but more difficult to control. The simple type is easier to control with diet and exercise. The genetic type requires medical assessment to correct metabolic or hormonal dysfunction. As the C. Everett Koop Foundation summary puts it, "For a minority of people, obesity is a genetic condition that can be extremely difficult to control." I know this difficulty firsthand.

b. Skinny people seem to be of two broad types as well. Those who can eat all they want, sometimes two or three times what average people eat, and balance it out easily with light physical activity; and those who must be constantly careful about what and how much they eat as they will gain weight if not balanced by heavy physical activity.

This subject is being researched at the Mayo Clinic. A study is being done on people who are able to eat as much as they want and don't gain weight.

c.  If the genetic control of body weight involves several genes, maybe one plays a role in the control of the elastic qualities of abdominal muscles. It seems that one common problem among overweight people is that the abdominal muscles can be stretched easily, but they don't have the normal elastic rebound. Maybe the Human Genome Project will soon shed some light on this.

d.  A quote from one of the articles from the International Journal of Obesity is very revealing:

"Of all the conditions for which a person may be stigmatized in our culture, the stigma of overweight may be the most debilitating. Since obesity is immediately visible to others, it can affect most social interactions. Furthermore, the stigma of overweight has two aspects: stigmatization of the appearance of the body and the stigmatization of the character of the person for the moral failure of not controlling one's weight."

In taking control of my medical condition of obesity, I had to push my physician. In fact, after a few years of being treated as if I were cheating on the diet and exercise plan, I had to defy the system of controlled access to a specialist and went to an endocrinologist on my own.

I was diagnosed as hypothyroid, and deficient in vitamins B-1, B-6 and calcium. I am now on thyroid medication, have corrected my nutrient deficiencies and now have the energy to exercise more regularly.

I had a chance to take part in a physician-supervised pilot study of a new meal replacement plan. The meal replacement plan was food-based with high, balanced nutritional content including all the vitamins, minerals and antioxidants. "Phytofactors" and herbal extracts were a part of the regimen.

After doing some checking with the USDA research library on things like bitter orange extract, we felt the regimen was safe and could be part of a long-term plan. The company supplied the product, and a group of physicians did the pretest and post-test evaluations.

Success breeds success. Small steps in gaining control over a chronic case of obesity led to feeling more enthusiastic and positive about the long term. My goal is to do what I now know I can do, to avoid negative health consequences and enjoy as many healthy years as possible. I have a lot to be healthy for.

My personal effort seems to take more work compared to other people I know. I have to have lower fat intake and have more physical activity more frequently than most people I know in order to control weight and maintain physical fitness. I believe that it will increase the healthy years as I begin to devote time to my grandchildren.

Since my 1997 pilot study of the alternative weight program, I regained what

I had lost. Several conditions led to a prolonged depression.

I believe I had some spiritual and psychosocial issues to deal with before I could really assert the control and discipline required. I think the knowledge and understanding didn't come to a level of strong belief until recently.

The final push that increased my motivation level came from two groups. the Rockville Full Life Fellowship (RFLF) and the Inner Visions Center. I took the "Wonder Woman Weekend" workshop with Iyanla Vanzant at the Inner Visions Center to work through a few issues. That new start with the support of the group at RFLF has given me a new outlook on the challenge. Only those who live the experience understand the issues.

I'll go the distance with a little help from my friends.

The sixteen pages of anatomy in this section are reproduced with the kind permission of The McGraw-Hill Companies. The source of this material is:

*The Student Art Study Notebook*
Copyright 1996 Times Mirror Company
ISBN 0-697-25381-3
Published in the United States of America by Wm. C. Brown
Communications, Inc., Dubuque, IA

The above book of anatomy illustrations is a study guide that accompanies the textbook *Hole's Human Anatomy & Physiology 7th Edition.*

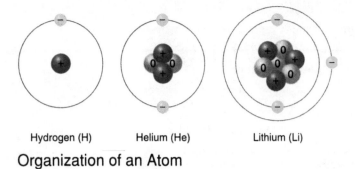

**Organization of an Atom**

Hydrogen (H)    Helium (He)    Lithium (Li)

The number of protons determines the size and properties of an atom.

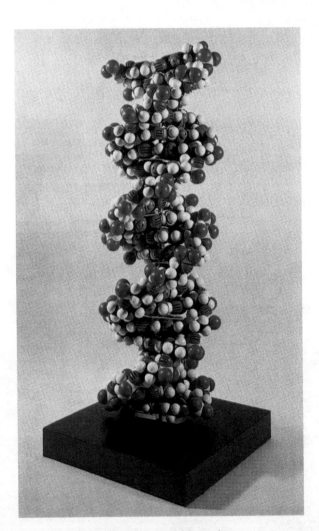

Portion of a DNA Double Helix

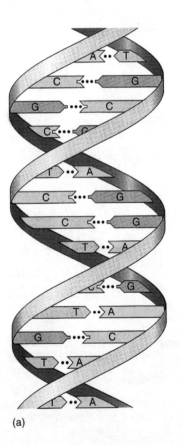

(a)

DNA (Deoxyribonucleic Acid) — The macromolecule that carries the genetic information in segments called genes.

**FIGURE 5-1**

A cell is the unit of structure and function. Each tissue or organ can do what it does because the cells are specialized for particular functions.

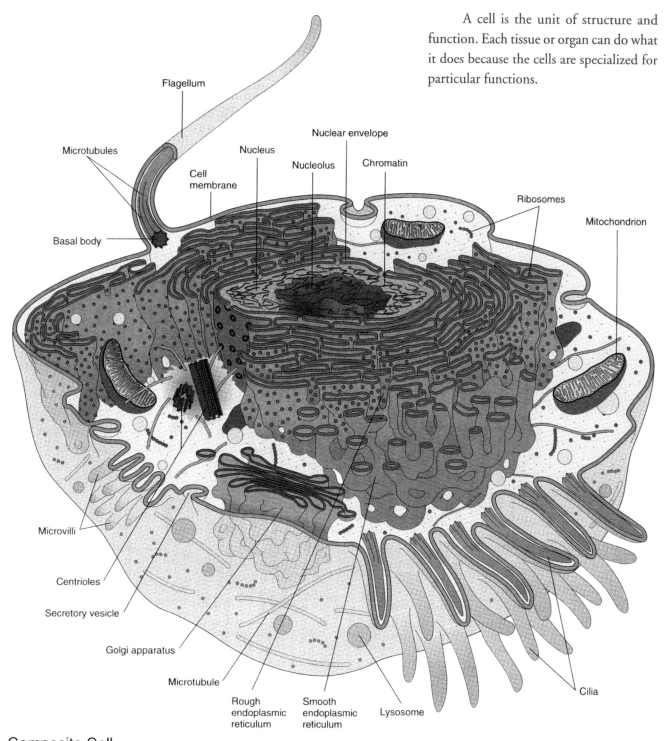

Composite Cell

FIGURE 5-2

The skin is the largest organ of the body. It helps regulate temperature, has sensory receptors, contains immune system cells and excretes small quantities of waste substances.

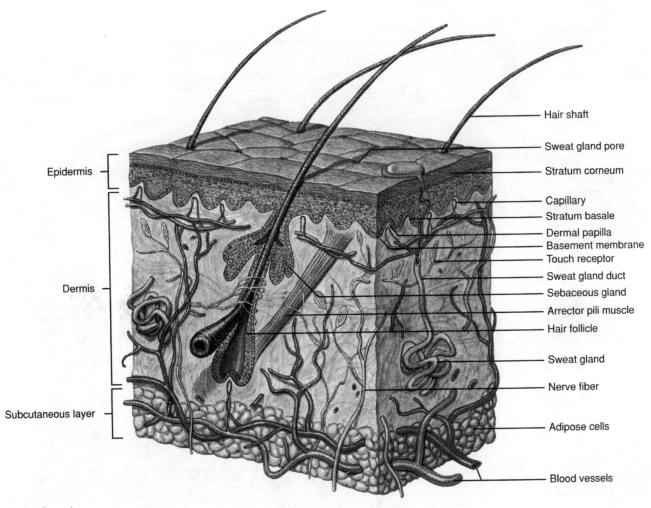

Epidermis

Dermis

Subcutaneous layer

Hair shaft

Sweat gland pore

Stratum corneum

Capillary

Stratum basale

Dermal papilla

Basement membrane

Touch receptor

Sweat gland duct

Sebaceous gland

Arrector pili muscle

Hair follicle

Sweat gland

Nerve fiber

Adipose cells

Blood vessels

Skin Section

FIGURE 5-3

The arrangement of the protein filaments and the connection of the whole muscle to bone enables contraction to produce movement. Voluntary muscles are stimulated by nerves before they contract.

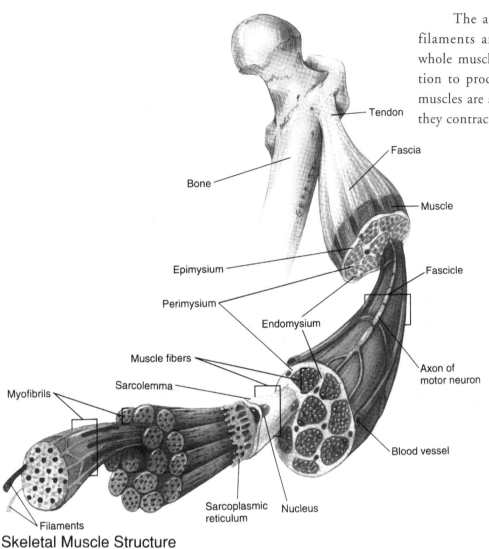

Tendon

Fascia

Bone

Muscle

Epimysium

Fascicle

Perimysium

Endomysium

Muscle fibers

Sarcolemma

Myofibrils

Axon of motor neuron

Blood vessel

Sarcoplasmic reticulum

Nucleus

Filaments

Skeletal Muscle Structure

FIGURE 5-4

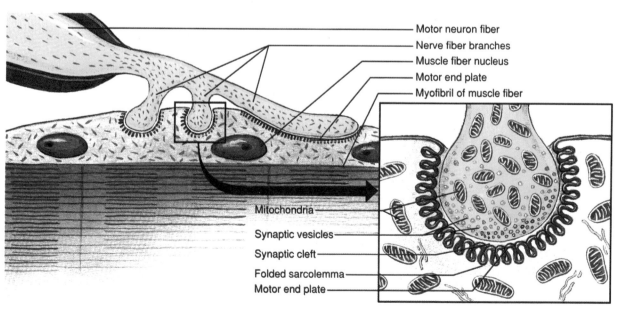

Motor neuron fiber
Nerve fiber branches
Muscle fiber nucleus
Motor end plate
Myofibril of muscle fiber

Mitochondria

Synaptic vesicles

Synaptic cleft

Folded sarcolemma

Motor end plate

Neuromuscular Junction

Bones provide support and protection, allow movement and are the site of blood cell formation.

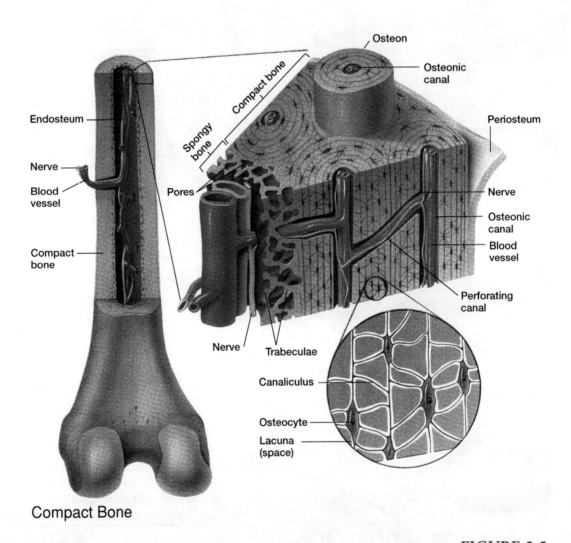

Compact Bone

**FIGURE 5-5**

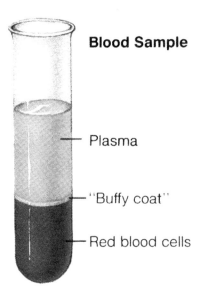

**Blood Sample**

Plasma

"Buffy coat"

Red blood cells

The liquid portion of unclotted blood is called plasma. The liquid portion of the clotted blood is called serum. Mature blood cells develop from a precursor cell called the hemocytoblast. (See Figure 5-12.)

**Peripheral Blood Smear**

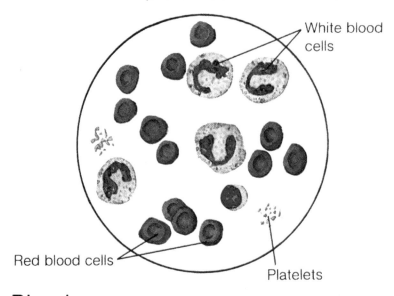

White blood cells

Red blood cells

Platelets

# Blood

FIGURE 5-6

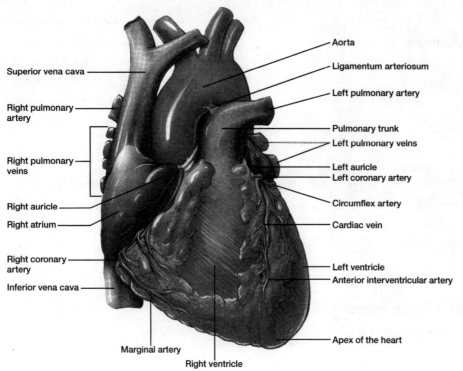

Heart and Coronary Vessels, Anterior

The heart muscle provides the force to circulate blood containing oxygen and nutrients to all cells.

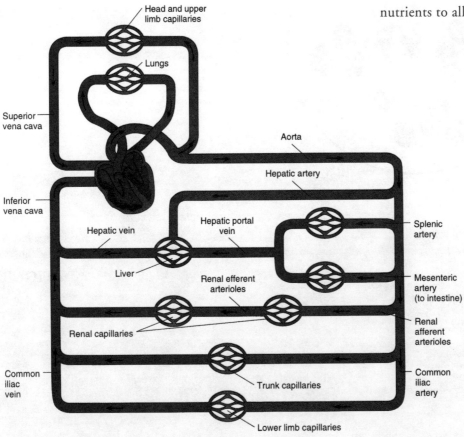

Circulatory System

**FIGURE 5-7**

The kidneys regulate volume, composition and pH of body fluids. Each kidney contains about one million nephrons, the unit's structures for filtration and reabsorption.

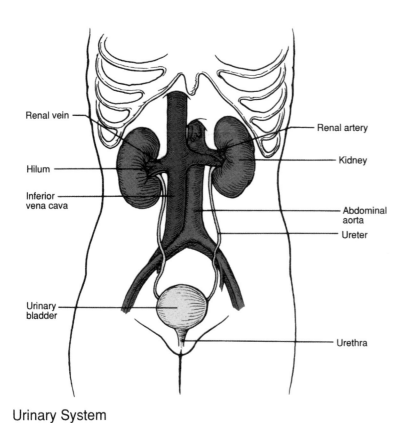

## Urinary System

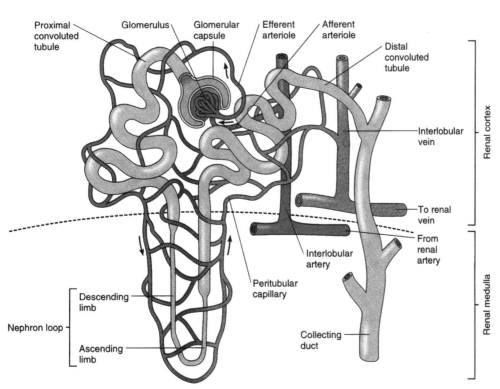

## Nephron Structure

**FIGURE 5-8**

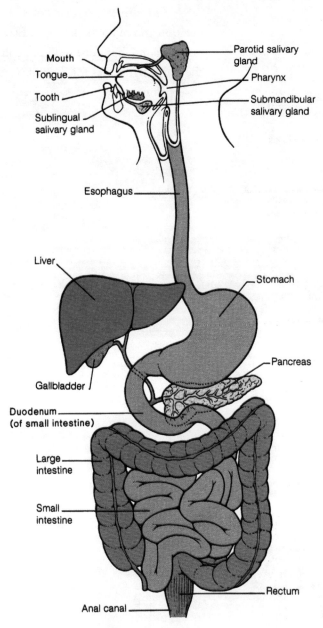

Mouth

Tongue

Tooth

Sublingual
salivary gland

Parotid salivary
gland

Pharynx

Submandibular
salivary gland

Esophagus

Liver

Stomach

Gallbladder

Pancreas

Duodenum
(of small intestine)

Large
intestine

Small
intestine

Rectum

Anal canal

**Digestive System**

The passageway from mouth to anus is called the alimentary canal or gastrointestinal (GI) tract. It is about nine meters long in adults.

**FIGURE 5-9**

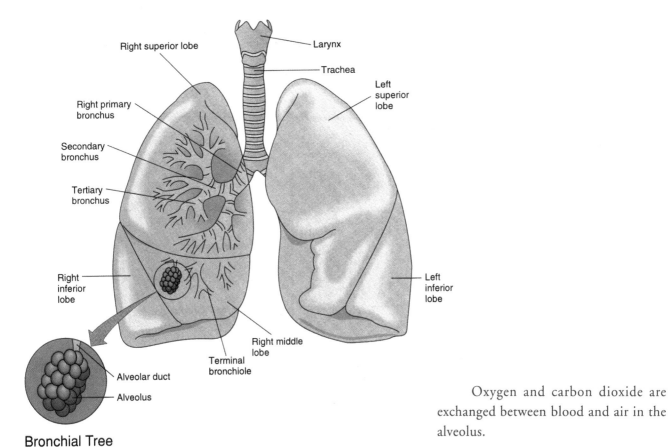

Bronchial Tree

Oxygen and carbon dioxide are exchanged between blood and air in the alveolus.

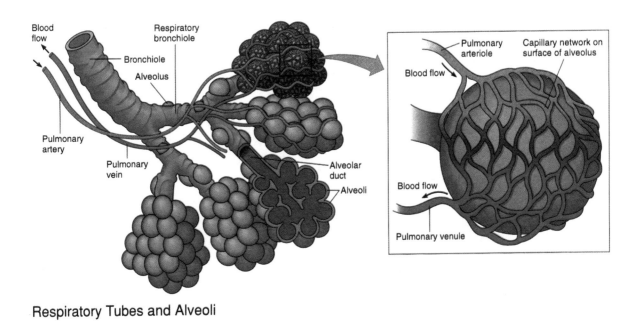

Respiratory Tubes and Alveoli

**FIGURE 5-10**

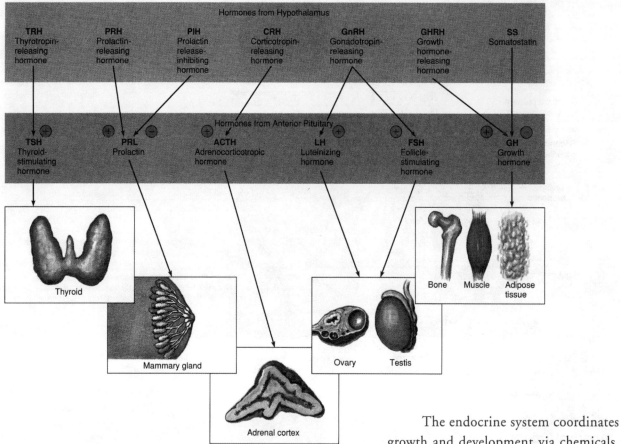

Hormones from Hypothalamus

| TRH Thyrotropin-releasing hormone | PRH Prolactin-releasing hormone | PIH Prolactin release-inhibiting hormone | CRH Corticotropin-releasing hormone | GnRH Gonadotropin-releasing hormone | GHRH Growth hormone-releasing hormone | SS Somatostatin |

Hormones from Anterior Pituitary

| TSH Thyroid-stimulating hormone | PRL Prolactin | ACTH Adrenocorticotropic hormone | LH Luteinizing hormone | FSH Follicle-stimulating hormone | GH Growth hormone |

Thyroid

Mammary gland

Adrenal cortex

Ovary     Testis

Bone     Muscle     Adipose tissue

**Hormones from the Hypothalamus and Anterior Pituitary**

The endocrine system coordinates growth and development via chemicals. The section of the brain known as the hypothalamus is the center for integration and control.

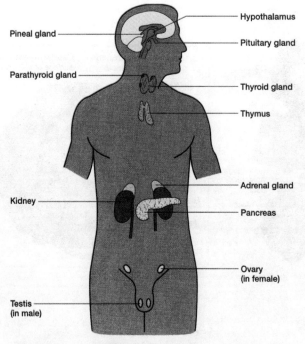

Pineal gland

Parathyroid gland

Kidney

Testis (in male)

Hypothalamus

Pituitary gland

Thyroid gland

Thymus

Adrenal gland

Pancreas

Ovary (in female)

**Major Endocrine Glands**

**FIGURE 5-11**

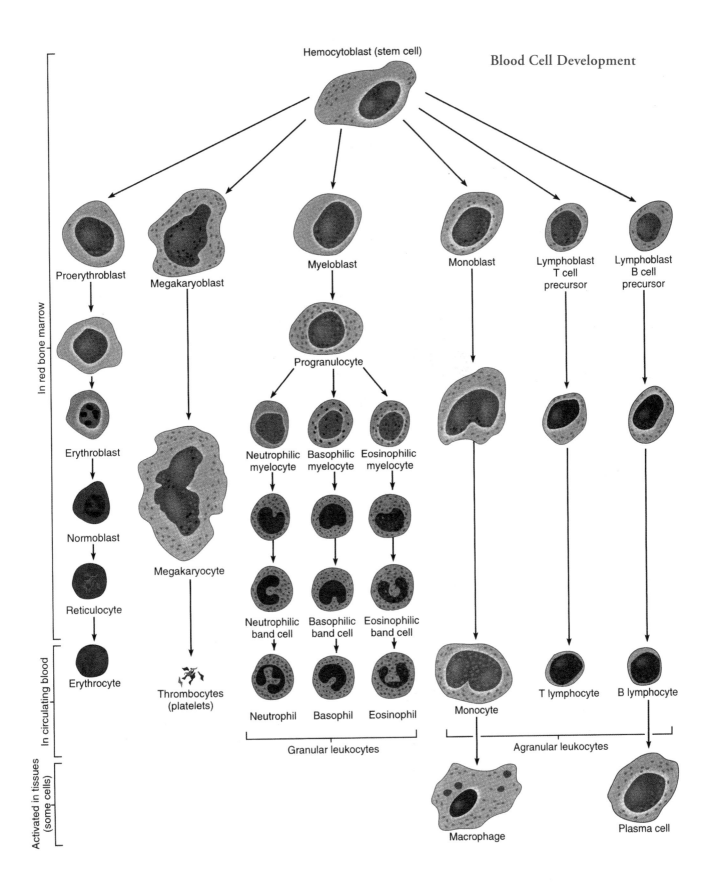

Hemocytoblast (stem cell)

Blood Cell Development

In red bone marrow

Proerythroblast

Erythroblast

Normoblast

Reticulocyte

In circulating blood

Erythrocyte

Megakaryoblast

Megakaryocyte

Thrombocytes
(platelets)

Myeloblast

Progranulocyte

Neutrophilic
myelocyte

Basophilic
myelocyte

Eosinophilic
myelocyte

Neutrophilic
band cell

Basophilic
band cell

Eosinophilic
band cell

Neutrophil

Basophil

Eosinophil

Granular leukocytes

Monoblast

Monocyte

Activated in tissues
(some cells)

Macrophage

Lymphoblast
T cell
precursor

Lymphoblast
B cell
precursor

T lymphocyte

B lymphocyte

Agranular leukocytes

Plasma cell

FIGURE 5-12

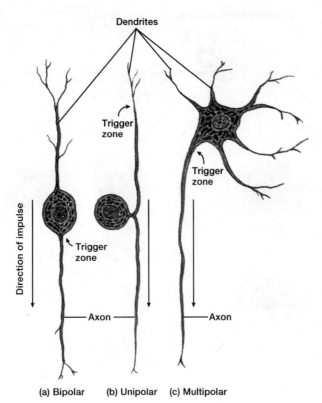

Dendrites

Trigger
zone

Direction of impulse

Trigger
zone

Trigger
zone

Axon

Axon

(a) Bipolar    (b) Unipolar    (c) Multipolar

## Types of Neurons

Neurons generate and transmit action potentials. The action of excitatory or inhibitory neurotransmitters at the synapse controls the flow of information.

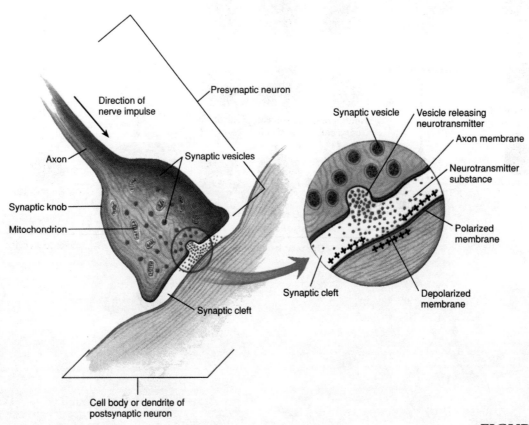

Presynaptic neuron

Direction of
nerve impulse

Axon

Synaptic vesicles

Synaptic knob

Mitochondrion

Synaptic cleft

Cell body or dendrite of
postsynaptic neuron

Synaptic vesicle    Vesicle releasing
neurotransmitter

Axon membrane

Neurotransmitter
substance

Polarized
membrane

Synaptic cleft

Depolarized
membrane

**FIGURE 5-13**

During stress, the hypothalamus helps prepare the body for fight or flight by triggering sympathetic impulses to various organs. It also stimulates release of epinephrine, intensifying the sympathetic responses.

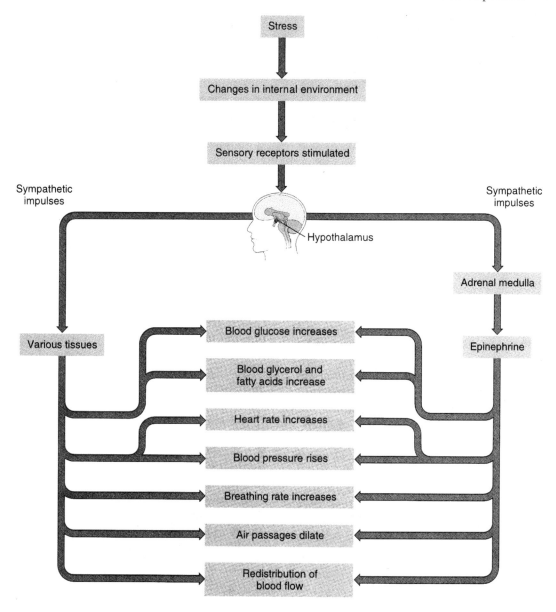

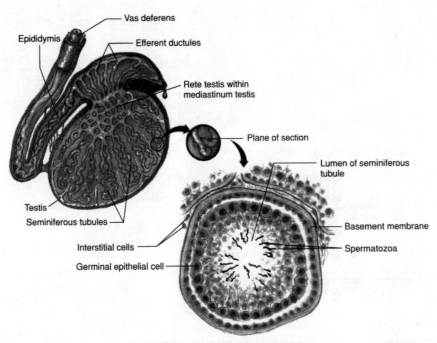

**Testis and Seminiferous Tubules**

The process from fertilization to implantation takes about 7 days.

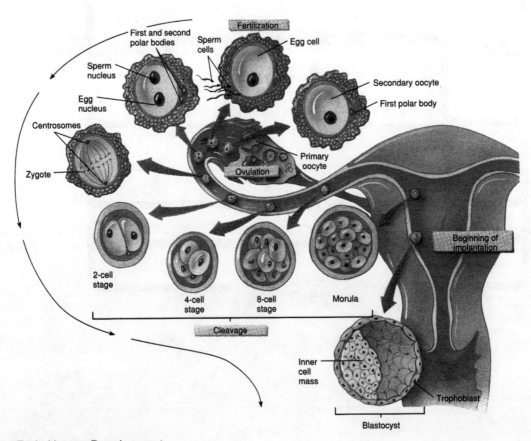

**Early Human Development**

**FIGURE 5-15**

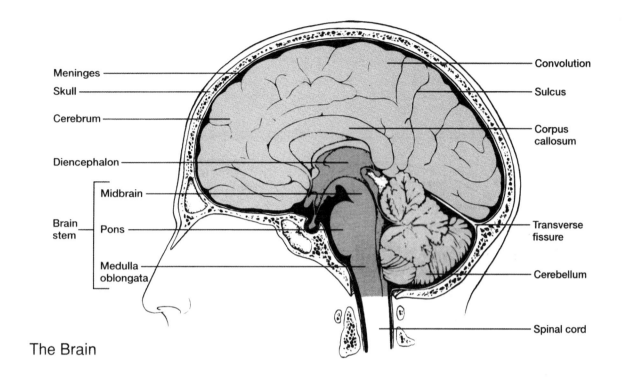

Mena, Menines · Skull · Cerebrum · Diencephalon · Brain stem (Midbrain · Pons · Medulla oblongata) · Convolution · Sulcus · Corpus callosum · Transverse fissure · Cerebellum · Spinal cord

The Brain

The brain is the ultimate control center for integrating function.

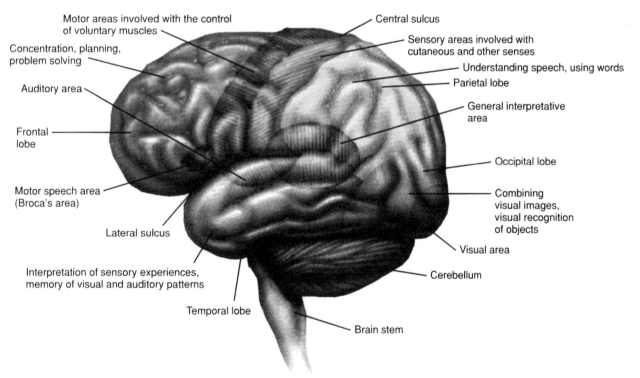

Motor areas involved with the control of voluntary muscles · Concentration, planning, problem solving · Auditory area · Frontal lobe · Motor speech area (Broca's area) · Lateral sulcus · Interpretation of sensory experiences, memory of visual and auditory patterns · Temporal lobe · Central sulcus · Sensory areas involved with cutaneous and other senses · Understanding speech, using words · Parietal lobe · General interpretative area · Occipital lobe · Combining visual images, visual recognition of objects · Visual area · Cerebellum · Brain stem

Sensory, Motor, and Association Areas

**FIGURE 5-16**

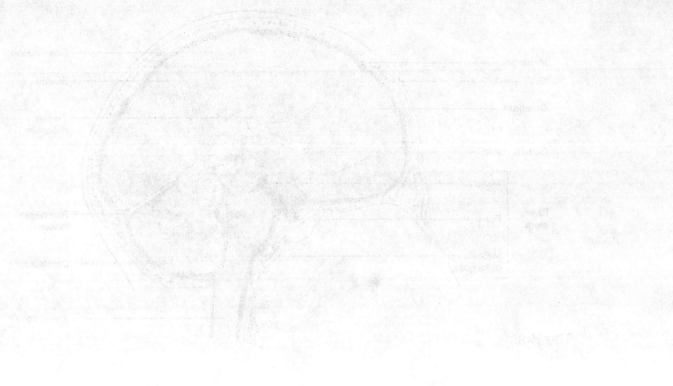

# Understand How the Mind Works as Information Processor

*"Heights that great men reached and kept*

*Were not attained by sudden flight.*

*But they, while their companions slept,*

*Were toiling upwards in the night."*

Henry Wadsworth Longfellow

Six

# Dedicated to


**Edward and Hetty Marcano, Al's grade school teachers**

*Thanks for the emphasis on basic skills.*

*Good teachers make all the difference in the world. It is a special privilege and pleasure to have you read the manuscript before publication.*

*I*s the human mind only a complex biological computer? Or does brain tissue give rise to some energy field that hovers above the brain and endows it with the remarkable capabilities of human thought, reason, memory and emotions? What do we know about the human mind, and how can we enhance the capabilities we have?

These questions lead to a review of what we know about brain function, and what we are learning about how to optimize our mental capacities for increased quality of life.

As we summarize this information, the aim is to form an overview of mental function. This then leads to a personal understanding of possible ways to harness our mental powers to promote personal wellness.

A few months ago, a two-year-old girl and her parents were being interviewed on national TV on the occasion of her being inducted into Mensa, the society for people with high intelligence. It was reported that she began to talk at one month of age, and her unique abilities were noticed even when she was only a few days old. Is this kind of ability inherited or learned? How rapidly does the brain learn?

Let us start with homeostasis. By analogy to what homeostasis means to the body as a whole, homeostasis of the mental dimension means the balance and integration of the factors involved in handling and using information.

# Mental Homeostasis

The brain is the central command center of the body. Brain tissue is the foundation of the processes that collect information and store, recall and use information in the way humans are capable.

The nerve cell, the neuron, is the unit of function. As nerve cells communicate with one another, chemical substances called neurotransmitters serve to pass information around.

For each neurotransmitter, neurons may or may not have the receptor to which the particular neurotransmitter may bind. Binding of a neurotransmitter substance may excite or inhibit a particular neuron. Examples of neurotransmitter substances are noradrenaline (norepinephrine), dopamine and serotonin. Amino acids from protein are the basis of many neurotransmitter substances.

Neurons form electrical circuits that become established and can be triggered repeatedly. This is the basis of memory.

Brain centers are specialized to receive specific information. For example, there is a center for sight, a center for hearing and a center for reasoning.

There are also command centers for control of actions such as speech and voluntary movements.

Information goes into the brain as nerve impulses — spikes of electrical energy. Responses from the brain are nerve impulses to influence functions of other organs. The higher functions of thinking, memory and emotions are all integrated within the brain.

The brain does what it does and creates mind by having all its parts and processes in some state of balance. The various anatomical structures play their part. The information handling processes have their role. All these work in harmony to give humans the capabilities of mind. The specific balance achieved is what makes an individual unique.

## Anatomy of the Brain

The brain is anatomically divided into the forebrain, cerebellum and the brain stem. All parts of the brain share information through nerve connections. The forebrain or cerebrum, the largest part of the brain, houses the centers for control, thought and reason. The forebrain includes the cortex, basal ganglia, thalamus, hypothalamus, pituitary gland and pineal gland.

The cerebellum is a smaller mass of brain tissue which integrates information about position, physical balance and posture.

The brain stem consists of the midbrain, pons and medulla. These are relay centers and automatic control centers for such functions as breathing, heart rate and reflexes. (See Figure 5-16 for details.)

The brain and spinal cord are referred to as the central nervous system. All parts of the brain communicate with the others. The channeling, processing, interpretation and use of information by the spinal cord and brain give humans the capabilities of mind. Thus, intellectual function, personality and the human spirit have their foundation in brain tissue.

## Input and Output

All input comes into the brain as nerve impulses. Touch, sight, sound, taste, smell, pain, pleasure and temperature have special receptors that transform the specific energy into nerve impulses. The impulses travel to specific areas of the brain where they are interpreted. The information is recorded and interacts at two levels, the conscious and the subconscious. The output is nerve impulses to take action or to store the information in memory for future use.

## Conscious and Subconscious

The level of consciousness is the level of awareness and perception. Information from all parts of the brain flows into the higher centers of the cortex (areas in the gray matter), and the mind becomes aware of the information. Conscious decisions and responses are coordinated in the cortex. Reflex or automatic responses are coordinated in the brain stem and spinal cord.

Below the level of awareness, storage of information is referred to as the subconscious. Psychologists have defined functions such as the unconscious, the ego, etc., but physiologists usually deal only with awareness (conscious) or below the level of awareness (subconscious).

## Left Brain, Right Brain

The two halves (hemispheres) of the brain are referred to as the left brain and the right brain. In about 90% of people, the left hemisphere is dominant for the control of language functions such as speech, writing and reading. The right hemisphere supplies the interpretation, emotion and intuitive functions.

Whether a person is left brain dominant, right brain dominant, or whether both sides share equally in the control of functions, everything that a person does involves input areas, association areas and control areas of both halves of the brain. It really doesn't matter to overall function which half is dominant. They both work together as an integrated whole.

Genetics and early programming of the brain determine how the functions are shared. Females were once thought to be mostly right brain dominant because of their greater capacity for intuitive reasoning and emotional integration. The debate rages on as to whether that is really a brain function or social conditioning.

Left-handers are right brain dominant for motor control of the left side of the body, but they can be left brain dominant for language. In about 70% of left-handers, the left brain is dominant for speech. In 15%, the right brain is dominant. In the other 15%, both left and right brains are equally dominant. This impacts the individual's expressiveness and the emotional tone that accompanies speech.

The balancing of control and coordination in the brain is a topic of continuous study and research.

## The Higher Functions of the Brain

Reason, decision-making, memory and learning are referred to as the higher functions of the brain.

The unit of activity of the mind is a thought — the simplest piece of information. It can be generated by any one or a combination of sensory inputs into the brain. The nerve impulses arriving at the level of awareness trigger a thought — a packet of meaning. It could come from any stimulus (light, sound, touch, etc.) and conveyed meaning through what it represents (words, music, objects, conditions, etc.).

Thoughts create ideas, which form the basis of information in the mind. Ideas form the basis for reasoning, learning, decision-making and control of self within the context of the environment. Memories are thoughts stored for later recall.

## Memory

Information is filed in the brain in several areas. Items such as names of objects, people, places and experiences seem to be filed first in broad categories, then more selective groups that contain the individual words. The first level of storage is called short-term memory.

Short-term memory seems to involve only electrical circuits. The information enters the brain, a set of neurons is activated and the electrical stimulation reverberates for some time in that circuit. The last neuron in the circuit has the ability to trigger the first to keep the circuit activated. After a while, the circuit stops and the information fades from the level of awareness.

Short-term memory gets transferred into long-term memory through a process called consolidation. The electrical circuit gets dedicated to that information through a change in the structure or function of control neurons in the circuit. Protein synthesis is involved. This establishes long-term memory which can be activated by an appropriate stimulus — from inside or outside.

It is thought that most of the information coming into the brain is lost. Some scientists describe another type of memory called immediate memory, which is thought of as the instant recording of all information entering the brain before it reaches the level of awareness. Much filtering takes place before passing on the stimulus to the cortex. It could be that everything gets recorded in the subconscious, and only what is necessary for decision-making or acquisition of new information is passed on to the level of awareness.

## Learning

Learning is the process of acquiring new information that is retained and can be recalled for use. The newly acquired information is filed to fit in with previously stored information. Learning involves cellular changes in neurons and establishment of electrical circuits.

## Reasoning

Reason is the ability of the mind to purposefully and consciously use information to derive meaning. This is one of the highest abilities of the human mind. Other abilities in this category are creativity, intuition, synthesis, inspiration and transcendental awareness.

## Mechanism of Processing

Is the mind only a biological computer? It seems to function as a computer — the most complex computer we can imagine. There is hardware, circuitry, software, central processing, input and output. But there are functions not understood in terms of computer language or capabilities.

Is the mind a photographic medium where nerve impulses create pictures of both real and abstract information? It seems to function that way. In some people "photographic memory" is highly developed. Sight and hearing create images in the brain. Hallucinogenic drugs cause sight and sound circuitry to get crossed, and sound produces visual images in the brain.

Is the mind a holographic plate that creates holograms of both real and abstract information? In a hologram created by laser energy, the whole object is coded in every point of the image recorded on a photographic plate. By contrast, a photograph is a reproduction of an object by coding point for point from the object to the film.

As we learn more about computers, photography and laser energy technology used for information processing, we gain a better understanding and greater appreciation of our minds — ourselves. Our minds create the technology that then gives insight on how our minds work! Mind is the greatest capability of all human functions — it studies itself and reveals itself. It is the communication center within and without — from self to the greatest, highest reaches of the cosmos.

In summary, homeostasis in the mental dimension refers to the balance and integration of all the processes concerned with collecting, processing, storing, recalling and using the information that comes into the brain.

By analogy to the physiologic dimension, the mind has certain needs. It must be supplied with "raw" materials to feed its functions, it must work, it is the stress adaptation center, it needs rest, it grows and it reproduces.

# Mental Nutrition

Food for the mind is the information that feeds the processing mechanisms. The quality ranges from "junk food," like the content of many television programs, to complex, abstract thought that is too heavy for some to digest. As the current debate over the influence of violent and sex-oriented content of literature, music and video points out, behavior is influenced by the quality of information fed to the mind. The evidence is abundant when the lives of individuals or groups are examined.

The "GI-GO" effect — "garbage in" leads to "garbage out" — is more than just humorous terminology. Research and observations on human tragedies such as serial killers, violent criminals and others who perpetrate willful acts of destruction and deceit provide evidence for a direct relationship between the quality of input into the mind and the behavioral output. The effect is not as simple as a computer response. Other influences include the physiologic (genetics), psychosocial (relationships) and spiritual (belief in higher powers) dimensions.

Processes involved in "mental nutrition" include the home environment, modeling of parents and other adults, formal education, experience and observation. Richness or poverty of mental stimulation affects the capacity developed.

# Mental Stress and Stress Adaptation

Stress is the excess wear and tear on the whole organism caused by excess demand. Stressors are the triggers of the stress response.

The mind is the center of stress adaptation and control. Mental stressors cause a response because of the interpretation and perception occurring in the mind. The thoughts then trigger nervous and hormonal responses that affect physiologic function.

The "fight or flight" response triggers the General Adaptation Syndrome (as described by Hans Selye) and the physiologic consequences of acute or chronic stress.

The benefits of stress include increased productivity due to increased mental alertness stimulated by the extra demand. The challenge produces the extra effort that enhances productivity.

The negative effects of stress are decrease in productivity and quality of life. The process begins in the mind. Perception and interpretation of the challenge may result in anxieties, doubts, fears, frustrations, guilt, feelings of lack of control and depression. In the process of experiencing these, nervous, endocrine and immune system mechanisms trigger responses that lead to organ malfunctions.

Stressors that trigger the negative consequences of stress include: under-stimulation of the mind, overstimulation of the mind (information overload), lack of control, mistakes, time pressures, financial pressures, career pressures, actual or potential loss and inadequate planning or organization.

Stress management has been one of the fastest growing fields of applied science in the past two decades. The techniques include: developing decision-making skills; assertiveness training; cognitive restructuring; techniques for handling guilt, doubts and fears; goal setting; meditation; time management; financial planning; self-management; dealing with depression; and futuring.

## Mental Work

Work is expenditure of energy. Mental work involved in thinking, decision-making and reasoning demands energy expenditure just as physiologic work. Increased brain activity during thinking can be observed with techniques that capture pictures (positron emission tomography — PET scans) of the areas of the brain involved as mental effort is stimulated. The increased activity is reflected by changes in glucose metabolism. This is use of ATP for brain activity.

*Nothing good, great or beneficial gets done without work.*

Is there another form of "energy" involved in mental functions? Does electrical energy in the brain produce a force field that extends beyond the brain? These questions are within the realm of serious debate, philosophy, scientific research and speculation.

As our understanding of the brain increases, and as technology sheds more light on the mechanisms of energy transformation, we will learn more about how complex the mind is. In the processes of understanding the laws of science and the intricacies of possible dimensions beyond the physical universe, the human mind learns more about itself.

Mental work includes cognitive processes and communication processes. Within these broad modes of function, work involves use of information and functions of the mind to control self and the environment.

What stimulates the drive to do mental work? What is the will? What factors contribute to success, failure, creativity, mental exhaustion, depression, achievement and exhilaration?

Techniques of planning and organization help to get work done. Methods such as Total Quality Management (TQM), Continuous Quality Improvement (CQI) and Strategy Change Cycle are recent efforts to develop methods to get work done more efficiently.

Nothing good, great or beneficial gets done without work. Sometimes, and to some individuals, work is easier, more pleasant or has a pull all its own. When factors combine to allow the doing of mental work with relish and concentrated effort, a person is described as "being in flow," "being in a groove" or "being in the zone." That is the preferred state of work as opposed to "whipping yourself to get the work done." Getting into flow involves understanding self and the fit between self and the work. We will discuss this more in Chapter 10 as we discuss motivation. One aspect of happiness (Chapter 11) is having interesting, enjoyable work.

## Mental Rest

Rest is a period of reduction of work. The mind finds rest in several ways. There is a neutral awake mode where wakefulness and awareness are present but the mind is not actively engaged. This is referred to as an "alpha state."

Active relaxation is a process of mentally triggering the physiologic response of relaxation. This was first researched and described by Herbert Benson, prominent Harvard cardiologist. We will describe the steps of this process later in this chapter.

Sleep has already been discussed. The major benefit of sleep may be to shut the mind off from outside input and allow time for processing the information accumulated during the previous waking hours.

Dreaming may be a form of relaxation of the mind. We know it is essential for a healthy mind. What goes on during a dream or maybe what creates dreams is the interplay of information as new items are filed into the previous storage. Many different and unrelated items, new and old experiences and knowledge get jumbled together, and the mind creates fiction with them.

Many dreams have meaning to the individual. One branch of psychology uses extensive dream interpretation. Dreams have played roles in major religious experiences and other human relationships. The recurring dream, when the mind repeats the same or very similar dreams over some period of time, has significance to the individual which may be of great or of little importance to everyday living.

Meditation, mental imagery, daydreaming and visualization are other modes of mental rest and relaxation. The mind needs the variety and periodic reduction of effort.

## Mental Growth

Researchers such as Jean Piaget, Lawrence Kohlberg and Erik Erikson have described the process and stages of mental growth and moral development. More recent theories use an information processing model.

Cognition is the term for the mental processes of acquiring and using knowledge. Language development has been the focus of the stages of cognition in childhood.

Problem-solving abilities and the outcomes of decision-making are common estimates of mental abilities. The measurement of intelligence (IQ) by standardized tests is widely used.

There are normal stages and capabilities for cognitive, as well as moral and social, development across the life-span. Mental abilities and vocational productivity seem to peak in the fourth decade of life, level off and then decline with further aging.

The main point of this section is that growth in mental abilities parallels physiologic growth — rapid changes in some stages and slower increases in others before eventual decline. Beyond the abilities of cognition, the development of conscience and wisdom are important stages in the process of mental growth.

## Mental Reproduction

Mental reproduction is analogous to producing offspring to continue the species. Here, a product of the mind perpetuates the individual. Creativity and creative products of the mind are "conceived," go through a stage of "fetal development," have a "birth process," are "born" and may go through stages of "maturing."

Products of the mind may survive the individual and serve as a legacy of the person. In many cases these products are good. In many cases the products are bad.

When we think of creativity, we think of poets, writers, inventors, discoverers, etc. However, there are many creative thoughts and ideas going into everyday living that may not be far reaching, earth shattering or monumental. They spring from the same creative processes that seek to leave something of self behind.

## The Major Mental Health Problems

The leading mental health disorders are anxiety disorders, depression, and feelings of guilt and failure, which may manifest in attempted or successful suicide.

How do we deal with mental health problems for health promotion, disease prevention and growth towards high level wellness short of going to a therapist? Can the mind really heal itself, and what can a person do to promote healing?

There are several things that an individual can do and should do to promote personal mental health. Again, self-examination leads to self-understanding. Increased self-understanding generates self-acceptance. Greater self-acceptance leads to devising a self-management plan to put in the work to reach specific goals. This process, as a byproduct, enhances the self-actualization dynamics and growth takes place — a higher level of wellness sets in. Self-honesty is necessary to produce the examination that leads to positive growth.

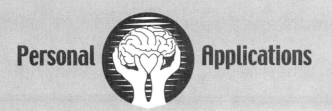

# Personal Applications

## Directions:

Complete the self-examination exercise in Section A. Look at the other sections and select those exercises that are of interest to you. If you want to practice the stress management exercises, doing them with a partner or in a group is helpful.

Simple assessments that facilitate introspection are helpful. Additional self-examination can be explored with instruments such as the anxiety scales, locus of control, depression scales and cognitive style evaluations. Use the following list of questions as a thought stimulating exercise, not as an attempt to measure, evaluate or label yourself in any way.

Use the self-contract document and the Vision-to-Action process as aids in your follow-through for taking action.

### A. Self-Examination II — The Mental Dimension

Check the most appropriate answer. Note that for each item your answer will be somewhere on the line between "T" for mostly true or "F" for mostly false. If you don't know the answer, check the "Don't Know" box. Check the "Don't Care" box if you believe that an item is not important to your personal health. Give the answers that you honestly think apply — not what you would like to be true.

# Mental Health Factors

| | True or False | Don't Know | Don't Care |
|---|---|---|---|
| 1. I feel mentally balanced and stimulated. | T———F | | |
| 2. I am comfortable with my mental capacity. | T———F | | |
| 3. I do not feel overloaded by information. | T———F | | |
| 4. My communication skills are good. | T———F | | |
| 5. I keep up with current affairs. | T———F | | |
| 6. My professional skills and qualifications are up to date. | T———F | | |
| 7. I have or am getting my desired level of education. | T———F | | |
| 8. I am not functionally hampered by anxiety. | T———F | | |
| 9. I am not burdened by major regrets. | T———F | | |
| 10. I am not burdened by guilt feelings. | T———F | | |
| 11. I experience normal doubts and frustrations. | T———F | | |
| 12. I feel in proper control of my life. | T———F | | |
| 13. I exercise adequate control over my use of time. | T———F | | |
| 14. My financial needs and plans are adequately aligned. | T———F | | |
| 15. I strive to develop my mental abilities. | T———F | | |
| 16. My reasoning and decision-making skills are good. | T———F | | |
| 17. I feel successful. | T———F | | |
| 18. I can deal constructively with failure. | T———F | | |
| 19. I am creative. | T———F | | |
| 20. I get adequate mental relaxation and rest. | T———F | | |
| 21. I have definite moral and ethical standards. | T———F | | |
| 22. I enter new experiences with calm and anticipation. | T———F | | |
| 23. I tend to procrastinate but get done what I have to do. | T———F | | |
| 24. I have good gut instincts. | T———F | | |
| 25. All in all, my mental pleasures outweigh my pain. | T———F | | |

**B.** Write short essays on the following four topics. (Write your first thoughts here and develop them into longer essays as you have the time.)

1.  My Ideal Career (include a career plan to achieve what you want in a specific time frame)



2.  The Lifestyle I Want to Live (with a sample two-week schedule)



3.  A Decision I Regretted and What I Would Have Done Differently



4.  Pleasant memories — from childhood to the present



5.  Write a letter of forgiveness to someone who has hurt or wronged you deeply. If you have never been hurt or wronged, compose a fictitious incident. If you use a real incident, concentrate on expressing your feelings of forgiveness, not on chastising, blaming or trying to hurt the other person with words. Express your choice in rising above a victim status and taking control of how the incident will affect the rest of your life. One week after writing this letter, decide whether or not to mail it.



6.  Describe any techniques you know that improve memory.



7.  My Financial Master Plan (include strategies for increasing income, debt management and retirement planning)



## C. Self-Management Skills

Several authors and researchers have developed techniques and processes that help develop skills for decision-making, goal setting, communication, time management, dealing with the effects of stress and creating optimism. Some general reflections and recommendations on these follow.

I am reminded of the student who, for one of our class activities in goal setting, shared with the class what I think is the most ambitious goal I have ever heard discussed in a health class. He was very serious when he announced that the goal he had charted was to "live forever." He had a plan outlined according to the techniques of goal setting with the steps and time frames for everything he had to do to accomplish that goal.

Most other goals may not be that ambitious, but the following techniques apply to the processes involved in "managing life successfully" as one of my colleagues has titled his program.

1. <u>Decision-making</u>. The steps in decision-making are similar to the scientific method: Gather information, list the options, project possible outcomes, test what is testable and select the option with the highest probability of producing the most favorable outcome. In decision-making, the gut instinct carries weight — how much weight depends on the individual. The best gut instincts are the instincts that arise after the process is followed.

   Among the decisions we make in life, the ones about careers, marriage, having children, where we live, and how we live are the major ones that influence our quality of life. How much of these decisions are left to chance, logic or emotions depends on the individual make-up.

   Intuitively, it seems that those who plan more and work harder at their plan should have greater success and satisfaction. This may be so if the information processing capacity of mind were the only function involved in determining success and satisfaction.

   An example of a practical application with life-changing impact is making career choices. Here is an abbreviated version of discussions with our older son as he explored his career choices.

   Mike always wanted to be a doctor. His skills and abilities were evident from grade school, but as he got older we discussed the negative as well as the positive sides of life as a physician.

   During his high school years, I was working for a group of heart surgeons at Washington Hospital Center, Washington, DC. I would share with him things about the hospital environment, heart surgery and a heart surgeon's lifestyle.

   I shared my reflections on being in the operating room observing a world-renowned surgeon perform coronary bypass surgery on a heart that was still beating. The skills in those hands had to be inborn. I wondered whether they could be learned. I had killed many dogs in similar operations in my research at the University of Virginia. I also knew a few surgeons who were struggling to get established in the highly competitive field of heart surgery.

   Mike met some of the surgeons for whom I worked, and by eleventh grade he was sure he wanted to be a heart surgeon. Later, I think his thoughts switched to sports medicine.

But we also explored what it takes to become a doctor, the financial investment, the risks, the demands of the years of preparation and the lifestyle. We finally got to the main question — why? Was the desire for the earning potential and prestige the leading reason? Was it the desire to fulfill a family imposed goal? Was it just to be employable? Was there any inner conviction that this was the best way towards personal fulfillment? Was it a task to do because you are capable of it? Will you really know if you are capable unless you try?

The answers to those questions finally led to choices in business and marketing, with a combination of practical experience (some dictated by circumstances, not entirely by choice), and an aim to finish college and go on to graduate school in the area he enjoys most — philosophy.

Rate your decision-making skills.

[  ] excellent        [  ] good        [  ] fair        [  ] poor

2.  Self-discipline. Self-discipline is one decision-making process that seemed to have been de-emphasized in the sixties and seventies when "feelings" were more of a guide than moral behavior. Getting things done; sticking to principles of a moral code; developing honesty, trustworthiness, dependability and other positive character traits are part of decision-making. They are actively cultivated. They do not develop by accident. How they develop is, of course, greatly influenced by the programming of the environment and the belief system modeled to the developing mind.

The concept of resisting temptations is involved in self-discipline. A temptation is a strong enticement to make a decision to act contrary to a belief or principle. Here is an apple. You like it; you want it. It will make you feel good. No one will have to know you ate it. It is a safe apple. There are no negative consequences except in your own mind.

Whether you believe in a devil or not, this is a mental phenomenon. When the decision is to violate a moral principle, that is what is classified as a sin. Whether you believe in a God or not, violation of a held principle is wrong. This is a good reason to examine the moral code you live by and keep the principles general, few and meaningful. When moral codes and principles are expanded to cover every possible decision and act, you set yourself up for guilt and neurotic behavior.

Temptations can strengthen self-discipline and the decision-making capacity. You never really know how honest you are until you have the opportunity to be dishonest and can get away with it.

Rate your self-discipline.

[  ] excellent        [  ] good        [  ] fair        [  ] poor

3.  <u>Communication.</u> Good communication skills are a major asset. A large percentage of employment ads say something about communication skills, even for positions not involving public contact.

To get ideas across to others in clear, concise language is a skill that can be developed from early childhood. Language development is one measure of brain growth and development.

The other important factor for good communication is listening. Effective listening skills may be even more important than verbal skills. Many interpersonal, interoffice and other relationships suffer from lack of effective listening skills — probably more than from lack of good verbal skills.

A skill that is important for good communication but that seems to be de-emphasized in our school curriculum is comprehension and summarization. In the high school I attended, we used to call that doing a "precis." You read a long passage and rewrote it to about one-third its length to convey the main points and the impact.

Rate your communication skills.

[  ] excellent      [  ] good      [  ] fair      [  ] poor

4.  <u>Goal setting</u>. A large goal has to be broken down into sub-goals. A goal has to start with a realistic, concrete, specific outcome defined in writing. The sub-goals serve to outline doable action steps, a time frame, concrete measurable outcomes, contingency plan, and reward for achievement.

Individuals modify these steps according to what seems to work for them. A self-contract (sample on next page) helps to make the goal a serious matter for persistent effort. "Futuring" helps to project success. A futuring process called "Vision-to-Action" was developed by the Search Institute in Minneapolis, Minnesota, and has been adapted for health promotion. It is described on page 162.

Some of the areas of life for a strong effort in goal setting are career, finances and control over lifestyle. Career goals should be compatible with abilities, desired earning and work that offers challenge and fulfillment. Financial goals must include budgeting, debt control, projections for family growth and inflation and retirement needs. These three areas alone are enough for an entire book.

Rate your use of goal setting techniques.

[  ] excellent      [  ] good      [  ] fair      [  ] poor

# Helps for Goal Setting:
# A Self-Contract and The Vision-to-Action Process

The following self-contract is useful in goal setting. After you write down a specific goal and define the tasks and time frame, use this to summarize your intent and give "official," serious status to your effort by signing the document.

## A. Self-Contract

I, _____, having given careful

consideration to all the factors involved in achieving _____

hereby establish this plan with full intention and desire to carry out the plan and provisions, as attested to by my signature below.

a. I will [write a concrete, realistic goal, such as lose fifteen pounds over the next three months]

_____

_____

b. The sub-goals and dates for accomplishment are:

_____

_____

_____

c. If I do not attain my goal, I will review my effort and find ways to overcome the obstacles identified. I will then rewrite this contract with the necessary adjustments.

d. When I reach my goal (or each sub-goal), I will reward myself with:

_____

_____

_____

e. My signature is witness that I believe that this goal is attainable, and I will put forth my best efforts to achieve it.

Signed: _____ Date:_____

## The Vision-to-Action Exercise Adapted to Personal Wellness

The Vision-to-Action process is a model developed and used by the Search Institute to help program organizational or group change. My exposure to this process came as a member of a school board at a time of extensive planning for change. I then contacted the Search Institute to learn more about the process and its history, and to get permission to adapt the exercise.

It is based on the concept of "futurism" or "futuring," as described by Ronald Lippitt, formerly of the University of Michigan. Futuring is the concept of choosing a preferred future, visioning that future and deciding what has to be done to create that future. It is not trying to predict the future. It is proactive planning with optimistic, desirable outcomes purposely pursued.

The process, adapted to Personal Wellness, involves writing an essay with the following directions:

a. Imagine yourself three years from now (or choose a time frame fitting to your view of your most optimistic future). You are celebrating a special occasion. Choose what that celebration is for, where it is held (place and building), when it is held (specific date and time of day), who is in attendance (how many and how selected) and what you are wearing. Describe that in one paragraph.

b. Imagine yourself floating freely above the crowd at your celebration event. You are able to get close enough to listen to anyone at anytime, and you are able to see the whole group at one time or to focus on specific individuals. Describe what you see and hear. Write one-sentence summaries of any speeches delivered by specific individuals, and bits and pieces of casual conversation. Begin each sentence with "I see..." or "I hear..." Use names of the people there to identify who is saying what.

c. You are giving the final speech at your celebration. You tell the group what you accomplished over the past three (or your time frame number of) years. You thank them for sharing this event with you. Describe what you say in one paragraph. Begin with "I am here today because..."

d. Review what you have written thus far. Now, write a list of the specific accomplishments you will have to achieve in specific time periods to bring that celebration event to reality.

e. Identify any obstacles that are in the way of bringing that celebration event to reality.

f. Write out a plan to overcome each obstacle identified, or how you will plan for your celebration if the obstacles cannot be removed or circumvented.

g. Take each specific accomplishment in "d" above and write out a self-contract to pursue it.

5. <u>Time Management.</u> You can't manage time. You manage yourself in the context of the same twenty-four hours each day we all experience. Stephen Covey, in his books, *The 7 Habits of Highly Effective People* and *First Things First*, describes four generations of time management techniques. His approach adds results and relationships as important considerations in prioritizing. He calls this the fourth generation time management technique. It is worth some study.

There seems to be a fifth generation of time management perspective developing. This includes energy and purpose in the factors involved in managing time. Sometimes you have the time but not the energy. Sometimes you find the time when you have the energy. Sometimes you have to suck it up and find both.

Every task has some connection to the short-term or long-term purpose of an individual's life. If it doesn't, don't waste the time.

In arranging these factors, Time, Energy, Results, Relationships and Purpose, the acronym TERRP became meaningful and appropriate since the idea was born in a classroom on the University of Maryland, College Park campus, home of the mighty Terrapins. The original intent was for use as a means of changing a tendency to procrastinate.

Used in conjunction with other organizing and task prioritizing methods, the TERRP component of time management asks the following questions about each task:

| | | |
|---|---|---|
| Do I have the Time? | ☐ yes | ☐ no |
| Do I have the Energy? | ☐ yes | ☐ no |
| Is the task necessary for the Results I want? | ☐ yes | ☐ no |
| Does the task help build Relationships? | ☐ yes | ☐ no |
| Does the task contribute to my Purpose in life? | ☐ yes | ☐ no |

The greater the number of "yes" answers, the greater the urgency to do the task now and not postpone it. You may set a predetermined cut-off. For example, three or more "yeses" will require the task to be done now or before the day is over. Two or less will mean the task can be postponed without guilt or anxiety over procrastination, if procrastination is viewed as a weakness.

Project management, project planning, career development, financial planning and life planning are examples where decision-making, goal setting and time management are put to use. One measure of success is how these skills are used to produce the desired outcomes.

However, the mind is not just a biological computer. Organized information processing is necessary to success and happiness, but it is still not the highest level of mind function. There is much more.

Creativity and wisdom may be the highest level of output from the information processing functions of the brain. What would our world be like without inventors, artists, philosophers, musicians, poets, playwrights, scientists and writers?

We all don't have to be acknowledged by others to be these things. In our own ways, we each have our creative functions, and we each have our personal wisdom.

Wisdom is our tested conclusions about life. In this definition, creativity and wisdom cannot be outputs of just the information processing level of mind function. The higher levels of psyche and spirit must be involved. These are whole-person phenomena.

Rate your time management skills.

[  ] excellent        [  ] good        [  ] fair        [  ] poor

6.  Stress Management Skills. There are five stress management techniques that I think everybody should know. They are widely used, and taught in college courses and numerous workshops. Their adaptation to the workplace is occurring, which will help to spread their use. The combination of these techniques helps to prevent the stress response, to interrupt the stress response early enough to short circuit the consequences and to build stress resistance, stress hardiness, or as some authors call it, stress inoculation.

These techniques are:

a.  Diaphragmatic Breathing. Breathing from the diaphragm is the most efficient. This deep breathing gets oxygen to the lower parts of the lungs where most of the air-blood gas exchange takes place. In diaphragmatic breathing, the abdomen rises as the breath is taken in.

    Practice taking four successive deep breaths by expanding the abdomen before the chest rises on inhalation. Do it slowly and comfortably. Don't do it too many times in a row as it may lead to hyperventilation and dizziness.

b.  Muscle Tension Reduction. Having a feel for where the tension is in our muscles is a help in reducing the effects of stress. Develop the habit of scanning your body mentally from head to toe to see where tension and soreness exist.

When the tension is discovered, consciously relax those muscles. A good way to practice relaxing specific muscles is to willfully increase the tension in them, and then let go. One of the principles of muscle elasticity is that they return to a greater degree of relaxation immediately after contraction.

Muscle tension is due to partial contraction maintained over a long time. This brings on soreness and fatigue. Many people find this tension in the facial, jaw, neck and shoulder muscles.

c. <u>Massage.</u> If you have never tried this delicious muscle tension reducer, learn to receive and to give a massage. The extent and degree of involvement will be determined by whom the other person is.

There are many books on massage therapy, or take a lesson from a certified therapist. The "feather-light touch" and the deep muscle massage are particularly enjoyable.

d. <u>The Instant Calming Sequence (ICS).</u> This process is aimed at stopping the stress response at its very beginning, before the whole nervous, endocrine and immune response is triggered. This consists of five steps. It has also been called the "Quieting Reflex."

At the very first sign of an acute stress event (such as a sudden verbal assault that triggers anger, or getting cut off in traffic when you are already late), the mind can reflexively bring to bear these five steps that have been shown to stop the stress response. These take a long time to build into a natural reflex pattern, but it can be done. Some people have habits that are similar to these. The steps, as outlined by Robert Cooper, are as follows:

i. Continue breathing evenly. (An acute stress event interrupts the breathing cycle for a few seconds. The reflex to continue breathing keeps the nervous system drive calm and even.)

ii. Maintain a positive face. Keeping a positive face, even a slight smile, tells yourself and those observing you that you are in control.

iii. Maintain a balanced posture. An acute stress event causes upper body muscles to suddenly relax, causing a slump in posture. A conscious resistance to this slump tells the mind and body you are not giving in.

iv. Do a quick scan of muscle tension, and send a wave of relaxation throughout your body. This increases focussing and centering.

v. Take mental control of the situation. Accept the reality of the event, and look for the best outcome. Decide how to apply your expertise, character and belief system to steer the outcome to a win-win situation. Give the benefit of the doubt to others. You can afford to be generous — that's just the way you are. You are in control.

The ICS, described by Robert Cooper in his book, *Health & Fitness Excellence: The Scientific Action Plan*, is an example of a broader process called "cognitive restructuring" which is beyond the scope of this discussion. It takes time and practice to change patterns of behavior. But it can be done. There are many examples of people changing hostile behavior, pessimism and helplessness. It can be done.

e. **Herbert Benson's Principle of the Maximum Mind.** This has been one of my favorites to use personally and to teach to others. Benson, a Harvard Medical School cardiologist, devoted much of his research to studying the physiologic relaxation response and a form of transcendental meditation that is adaptable to all belief systems. This combination he called "the Principle of the Maximum Mind" in his book, *Your Maximum Mind*.

There are two phases to this process. The sequence takes about fifteen to twenty minutes altogether. Preparation for the sequence is to choose a place and time away from noise and distraction. Select a word or phrase that you can repeat — this word can be something abstract such as "one," or meaningful as in "peace" or even religious as in "The Lord is my Shepherd."

The second phase of the process calls for feeding the mind something positive, uplifting and inspiring. So, before starting the process, select a passage of inspirational writing, scripture or poetry to use.

Phase one is to elicit the relaxation response as follows:

i.   Sit in a comfortable position. Close your eyes. Relax all excess muscle tension. Breathe deeply, evenly and regularly without hyperventilating.

ii.  Each time you breathe out, say your selected word or phrase silently to yourself.

iii. Continue in this position with deep breathing for about ten to fifteen minutes. If your mind strays, as soon as you catch yourself, recall your word or phrase to refocus yourself.

In phase two, when you feel relaxed in body and clear in the mind, open your eyes and read the passage selected. Meditate on the passage for personal applications. Make some decisions to use whatever practical ideas arise from your meditations.

The Benson relaxation/meditation technique is what I use most often. It has helped me to control a spastic colon and quit using Librium and tincture of belladonna alkaloids. I think medical practitioners will get to the place where they understand these techniques, have someone to teach them to their patients and recommend their use before prescription drugs. I see a move on the part of consumers towards this model.

New research in stress management is leading to the development of more specific techniques, which lead to quieting the nervous system traffic between the brain and the heart. This balances the sympathetic and parasympathetic nervous systems.

The "Freeze-Frame" technique is researched and taught by the Institute of Heart Math in Boulder Creek, California. It holds great promise as a tool to be incorporated into conventional medical practice. Its effects can be measured by recording the electrical patterns of the heart.

Other cognitive skills that reduce stress and increase the power of the mind include the decision to forgive self and others, to deal constructively with change, to accept what cannot be changed, to change what can be changed, to reason through past mistakes and handle regrets, to think through the things about the present or future that are the causes of anxiety, to plan for financial security, to understand our locus of control, and to understand and deal with depression.

These skills are very individualized. However, there are some general guidelines that apply. Understanding depression, for example, can lead to prevention or faster recovery for self or a loved one. Everyone needs to have a financial plan. Left to chance and unplanned process, financial problems quickly become a disaster.

Depression has both physiologic and cognitive causes. An imbalance in neurotransmitters is always a primary or secondary cause of depression. That is why drugs help. Effects on the circadian rhythm of the body are involved. Seasonal Affective Disorder (SAD) is a form of depression related to the length of daylight exposure on susceptible individuals. Psychological and spiritual processes are involved. Depression is a whole-person phenomenon.

Financial planning has to include generating maximum income within the limits of health, education and skills; debt management; savings and investment; projection of future needs for family growth; and retirement planning.

The details of these skills are beyond the scope of this book. Resource material on some of the above include Dr. Glenn Shiraldi's *Hope and Help for Depression*, and *Your Money or Your Life* by Joe Dominguez and Vicki Robin.

Rate your stress management skills.

[ ] excellent      [ ] good      [ ] fair      [ ] poor

## Carol's Turn

My thoughts on this chapter are about creativity, decision-making and memories. My creative instincts are directed towards family and homemaking. Al has more creative abilities in the use of language and ideas. It has been fun to share in some of the output as we put this book together.

Several years ago, he shared with me a short prayer he composed as a teenager. It brings back good memories for him since it was at a meal with friends whom he had not seen for many years — Percyval Lewis and Jeremiah Cox. All three were teachers at the same high school and lunched together. It was Al's turn to say the grace before meal and, as he tells it, these words came to his mind:

*Author and Source of every good,*
*Dear Lord, we thank Thee for this food.*
*May health and strength to us it give,*
*And may we for Thee always live. Amen.*

Nothing earth shattering. Just a simple rhyme. Could he have cultivated this into writing and publishing poetry? He says no, it was probably just a one-time "burp of the brain."

I believe that everyone has creative abilities in many ways. Sometimes it is just that the definition of "creative" is other people's expectation. Creative, to me, means an individual way of doing something or looking at something. I find creative fulfillment in organizing a household, planning a menu (especially when one's husband calls on the way home to lunch to say that he has just invited twenty people to join us), caring for plants and flowers, and entertaining guests.

I admire those who write music, poetry, books and plays, etc. I enjoy their compositions without feeling any less adequate or cheated. If I use and work with what I believe are my creative abilities, I accept my gifts or lack of gifts.

However, sometimes, just sometimes, I get the thought that "it would be nice to put these feelings into words, or music, or poetry, or a painting, or something to become a concrete product of what goes on in my mind. Contributing to this book has been a most enjoyable mental effort for me.

Carolyn Staub, one of the students who took Al's course in 1987, composed the following during some of the writing exercises in the class. She gave copies to us with permission to use them if ever we wanted. I want to include them here as an example of some creative writing from a friend whose life touched ours nine years ago.

*Your world looks rather bleak today*
*People telling you how to live your life*
*Telling you who you should be*
*Trying to make their truth yours.*

*Look inside your own reality*
*You'll find life there*
*Life that thrives with pleasure*
*Life that reaches out*
*Life that dreams freely.*

*A life that binds*
*Is not worth living.*
*You are who you want to be.*
*Surely, each choice is yours to make.*

*So if you feel your world is bleak*
*Then it is only because you follow.*
*Follow the words that others choose*
*Without regard for your own truth.*

Carolyn shared other pieces of her writing which we have kept. One, shared towards the end of the course, was especially meaningful:

*A feeling of fullness has come over me*
*Even though I am hungry*
*My hunger for security has subsided*
*But now my mind is spurred by challenge*
*My heart beats irregularly*
*Not as much from fear as from excitement.*

Another piece was shared as part of an exercise to bring samples of inspirational/motivational quotations to class. She composed her own:

*Rather than trying to see through the darkness*
*... embrace it.*
*Once the fear of darkness is transformed into acceptance*
*... the darkness fades.*

These need no further comments.

I think Albert Einstein is widely regarded as one of the most creative human beings. His theory of relativity is one of the great theories of modern physics. Al delights in telling the story of how Dr. Einstein conceived this theory. Since Al didn't use this in his portion of this chapter, I am going to.

It seems that Dr. Einstein was lying out in the fields one day looking up at the sun. He began to imagine that he was riding a beam of light that left the sun and traveled to other planets. This imaginary journey at the speed of light led him to develop the special theory of relativity and the general theory of relativity. His creative imagination mixed with his mathematical genius to discover new knowledge.

It is said that most people don't understand the theories of relativity. I didn't. But Al has explained them to me this way: The special theory of relativity says that time is dependent on the position of the observer. That is, two observers at different distances from an event will see the event at different times — even hundreds of years apart. The greater the distance, the greater the time difference. This makes sense on earth between time zones. At the speed of light and on planets at different distances from the sun, it seems to make sense too.

The general theory of relativity is easier. It says that time is dependent on mass. That is, if the earth were bigger, time would be slower. I don't understand why.

Al says that one of these days he will ask a physicist this question: If time is slower as things get bigger, does it mean that time stands still at the level of the largest unit — the universe? Is that what eternity means?

Those things are too deep for me. I don't care to even think about them. Al thinks it's fun to speculate and fantasize in these areas.

The other question that I sometimes wonder about is the question of "What if we had made a different decision?" I think about several major turning points in life and wonder how things would have turned out if we had chosen a different option.

Two of the most memorable of these decisions were before major relocations. One, a move from Michigan to Virginia. When Al finished his doctorate at Michigan State University, we had a choice to stay in Berrien Springs, Michigan, where we owned a lot of land ready to build our first house. He was accepted for a post-doctoral fellowship in the Department of Physiology at the University of Virginia. All our closest friends were in Michigan. What did we do? We sold the land and moved to Virginia. How would our lives be different now if we had stayed in Michigan? We have settled that question.

The other turning point was the decision to leave Virginia. One option was to accept a fully supported fellowship from the University of North Carolina, Chapel Hill, where Al would take an MPH in cardiovascular epidemiology. The other option was to move to Maryland to teach college biology at Columbia Union College. We moved to Maryland. We have settled our questions about our choice at that turning point.

Looking back, it seems that emotions and gut feelings were a larger part of our decision-making than the cold, hard facts. Both of us seem to make decisions this way. We have become comfortable with our style. The outcomes have been mostly good. The bad that came brought many important good insights and enough good results to outweigh the bad.

As we see our three children reach adulthood, we often wonder if we helped them to form good decision-making skills, or how much of their decisions are left to feelings and emotions. Each one is so different.

Our oldest son is the logical thinker and planner. I remember our several discussions about his career interests and how he came to choose between medicine and business. He has the ability to do anything he sets his mind to.

Our second son is the emotional decision-maker. Things must feel right. He brought us a granddaughter before any of us was ready for such an event. How he is dealing with this situation and how we feel and relate to everyone involved in these relationships has brought some new insights to us.

Our daughter, youngest of the three, is the balanced decision-maker. She seems to have her logical and emotional parts equally involved. No wonder she is looking at a career combining computers with photography and health and fitness.

Reviewing how we have made decisions over the years, we see, understand and accept our children and ourselves for who we are individually. I wouldn't want to be totally a biological computer.

In talking about memories, we had a family ritual when the children were growing up. Almost every Friday evening we would have a candlelight dinner. Everyone at the table, including any visitors, would tell about their "highlight" and "low light" of the week. Many times this would be followed by Dad pulling out the slide projector to show the old family pictures.

We have had good times and bad times. The good times and the pleasant memories have always outweighed the bad.

To go the distance, the brain must be actively engaged in charting the path.

# Understand How the Mind Works as Psyche

> *"I want to be the white man's brother, not his brother-in-law."*
>
> Martin Luther King, Jr.

> *"Remember, no one can make you feel inferior without your consent."*
>
> Eleanor Roosevelt

Seven

*Dedicated to*

**Intercultural families everywhere**

*We are rooting for you. The way you meet challenges in integration gives us all hope for the future.*

When Carol and I decided to marry twenty-nine years ago, we received some interesting advice and opinions. One was from a person who felt she knew broad characteristics of different peoples. "Don't do it," she advised the bride-to-be. "Indian men are too sexually demanding."

Another piece of advice came from a highly respected counselor in our church organization. "Don't let her do it," she wrote to Carol's mother. "They will not be able to travel in the Deep South." Traveling in the Deep South was not a high priority item for us at that time.

One of Carol's girlfriends put the situation this way: "How can you even think of getting close to a dark-skin man, much more being intimate with one?"

One of my friends gave me a history lesson on race relations in America. At the end he said, "Sammy Davis, Jr., was attacked and threatened with castration for dating a white woman." I never checked on the historical accuracy of that one. I believe much worse than that has happened to non-whites in the past.

A budding psychologist gave the most comprehensive advice. Here is that story:

• • • • •

He came for a visit and outlined for us what we were getting into by establishing an interracial home. I believed he was sincere and well intentioned.

"It's like this," he counseled. "There are three racial lines in descending order of value ascribed by society at large — white, brown/yellow and black. Within each racial line there are three classes of people — upper, middle and lower class. To complicate things further, a secondary factor within each color line is the value placed on the degree of paleness, brownness, yellowness or blackness. In whites, the value increases for having a tan upon the paleness. Among the other colors, the value decreases for increasing intensity of color."

• • • • •

He then went on to explain who marries whom depends on the level of self-esteem within one's racial and class categories. The gist of his lecture was:

1.  Upper class whites only marry whites.

2.  Low self-esteem upper class may marry lower class but mostly stay within the same racial group.

3.  Lower class whites, especially with low self-esteem, are the ones who marry outside of their racial line.

4.  Low self-esteem black and brown/yellow men of any class feel they are moving up the scale by marrying white women. They usually end up with low self-esteem, lower class white women.

5.  Among whites, women have lower self-esteem, so you will find more white women marrying brown/yellow or black men than white men marrying brown/yellow or black women.

6.  The children of interracial marriages always suffer psychologically.

7. Before you make the decision to marry interracially, you should carefully consider the reasons, the possible effects on your future and the consequences to your children.

We emerged from that lecture with sober thoughts about our situation and ourselves. Was this research, observations, speculation, unchangeable nature or a condition predetermined in the stars? Can people of different color just be in love? Can they have the freedom to co-exist with others without being the object of abuse or disapproval?

The history of racial discrimination and intolerance has basis in color, class and value of self and others. This was the end of the decade of the sixties when civil rights and race riots were fresh in the American consciousness.

The thinking stimulated then, and the observations of other interracial families over the last twenty-nine years, have contributed to some of the thoughts that guided the development of this chapter. This is an overview of functions in the psychosocial dimension. Let's start again with homeostasis.

## Psychosocial Homeostasis

Psychosocial homeostasis refers to the maintenance of balance within self, and between self and the rest of the environment. The factors within self deal with the personality and behavioral dynamics.

The balance within self has to do with self-value or self-esteem, the private versus the public self, the facade we project to fit the occasion and how authentic we are — how real, or how well the person we portray to others fits with the person we know ourselves to be. The evaluation produces a "feeling" in the mind. This feeling state is the barometer of psychosocial homeostasis.

The balance between self and the rest of the environment has to do with the social roles we fill and the relationships we have — including processes and things outside of ourselves. In these relationships, we have to deal with social stratification, cultural conditioning, ethnicity, and beliefs and attitudes of others.

The demands of our social roles; the impact of other people; cultural, societal and religious standards; and level of self-worth or self-confidence all interact in setting the balance within which we function. Achieving a comfortable balance within which we find a place to make our mark in life, whether small and unnoticed or large and impacting others, is what homeostasis of the psychosocial dimension is all about.

Within this homeostasis, there are forces that regulate. There are forces that push towards isolation and individualism. There are forces inside and outside that push towards connectedness and belonging. The test of these forces is mostly subjective and measured in feelings.

These "feeling states" — high or low self-esteem, self-confidence, self-worth, call it what you may — are major determinants of satisfaction in life. The objective data, coming from the information processing part of the mind, may say otherwise. But the conclusions drawn by the psyche are those of the feelings generated.

Personal growth is the pathway to understanding self, achieving balance and feeling full satisfaction with life. This cannot be completed without the higher dimension of spiritual homeostasis, which we will consider in Chapter 8.

## Psychosocial Nutrition

The factors that feed the development of the psyche have effects beginning in the womb. The comfort, safety and security of being nurtured and cared for register on the developing nervous system. However, I believe that the factors of chemistry and genes during fetal development are not as important as the factors after birth.

How the newborn is regarded, touched and treated lays the foundation for the major qualities of the psychosocial dimension. It is how the infant and growing child are surrounded by a nurturing, caring, loving, encouraging, value reflecting and affirming environment that is the key to high self-worth.

Development continues through responsibilities and challenges met successfully. Learning to deal with setbacks and overcoming difficulties nurture and build a strong, positive psyche.

This kind of growth cannot be ordered, legislated, dictated or forced. It has to be nurtured with the proper "nutrients."

Through this process, people move through stages, as one writer puts it, "from dependence to independence then on to interdependence." People find their proper places in the larger scheme of things.

It is far easier to provide physical food (though sometimes that is the greatest immediate challenge), shelter and clothing for children than to provide the "nutrients" for psychological growth. Feeding the psyche is of a higher order of "nutrition" than feeding the body. Feeding the psyche is even of a higher order than feeding knowledge and information to the mental faculties. This is a matter demanding emphasis in planning homes and families, in education, in social programs and in churches.

## Psychosocial Stress and Stress Adaptation

Common psychosocial stresses are social anxiety and shyness. Everyone has some sense of being evaluated by others. When this sense of being evaluated is at the level of awareness and causes one to feel uncomfortable, the discomfort influences behavior and feelings. This produces anxiety about how one is perceived, accepted, valued and evaluated. The anxiety leads to shyness.

Causes of shyness may relate to self-esteem, peer pressure, social role and unrealistic expectations — by self or others. There may be a genetic predisposition, and recent studies show that characteristics of shyness can be detected very early in a child's life. The behavior seems to get accentuated when the individual gets into patterns of self-perceived social failure.

Stress management for social anxiety and shyness depends on the extent of the problem. In many cases, self-help books and lay counseling in an individual or group context are successful. In cases where more severe dysfunction is present, professional therapy may be indicated.

Some of the techniques available include cognitive restructuring (involving thinking processes, perceptions, adapting to change, rational reappraisal of situations), raising self-esteem and building a social support system.

## Psychosocial Work

Is there such a thing as "psychic energy?" How about "ego strength?" Does the psyche "exert effort" to accomplish certain tasks? I believe that a case can be made for work, effort and expenditure of energy by the part of the mind we label as psyche.

Psychic energy in this context is not the ability to read other people's minds or send telepathic messages. I believe that, subconsciously, the part of the mind that holds the knowledge of our innermost self has a program that tells it what is the preferred feeling state — one of comfort with self. The mind then tries to heal things that have gone wrong, or tries to defend from any further hurt and damage, and tries to push towards achievement of the desired state. The conscious part of the mind then seeks to acquire information and make decisions to fulfill the effort of the psyche.

In this context, "ego defenses" and "ego strength" are meaningful terms. I don't think that the "psychic energy" expended can be measured in terms of ATP expenditure, but there is effort put out. (Maybe the relationship between glucose metabolism and psychological states will be explained someday. One of the difficulties with this type of research is that for some brain activities, electrical discharges decrease as the brain is engaged — some processes go on by inhibiting other activities.)

One of the ways we feel the output of psychic energy is the experience of being in caretaker roles. Whether it's caring for children, the sick and bedridden, or the elderly, caretaker roles have a demand on total energy output that is more than just physical energy. Exhaustion and burnout in these roles is as much or more a psychic exhaustion as it is physical exhaustion.

Some people are more caring in general. Caring for others as friends, loved ones, or just caring for humanity as a whole has its point where a degree of caring is growth promoting, and a further degree of caring can lead to overdemand on the psyche.

## Psychosocial Rest

The psyche needs reduction of effort, variety, change of pace and relaxation similar to the need for physical rest and relaxation. This rest comes in the form of personal space, privacy and solitude.

Each one has a comfort zone around their person that determines how physically close and how psychologically close another person can be. This personal space ranges with the quality of the relationship — from intimate to distant.

Everyone needs a certain degree of privacy. This privacy is to establish ownership, control and identification with some part of the surrounding where communication with self is the dominant activity. The circumstances and personality dictate what degree and extent of privacy is possible, but it seems that there is some minimum privacy necessary for growth and comfort.

Solitude is time and place to be alone, but not being lonely. This is aloneness desired, chosen and enjoyed. This rest and relaxation for the psyche contributes to psychosocial strength and growth.

Psychosocial rest also comes when we have settled the question of who we are ethnically. This includes how our personal value stacks up with others; how equal, superior or inferior we feel; and how much of a "citizen of the world" we truly feel, as opposed to belonging to just a small subgroup of humanity. For those troubled by these questions, rest comes when the matter of roots, trunk and branches is settled in the psyche.

The first broadcast of Alex Haley's "Roots" as a mini-series on network television is rated as the most watched TV event of all time. There seems to be something in us that wants to connect to our past and settle some restlessness about belonging.

# Psychosocial Growth

Freud was the first to describe stages of psychological development. Other theorists have provided us with descriptions of normal and abnormal psychological development. To bring this discussion to a lay perspective, I like to consider psychosocial growth simply as the process of maturing socially.

Growth then would mean the process of developing appropriate behavior and feeling states for the appropriate stage in life. Who determines what is appropriate or normal? Each culture has established guidelines and traditions.

Appropriate behavior may be codified as in standards of etiquette, or just handed down in unwritten guidelines. How people treat, value and regard one another is the basis for balance in the psyche.

Psychosocial growth, then, is the process of getting to know, understand and cultivate the standards of treatment, valuing and regarding other people to produce the greatest comfort level for self and others. It is an interactive process.

Examples of psychosocial growth are seen in people moving from shyness to pleasant assertiveness, from anxiety to calm, from a feeling of needing other people's approval to confidence in their own ideas, from broken and damaged relationships to healing and restoration.

*Solitude is time and place to be alone, but not being lonely.*

# Psychosocial Reproduction

The process analogous to the physiologic event of producing offspring is the process of being perpetuated through relationships. The ties formed with other human beings, which endure time and distance, and which survive in the minds and hearts of the individuals, constitute psychosocial reproduction. These ties are left behind when we depart this life and perpetuate us in the minds of others.

These ties are beyond genetic and blood ties. They are forged in shared experiences, shared values, unconditional acceptance, willingness to forgive and purposeful planning to interact.

In this way, people who may or may not have produced offspring, or created mental products as evidence of having lived, can leave a legacy in the lives they have influenced, in the caring they have shared, in the memories they have created. May that legacy be only a positive one.

# The Major Psychosocial Health Problems

Low self-esteem, social anxiety and shyness and broken relationships are the major health problems in the psychosocial dimension.

How does the individual deal with these problems from the viewpoint of prevention, diagnosis, treatment and rehabilitation? From a layperson's perspective, knowledge and awareness of how these conditions are established seem to help. An understanding of personality dynamics, the effects of genetics, child raising practices, interpersonal dynamics, and religious belief systems impact on the comfort level one establishes with self. This personal comfort level sets the tone for dealing with other people.

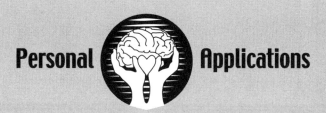

# Personal Applications

## Directions:

Complete the self-examination exercise in Section A. Look at the other sections and select those exercises that are of interest to you.

Other assessments that may be a part of a helpful self-examination exercise are measures of self-esteem, the anxiety scales and quality of relationships. These are more structured and many are used in research and clinical assessments. The purpose of the exercises given here is introspection and self-understanding,

A. **Self-Examination III — The Psychosocial Dimension**

Check the most appropriate answer. Note that for each item your answer will be somewhere on the line between "T" for mostly true or "F" for mostly false. If you don't know the answer, check the "Don't Know" box. Check the "Don't Care" box if you believe that an item is not important to your personal health. Give the answers that you honestly think apply — not what you would like to be true..

## Psychosocial Health Factors

| | | True or False | Don't Know | Don't Care |
|---|---|---|---|---|
| 1. | I am comfortable with the way I behave. | T———F | | |
| 2. | I feel in balance with my total environment. | T———F | | |
| 3. | I have a good sense of who I am. | T———F | | |
| 4. | I am comfortable with my role in life. | T———F | | |
| 5. | I adapt to change fairly well. | T———F | | |
| 6. | I have a strong feeling of positive self-worth. | T———F | | |
| 7. | I am not overly self-conscious. | T———F | | |
| 8. | I get along well with most people. | T———F | | |
| 9. | I enjoy close personal relationships. | T———F | | |
| 10. | I have a comfortable circle of friends. | T———F | | |
| 11. | I am not easily offended. | T———F | | |
| 12. | I am socially mature. | T———F | | |
| 13. | I have adequate privacy and personal space. | T———F | | |
| 14. | I handle problem relationships satisfactorily. | T———F | | |
| 15. | I understand my people preferences. | T———F | | |
| 16. | I feel connected to all humankind. | T———F | | |
| 17. | I treat other people with value and dignity. | T———F | | |
| 18. | I feel that I contribute to the good of others. | T———F | | |
| 19. | I enjoy making other people happy. | T———F | | |
| 20. | I have experienced the pain of self-doubt. | T———F | | |
| 21. | I have known pleasure in self-improvement. | T———F | | |
| 22. | I have experienced pain in relationships. | T———F | | |
| 23. | I have known the pleasure of love and caring. | T———F | | |
| 24. | I help to generate peace, love and optimism. | T———F | | |
| 25. | My psychosocial pleasures outweigh my pain. | T———F | | |

B. Write short essays on the topics below. Write down the first thoughts that come to mind after you read the topic. Develop those you choose into longer compositions.

1. How I Became Who I Am — The Most Significant Influences

2. The Pleasures and Pains in My Relationships

3. The Things I Like About Myself, the Things Other People Like About Me

4. My Role in the Lives of Others

5. My Successes and Failures as an Individual

6. Psychosocial Growth in Myself and Others

7. Take one side in the debate, "The Government Should Establish Licensing Requirements for Parenthood"

8. Social Stratification, Class Structure and Categorization That Affect My Life

9. The Most Embarrassing Incident in My Whole Life

10. Taking Care of the Elderly

C. On a blank sheet of paper, draw a small circle at the center of the page. Label that "ME." Around that, draw concentric circles to represent each of the relationships in your life from intimate to distant. The first circle next to "ME" is the most intimate relationship. Label each circle with the name of a person or a group (e.g., co-workers, team members). Examine each relationship circle by asking yourself the following questions and writing out the answers:

1. What is the quality of this relationship?

2. Am I satisfied with the quality of this relationship?

3. Do I want to improve this relationship or should it become more distant?

4. What do I need to do to move this relationship to the desired level, closer or more distant?

5. Would this relationship be richer, more fulfilling and mutually more beneficial in the future?

6. What realistic steps do I now take?

D. Discuss the role of a good sense of humor in everyday life. How is a good sense of humor cultivated?

E. Self-Management Skills

There are skills that can be learned to promote growth in psychosocial dynamics. Confidence and success can be enhanced through self-assertiveness balanced with consideration for other people's value and feelings. Visualization of performing a task successfully has been shown to improve performance. Planning and rehearsal help to inspire confidence.

If the need is recognized, self-help guides can contribute to overcoming anxiety, shyness, panic disorders, low self-esteem, and poor intra- and interpersonal relationships. More dysfunctional states may require help from a therapist.

List skills you may be interested in improving:

# Reflections

I started this chapter with some viewpoints about how people value one another. The history of how human beings have treated one another is replete with examples of class structure and dehumanizing treatment.

Should we accept that history as our lot and just find a comfortable place in the scheme of things as they are? Or, when the circumstances place us in a certain place at a certain time, can we contribute to promoting understanding among peoples and lessening the feelings of devaluation of one another?

A psyche that has the need to devalue and mistreat others in order to demonstrate its higher value is warped. Whatever the causes or the background, that psyche needs

to grow beyond bigotry and prejudice. The feelings of being treated as having less value than someone else have to be experienced to be understood. I know what it feels like to be a minority.

In understanding ourselves on the question of how we value and treat other people, here are some observations to stimulate thinking:

1. Some of the common causes for discrimination are ethnicity, skin color, religion, gender, language, age, size (short/tall, fat/skinny), economic class, social class and behavioral type (leader/follower, etc.).

2. We are unable to ascribe identical personal value to everybody. The mind seems to attribute value based on knowl-

edge and experience. Our individual tastes and comfort level vary. We are not called upon to be close friends of everybody. What equality of value requires is positive regard for everybody and zero tolerance for willful devaluation. This applies in all directions, along all scales.

3. Patience, the legal process in a system of democratic justice, and tolerant exhortation to growth in regard to valuing others are better methods of change than violence and death. But sometimes it is difficult to see changes occurring without confrontation. What is the solution?

4. Non-violent protests, civil disobedience and passive resistance are better means of forcing change than rioting, wounding and killing one another. These are lessons from our human history.

5. Parents are entitled to their preferences about whom they are comfortable with as friends, companions or spouses for their children. If the reason for the preference is based purely on lower or higher valuation of the other person, then there is room for growth. Bigotry should be respectfully addressed. Discussions and agitation for change may help.

If the preference is based only in social discomfort generated by lack of exposure or dissimilarities in language, behavior or social tastes, there is, again, room for education and growth.

Only the person expressing the viewpoint can truly know the real truth of the matter. Some people may come across as bigots when they are not. Some people may disguise bigotry under a cloak of false acceptance and pretended understanding. Only the person knows for sure.

6. Our mistreatment of one another usually reflects our unsettled valuation of ourselves.

7. Friends give one another unconditional acceptance and social support without expecting equal in return and a place to feel unashamed, regardless.

8. In many cases, people's feelings about how other people are treating them are only a reflection of their own fears, apprehensions and expectations.

9. In the world as a whole, and especially in the West, we have made much progress in race relations, accepting differences and treating one another with dignity and respect.

10. In the world as a whole, and especially in the West, there remains much hurt and sadness about race relations, accepting differences and treating one another with dignity and respect.

11. What responsibility do I, as an individual, have for helping others to grow psychosocially? As a parent, as a spouse or as a friend, there is responsibility. It has to be approached with love and patience.

We have the capacity to evaluate ourselves through our feelings. Hurt and embarrassment, shame and disgrace, failure and social ineptitude create feeling states that are negative. These negative states have negative effects on the physiology — nervous, hormonal and endocrine functions are affected and may precipitate illnesses.

On the other hand, feelings of accomplishment, pride, success and social acceptance are positive feelings that radiate into physiologic function and enhance health. These positive states are preferred, naturally. To be truly positive and health promoting, these feelings are not based on devaluing, discrediting or putting down others. In fact, these feelings are heightened when the help and contribution of others is acknowledged.

The feelings of a middle-aged man seem to be positive or negative based on his evaluation of his accomplishments and how he perceives other people evaluate his accomplishments. The key areas of evaluation are personal income, job or position, kind of home he lives in, status in social circles, his physical shape and the physical shape of his wife, the position and accomplishments of his wife and children, and his ability to provide for the future needs of his family. If the objective evidence does not support positive feelings, he finds a way to bolster his pride or limit the stress of the negative feelings.

Whether young, middle-aged or elderly, we know that some accomplishments, some insights and some successes come only through a path beset with failures, hurt, shame and disgrace. The ultimate failure is failure to use these events as springboards for accomplishments. Within most things bad, within most mistakes, the seeds of something good lie waiting to be watered and cultivated.

The psyche — the psychosocial dynamics of the mind — is even a more complex mechanism than the information processing dimension. The psyche depends on the information processor, which in turn depends on the physiologic dimension. This connection is becoming clearer as we study and understand more about the human mind.

The relevant application here is what I, as an individual, am learning about myself in terms of worth, capabilities, influence, creativity, value to others and valuation of others. Why do I treat other people the way I do, and how do I feel about myself as a result?

## Carol's Turn

My thoughts on this chapter are about feelings: feeling loved, feeling accepted, feeling embarrassed, feeling lucky, feeling hurt, feeling devalued, feeling assertive, feeling a surge of pure joy generating a high lasting for several weeks. These are the joys and sorrows that are a part of living, a part of raising a family.

• • • • •

One of my embarrassing situations was a social occasion to see the play *Les Miserables* at the National Theater in Washington, DC. Our daughter had purchased tickets as a birthday present for me to take Al and four friends to the play. We got to our seats and were just commenting on how good the seats were.

An usher came over to let us know that we were in the wrong seats. After some checking and the commotion of moving, we were informed that we should be in the standing section. I stood through the entire *Les Miserables* performance feeling quite miserable. Our daughter had asked if any

*Within most things bad, within most mistakes, the seeds of something good lie waiting to be watered and cultivated.*

seats were still available and was told "the only seats remaining are in the standing section." She heard "seats" and thought that meant chairs, not space. It now remains a memory over which we share a laugh every now and then. I believe that the play and the occasion became more memorable because of the embarrassment. After the initial embarrassment and profuse apologies, our daughter laughs about it too.

• • • • •

The main character in Victor Hugo's *Les Miserables* is Jean Valjean who has to deal with shame and disgrace when he is required to carry a yellow slip of paper with his less-than-perfect record.

Al has had his fair share of embarrassing situations. He tells about them in class, so I feel free to share them here. One was the occasion of the ordination of Dr. Theodore Chamberlain when we were at the University of Virginia.

• • • • •

Dr. Chamberlain was our minister then, and he invited Al to be on the platform with him during the ceremony of ordination. At that time, we could be classified as poor — Al was on a post-doctoral fellowship at $10,000 per year, and he still clung to the ideal of having me at home to take care of our three children.

At the ordination ceremony, he didn't have the customary dark wool business suit worn on such occasions. He didn't think about it until the day of the ceremony when he showed up in a light-blue polyester suit!

To this day, I think he feels that he spoiled the official photographs of the occasion. There was Dr. Chamberlain, Ron Wisbey (presently one of the leading executives in the Adventist Healthcare System) and Dan Matthews (now a television personality) in their business suits, and in the middle of the group, Al in his light-blue polyester! Ted and Faye, if you ever read this, I apologize again on his behalf! He has given up being a one-man protest against fashion.

• • • • •

The other time that dress was an embarrassment to us was at a party at the Marriott Hotel on Capitol Hill in Washington, DC. We were invited to the black-tie affair sponsored by the heart surgeons for whom Al worked.

That year was hard on our entertainment budget because our sons each had two school banquets for which they just had to have rented tuxedos.

Al showed up at the black-tie affair in an old white dinner jacket which we had carried around for years. He still talks about the feeling of the occasion when everybody was decked out in their tuxedos and party dresses, and he and the waiters had on white jackets.

• • • • •

He is a little better now about dressing for the occasion, but he still doesn't get overimpressed with dress and external show. He seems to survive this kind of embarrassment very well. I just hope he is through with it. Luckily, our daughter has taken on the responsibility to see that her Dad is appropriately dressed when he leaves home.

He pays more attention to her wishes than to mine. She is his fashion police.

There are two occasions when what seemed to be a major disaster for us became insignificant by comparison to what other people were going through at the very same moment. One was when the water pipes in the bathroom of our house froze and burst.

• • • • •

It was one of the coldest, winter days in January 1982. We stood looking on as the plumber from Johnny-Be-Quick tore out the walls to get at the frozen pipes. We were feeling rather sorry for ourselves. Sorry over the decision to buy that house. Sorry over the huge emergency plumbing bills, and sorry for letting other people push their problems off on us.

As we stood there wallowing in sorrow and regret, we turned to catch the news on TV. An Air Florida flight taking off from National Airport in nearby Washington, DC, had crashed into the frozen Potomac River. People were dying, struggling for their lives in a frozen river. Our problems didn't appear to be that big anymore.

• • • • •

The other incident was just last summer. The rains were heavy and the basement leaked again. We had to mop up about twenty gallons of water — maybe one-quarter inch in a fifty square foot area. Again, we were lamenting our lot — our decision-making, our expenses. But the TV pictures of the floods in the Midwest with homes and entire towns being washed away or completely flooded showed us how lucky we were. We didn't feel like being sorry for ourselves just then.

I have always been a person to look out for the needs of others. My training and experience was to always put other people's needs and comforts before my own. I felt good doing that. It seemed to be fulfilling. Then I learned about assertiveness training. I took a course. It seemed to emphasize what I used to call "selfishness."

The one part of the course that was helpful was to come to realize that a balance between doing for others and taking care of yourself is essential. I had to find my own balance. It is still more of a joy to serve than to be served. By understanding my own make-up, I adapted the assertiveness principles to fit with my own belief system.

There is great joy in giving yourself permission to do something you feel you want to do but were always inhibited about. At our first son's wedding, Al and I danced in public for the first time. We both had grown up believing that dancing was sinful. I had always had dreams of being able to waltz around a ballroom floor at some formal occasion. But believing it was a sin and not wanting to commit sin or disobey parents and church leaders, I never learned.

Preparing for that wedding was great fun. The bride-to-be and her parents engineered the dance lessons, and we were ready and well rehearsed when the big day came. Stepping out on the ballroom floor with my son and later with my husband was a thrill I will always treasure. I didn't feel sinful. I felt assertive, liberated and exhilarated. I don't believe that God will count that against me in His book of records as sin!

These stories, to me, are examples of growth. I share them to serve as a reminder that each one has evidence of positive growth in life. It also feels good to share some highlights of my family!

Feelings seem to create stronger memories than just the knowledge alone. Feelings of love, peace and joy, feelings of pride and liberation, feelings of being valued just for myself are good feelings. They outweigh the negative feelings of being unwanted, feelings of being devalued, feelings of shame and disgrace, and feelings of broken relationships. I have known a wide range of feelings. I look forward to more good feelings, but I believe that I can handle anything life brings.

The treatment of women throughout history has been rotten. Both in value and freedom of expression, most cultures have oppressed women. Things are changing through the hard work of pioneers for social change. Equality and equal value for abilities and work are achievements of most Western countries. Women have more freedom to carve out their own careers and to choose the best combination of career and motherhood. This is major social progress.

Some of the tragedies of the past were the practices of discarding female babies and female circumcision. Female circumcision is still a major problem in some African countries. Discarding of female babies is still part of life in some regions in India.

There is a clinic compound in Hosur, India, where there are homes established for abandoned children — Anantha Ashram it is called. This small effort to address a great need in a big country was the dream of a retired World Health Organization worker, Samuel Koilpillai. I plan to spend some time in the near future working in those homes for abandoned children.

I know what it feels like to be unwanted. But I know also what it feels like to be wanted and valued and treated as equal, even at times when I feel I don't deserve it. Dreams can come true. Sometimes, however, before dreams come true, you may have to suffer through a couple of nightmares.

To go the distance, the heart must know the pull on its deepest strings. Feelings count.

# UNDERSTAND HOW THE MIND WORKS AS SPIRIT

*"In matters of conscience, the law of the majority has no place."*

Mahatma Gandhi

Eight

*Dedicated to*

**Sunderan and Evangeline Moses**

*The couple with whom we can share our deepest suffering and our greatest joys, and together explore the healing power of music.*

There are times in my life when I witnessed the power of a ritual to change circumstances and lives. The ritual with which I have some firsthand experience is called "the Ordinance of Humility." The ordinance ends with a foot washing ceremony and singing. Here are three examples of its effectiveness.

. . . . .

The first involves my dad and one of my uncles involved in a major interfamily feud. At least, that's how it appeared in the eyes of a ten-year-old. Uncle Fonso was the most educated of my uncles and was good at making speeches and strong arguments for his case.

I remember well the circumstances, but they don't need to be detailed here. This break in relationships lasted for about six months with neither side even acknowledging the existence of the other, though we lived only a few hundred yards apart.

One day, during the Ordinance of Humility, the two fathers, leaders of large families and leaders in their church, sought each other out and washed each other's feet. The healing and reconciliation broke into both families like a fresh breeze into a hot and stuffy building, like the relief when a festering wound is suddenly lanced and purged of pus. It made an impression on a young mind. There must be something to this ritual if it can affect people's lives in such a practical way.

. . . . .

Several years ago, Larry and I were involved in a business transaction which went sour. We blamed each other for derailing each other's career. "If you had not said or done..." "If you had done thus and such..."

We both knew there was much personal hurt and family disappointment remaining on both sides, and that what happened couldn't be undone. Many months passed, and we didn't communicate.

At one of the seasons for rituals in our church, we found ourselves heading to the same room for the Ordinance of Humility. We engaged each other in conversation and washed each other's feet. Healing began. It felt good.

"Maybe, there are other therapeutic systems that could be engaged in to heal relationships. But if effectiveness and price are considerations, this experience could be highly recommended." We both agreed.

. . . . .

A homeless man showed up when the Ordinance of Humility was just ending. We met at the door. "Dr. Bacchus," he said, "I want to take part." I had met him a couple of times before when he made his daily trek through the streets of Takoma Park, MD.

My initial reaction was to find a deacon who should be on the lookout for people who show up late or who didn't have a partner. I had some preconceived notions about the feet of a homeless person who walked the streets as an occupation.

I was glad that I stifled my initial reaction and offered to wash his feet. Those feet were the softest feet I have ever touched. And they were not any more "smelly feet" than others in the room.

This gentleman, a truly brilliant, gentle person suffering from mental deterioration, died some months later. Instead of my doing him a courtesy to wash his feet, I felt honored to have had a moment of soul-to-soul communication with him.

• • • • •

I share the above stories not to show how good anybody is, but to illustrate the effects and potential growth stimulation in some common rituals. Wellness includes experiments with things like these. There might be rituals that you once knew and don't use anymore. Part of the personal exploration in this chapter on spiritual wellness is to connect or reconnect with beliefs and practices that build up the spirit.

The summer of 1999, I participated in a twelve-week group session for mind/body skills at the Center for Mind/Body Medicine in Washington, DC. The exploration and the reconnection with lost anchors of spirituality had been refreshing for me. The closing ritual for the group was to pick a polished stone from a small box and have each member of the group hold it and place their love and best wishes for you on that stone. Now, I am still a scientist by training, and I don't believe that any physical waves went from the mind of the person into the stone. But the symbolism of the act and the tangible memory of a most pleasant experience seemed to bind the group together better than if we had just left without doing that. I have on my desk a shiny, two-toned stone resembling a Siberian tiger that reminds me of the group.

Then there are other kinds of spirit. There are two of my graduate school professors who were remarkable and memorable for their different spirits. The professor I remem-

*But the symbolism of the act and the tangible memory of a most pleasant experience seemed to bind the group together better than if we had just left without doing that.*

ber most vividly at one university is remembered for his free-spirited living. He was the one caught making love to his laboratory assistant on the desk in his office!

Another professor at a different university stands out in my memory because he believed that the human spirit was an entity separate from brain function which presided over the brain during life and which departed at death. This was not just a personal religious belief. This was a philosophical and scientific viewpoint which he endeavored to study.

The spiritual dimension of humans is the most difficult to define and study. It has gained greater scientific attention during the last fifteen years, but since it is not possible to study it by objective means, the definitions may vary from one study to the next.

The one thing that is agreed on is that there is some part or function in the human machinery that deals with the higher needs. These "meta-needs" involve the highest levels of desire and drive to find full satisfaction with life and with existence as a whole. These needs and functions are universal and are not just religious. They touch on the largest questions of life — the questions that transcend the physiologic, the mental or the psychosocial dimensions.

The human spirit may be defined as the capacity to seek meaning and purpose in life. Meaning and purpose involves the ability to explore the depths and height of human existence. It means the capability to make sense of the past, present and future. It also means the capacity to feel connected to the rest of humanity and connected to powers higher and greater than anything known within the "real" world.

On one level, spiritual capacity is a product of beliefs, feelings, knowledge and emotions. The common terms for the entity embodied by this capacity are soul, spirit and heart. Here, all the good and bad in us, all the forces that drive, pull or push us, are integrated into the dynamics we define as spirit. When we say, "you gotta have heart," when we say "keep the spirits up," when we say "put your heart and soul into it," when we say in the world of business and career "do it with passion," we are addressing the human spirit.

So the contribution of physiology (brain cells and neurotransmitters), the mental abilities to make decisions, the ability to experience emotions and the ability to feel connected to things far removed from earth are all part of spirit.

It is important to our definition to keep "human spirit" separate from other spirits. Various religious and philosophical systems define entities, powers and beings that are referred to as spirits. Other philosophical viewpoints hold that these other entities are nonexistent and just beliefs present in the human mind. The relationship between these spirits and the human spirit is a matter of individual belief. The interaction of the other entities with the human spirit is also a personal matter. This is why spiritual wellness is the most individualized of all the aspects of health and wellness.

However, we are able to study, observe and research some of the functions of the human spirit. This is one of the most exciting frontiers of science. There are studies demonstrating the effects of faith, prayer and belief on the biology of the body.

Herbert Benson's recent book, *Timeless Healing: The Power and Biology of Belief*, is just one title among many that reviews the studies of the spirit/body connection. Benson reviews the science of how the chemistry of the brain is affected by belief. His review of the many studies of healing and pain relief with the use of placebos leaves no doubt that the phenomenon is real. People change their physiologic state because they believe it will change. In describing the placebo effect, he offers another name for it — "remembered wellness."

Maybe for spiritual wellness to be real, you first have to believe that there is such an entity as the human spirit!

With these types of studies accumulating daily, and with observations and personal understanding of the human spirit, we are able to draw some general conclusions and use these to promote spiritual wellness. It is in the spirit that the final and most important conclusions about life are made. This is the function that draws the ultimate evaluation about happiness, satisfaction and fulfillment. A fully actualized life, a totally fulfilled life, self-realization, may not be possible without the spiritual dimension.

*The relationship between these spirits and the human spirit is a matter of individual belief.*

## Spiritual Homeostasis

There are two types of balance to be considered. One has to do with the personal, internal balance of the emotions and beliefs. The other has to do with the outward direction of the personal beliefs and emotions. This outward reach is the interaction with other people within the earthly environment, and the interaction with the other forces in the universe — whatever that universe is to the individual.

The heart, soul, spirit and emotions find a balance between positive and negative states. The core beliefs serve as the anchor to maintain this balance. The final internal balance is an integration of the physiologic drives, the mental capacities, the psychosocial dynamics and the capacity to generate emotions. This is the full personality and character of the person.

Some of the positive and negative states that express spirit (heart, soul) are:

purposefulness : purposelessness

meaningfulness : meaninglessness

hopefulness : hopelessness

faithfulness : faithlessness

joyfulness : joylessness

peacefulness : peacelessness

lovingness : lovelessness

As I look at the list above, the question that comes to mind is not whether there is scientific proof that these factors affect health, but rather, is it better to be positive than negative? I believe that one aspect missing from our attempts to harness the power of the spirit to promote health is that we are searching for the answers in science before we understand what we are looking for.

The primary search is to probe our personal philosophy first and then see how the science stacks up. So that if one study comes out that says optimists live longer, healthier lives, it does not surprise you. It confirms the internal wisdom.

If another study says that pessimists live longer, healthier lives, you don't throw out your previous belief and live in doubt till you see a third, definitive study. You hold the second study suspect.

Why? You have had experience with optimism and pessimism, and your whole person has drawn a conclusion from that study over a lifetime. In the personal experiment, you can't be objective. You are not allowed to be objective. Too much subjective programming has been done. So what if the science proves that a pessimistic way of life is better? Do you try to change yourself from an optimist to a pessimist? Do you establish a self-help group for recovering optimists?

And suppose you are a pessimist and the science says that optimists live healthier, longer lives. Do you try to change? Not if you really believe that it is better to be a pessimist. Not till some personal precipitating factor drives you in that direction.

In the realm of the spirit, we tend to look for confirmation of what we already believe.

I was trained in research methods and believe in science. But in matters of the spirit, I think that philosophy matters more than science. You see, from the time we enter the world, we have been conducting our personal experiments and drawing conclusions about spiritual things.

If optimism and pessimism were two new drugs, you would have to approach the evaluation purely on a scientific basis. You would believe what the first study shows till the second study comes out, then believe what the second study says, or throw out both till the definitive study comes out. Or you examine the details of the two studies and find the flaws in the design. How many of us have the time, energy or expertise to do that?

The following discussion focuses on the philosophy of spirit rather than the science of spiritual effects on health.

Purposefulness is the state of not just having a purpose, but knowing what that purpose is and actively seeking to fulfill that purpose. Purposelessness is the lack of a purpose, and being directionless and dispirited as a result.

Meaningfulness is the state of knowing, feeling and acknowledging with conviction that life is worthwhile and the individual has special value and worth. Meaninglessness is the feeling and conviction that life is not worthwhile and the individual doesn't count for much, if anything at all. This leads to lack of desire to go on to meet life's challenges and to looking for a way out. This is one of the conditions that bring on suicidal thoughts.

Hopefulness is the active state of looking ahead for better things, dreaming realistic dreams and seeking out the best and highest possibilities in life. Hopelessness is lack of conviction about the great good that is possible in the next moment, the next day, the next week, or month, or year or for eternity. This leads to despair.

Faithfulness means not only to put trust and belief in future outcomes, but also to maintain trust and integrity in the principles you claim to live by. Faithlessness is lack of conviction that what you hope for will happen. It is also loss of trust and integrity. Faith is both conviction of the reality of things to come and maintenance of firm adherence to core principles.

Joyfulness is the expression of pleasure and heartfelt goodness. A sense of humor and the ability to laugh with soul-racking mirth is part of this quality of the spirit. Joylessness is absence of the capacity to experience pleasure and sense the goodness of life. Severe clinical depression is one cause of joylessness.

Peacefulness is the quality of serenity of soul that settles the questions of security and belonging and contentment — calm, quiet surrender to the anchor of the soul, inner peace. Peacelessness is being devoid of the assurance of rest and contentment for the here and now and for whatever is to come — the state of being haunted by insecurities with no anchor to bring rest to the soul.

Lovingness is the attribute, the capacity, that is the umbrella for a lot of positive qualities. To have love is to be caring and compassionate and patient and kind and tolerant and humble and loyal and not boastful, not jealous, not envious or devaluing of other human beings. Lovelessness is the inability to love, the lack of love, and therefore the lack of the positive qualities under the love umbrella.

Love has to be programmed into the mind and cultivated with hope and faith. The key factor in setting the capacity to love may be the quality of parenting in early life.

There are many operational words that express the impact of the above seven pairs of positive and negative states on the personality and character. Here are some examples.

*Hopefulness is the active state of looking ahead for better things, dreaming realistic dreams and seeking out the best and highest possibilities in life.*

*Love has to be programmed into the mind and cultivated with hope and faith.*

## Drive

A person's drive or degree of motivation has to be related to a sense of purpose and meaning. This is also called passion — the excitement and enthusiasm (or lack thereof) with which we approach a task or life as a whole. Passion is drive enough to lend the right amount of spiritual energy to a task, to be contagious enough to energize others as needed to get the best job done — whether the job at hand is a specific task or the job of everyday living.

Overdrive and overhype can be destructive to true passion. True passion is deeper than knowledge and intellectual decision, but it needs these too. True passion is the drive and determination to go on against all odds, to dig deep down to find one more gut-wrenching surge of energy for another try.

*Faith is the foundation of dreams. But faith is not delusional.*

Regardless of the desire, the passion or the drive, the human spirit has limits. A part of passion is to know when you have tried your best, with pride for the effort and comfort in having tried.

## Optimism

A positive outlook is more productive than a negative outlook. This has to do with belief, expectations and what Albert Bandura calls "self-efficacy." The basis for these dynamics is hope. "Hope springs eternal" only in those who have a basis in their beliefs for hopefulness.

Hopelessness is debilitating and destructive. Ungrounded and unfounded hope is delusional. The basis of the personal hope is the key to this dynamic.

## Security

The human mind is beset with fears about the future because it cannot know exactly what is to be. We can speculate, project, infer from the past and "vision" the future, but we ordinarily cannot know definitively. This leads to varying degrees of insecurity, uncertainty, apprehension and fear.

Faith is the degree of confidence and belief that things will work out. Faith may look to power beyond the known or the obvious. Faith acts with this combination of personal and "other" sources of power and moves into the future with confidence, security, certainty and hope for the most optimistic outcomes.

Faith works by planning, projecting and giving the benefit of doubts to hope for the best. Faith is the foundation of dreams. But faith is not delusional. It is not unrealistic fantasizing.

Faith to one person may involve belief in karma; to another, belief in fate and chance. And yet to another, belief in a personal, self-existing God. Can our science differentiate? Why not? Why would we want to differentiate?

## Joy and Happiness

A few weeks ago, I heard a presentation on happiness and joy. Happiness was defined as the surges of pleasant feelings and thrills we experience when things are good. Happiness was thought of as a transient feeling. The speaker's main point was that since happiness is not mentioned in the Christian Bible, it is not as valued an experience as joy.

Joy, on the other hand, was described as the better state of emotions, since joy is mentioned hundreds of times in the Bible.

This was excellent food for thought because happiness was the topic to be discussed in the next lecture I was giving in my class at Andrews Air Force Base.

Sometimes we get caught up in definitions. Are joy and happiness the same thing? I have discussed and read about happiness over the last fifteen years, and the distinction that I have come to accept is that joy consists of the surges and peaks of happiness, while happiness is the core state of positive feelings — the foundation of joy.

By this definition, a person is either basically happy or unhappy. The summation of life, which the brain makes moment to moment, is a conclusion about happiness or unhappiness. Within both states, there are upward surges of joy and downward surges of sorrow. In a basically happy person, the sorrow is appropriate for the event but most often short-lived. The return to happiness is fairly quick.

Surges of joy are peaks of happiness. The return to a basic state of happiness varies with the intensity of the peak. The basic state of happiness is deepened after coming down from the peak.

In a basically unhappy person, surges of joy are often short-lived. The return to unhappiness is fairly quick. Sorrow is indulged and overemphasized. The return from the depths of sorrow is slow. A dip into sorrow deepens the unhappiness.

Joy and happiness are accompanied by laughter. A sense of humor — good, clean humor — adds to the expression of joy. Great humor is reflexive and involves no devaluation of others, their beliefs or practices.

## Peace

Inner certainty, personal harmony and deep contentment — this is personal peace. It seems to be rare. There is so much to be concerned about, so much to be responsible for, so much that you cannot put your trust in and so much that is variable about human relationships. Yet the soul desires "settledness" — peace, tranquillity, quietude, spiritual rest.

Human history is replete with wars and discord and anger. Inner peace is the only antidote. How do we find this inner peace? Again, the personal belief system, the anchor to the soul, and the connectedness to others and to higher powers seem to be the sources of peace for the human spirit.

## Love and Caring

The capacity to feel value and impart value is the basis of love and caring. Physiologic love is romantic love based in hormonal and brain mechanisms. The mental component of love has to do with decisions, and vows and promises. Psychosocial love has to do with the value of self and other persons in intimate to distant relationships. Spiritual love is the deepest, most heartfelt, most soul-connecting love which enhances the other capacities. It is not so much a surge of emotions as a settled philosophy. It is the core belief and anchor to the soul.

When this love based in the spirit reaches beyond self and others to higher "other worldly" beings according to the personal belief system, it plumbs the depths of the capacity to love. This spiritual level of love then

*...happiness is the core state of positive feelings — the foundation of joy.*

flows down to the other dimensions and makes caring, empathy, kindness, patience, long-suffering, meekness, gentleness, faith, hope, tenderheartedness, respect, tolerance, humility, compassion, graciousness, joy, and any other endearing and positive-value-imparting capacity more effective and real.

*Hate is the opposite of love. It is action counter to what love engenders. It is not just the absence of love.*

Hate is the opposite of love. It is action counter to what love engenders. It is not just the absence of love. It is more than lovelessness. It is a destructive force in the human spirit. It is the source of violence and crime and wars and discord. It consumes self and others in bitterness, bigotry, rage and anger. It destroys caring, empathy, kindness, patience, long-suffering, meekness, gentleness, faith, hope, tenderheartedness, respect, tolerance, humility, compassion, graciousness, joy, and any other endearing and positive-value-imparting capacity in human nature.

So, of all the dynamics of the human spirit, love is the greatest, the most positive force, and hate is the most destructive. The highest accomplishment in life is to truly love. The worst fate in life is to be fully consumed and controlled by hate.

One of the best definitions of love that I remember hearing from one of my favorite speakers was that love includes all the other attributes such as caring, compassion, patience, gentleness, etc. The illustration of compassion is what stuck with me. He said that the Hebrew word for compassion paints the image of the relationship between the fetus and the womb. The womb protects, nurtures and provides warmth and life to the developing fetus. This is a powerful analogy for the call to live the compassionate dimension of love in our dealings with one another.

Spiritual homeostasis is the maintenance of balance — not to keep things evenly distributed between the good and the bad, but to actively promote the good and purposefully eradicate the bad. The ceiling for good qualities is limitless. That is the human spirit with its anchor in a grounded belief system.

The other part of spiritual homeostasis has to do with the balance between the human spirit and the higher power. What is the nature of the higher power in which you believe? How does this higher power interact and communicate with the human mind? If your higher power is a sinless being, can that being become part of, enter into or inhabit the mind of a sinful being? Is there a type of energy that passes from the higher power to humans? Is the higher power a rational being, or an undefined cosmic force or the great evolutionary force of chance and random events?

Spiritual balance calls for some degree of resolution to these questions.

## Spiritual Nutrition

What are the ingredients that nurture the human spirit? What inputs shape and provides fuel for the growth of the spirit? There seem to be four sources of nourishment for the spirit.

The first level is principles and values passed on by teaching and instruction. This occurs in the home, the school, the church and the society.

The second level is the example left in the history of highly spiritual persons — individuals who exhibited courage, heroism, altruism, sacrifice and drive to go on against all discouragement — people who were of deep convictions, integrity, honesty and trustworthiness.

Stories of people like Albert Schweitzer, Mahatma Gandhi and Martin Luther King, Jr., who modeled love and helped to extinguish hate; people who built faith and cast out doubt; people who strengthened hope and chased away disappointment and despair; people who lived tolerance and broke down bigotry; people who found deep fulfillment and satisfaction in life. We assassinated several of them before their full contribution to the world was completed. These true stories need to be told and retold for inspiration to each new generation.

A third level of nurturance of the spirit is to actually know and associate with individuals described in the paragraph above. To walk with, visit with and converse with; to share their wisdom and humor; to be befriended by positive, upright and saintly persons — this is a special richness in life. This is food of a higher order — food from a higher table, meta-nutrition.

The fourth level of nourishment for the spirit is the wisdom obtained with personal experiments with the great truths of life — experiments with faith, hope and trust; experiments that resolve questions that are resolvable and settle the unsettled ones. This is the pathway of finding one's own truth within the belief system upon which the soul is anchored. Within this level of nourishment, many people find a belief in a personal, self-existing God to be a powerful force for growth.

# Spiritual Stress and Stress Adaptation

The physiology of the body responds to the dynamics of the spirit in the same way it responds to other inputs on mind function. Positive stresses raise heart rate, nervous system drive and hormone levels. However, it seems that the positive events have some accompanying "happy hormones" that strengthen the physiology against excess wear and tear. Joy and faith and prayer seem to promote health and healing.

Hopelessness, helplessness, purposelessness, meaninglessness and lack of inner peace seem to promote illness and disease. The wear and tear on the body is accelerated.

Stress management and stress resistance are strengthened by consciously seeking to cultivate the positive qualities of the spirit and consciously seeking to eradicate or counter the negative qualities. How is this accomplished? The answer offered by Hans Selye is to "Do good and kind things for others when you don't have to, especially to those who cannot in any way repay you."

*"Do good and kind things for others when you don't have to, especially to those who cannot in any way repay you."*

## Spiritual Work

Does the spirit exert or expend energy to perform work? I believe that a good case can be made for this. The energy may not be measurable in the ATPs or glucose metabolism of the brain, but force is exerted and things are accomplished. Some day we may be able to measure this energy.

Think of some well-worn phrases: the "search for meaning," the "pursuit of excellence," the "cultivation of beauty," the "holding on to truth though the heavens fall" and going for it "against all odds." These take spiritual work, drive and exercise of faith, hope and love. The energy may be reflected in the other dimensions of function. But the source of the drive is the spirit.

*...liberation from the shackles of narrow and neurotic beliefs, liberation from exclusivist and bigoted viewpoints, liberation from guilt and fear and anxieties.*

## Spiritual Rest

Spiritual rest is personal peace and inner security. When everything around you may be crumbling, when loss and tragedy (accidental or through miscalculation) are present in your life, can you have peace and security? This is possible. This is the rest the human spirit needs. This is what the human spirit is capable of finding.

Spiritual rest is also personal liberation and freedom — liberation from the shackles of narrow and neurotic beliefs, liberation from exclusivist and bigoted viewpoints, liberation from guilt and fear and anxieties. Liberation from tyranny and repression. This is the rest the human spirit needs. This is what the human spirit is capable of finding.

Spiritual rest is resolution of the larger questions of life — settledness in the core beliefs about origin, purpose, the right way to be, responsibility for others, final destiny. This is the rest the human spirit needs. This is what the human spirit is capable of finding.

If religion is the pathway to this rest, then practice that religion with all your heart, soul and body. The evidence of this rest will be in the way you value and treat other people, and yourself.

## Spiritual Growth

The stages of spiritual growth may be analogous to the stages of physical development — infancy, childhood, youth, adulthood and age. In infancy, the spirit is provided all its needs, cared for and made to feel secure by others.

In childhood and youth, the spirit is being weaned from dependence to independence. The adult stage is spiritual maturity. The spiritually aged is the highest level of growth — this is when the qualities of the spirit are most fully expressed. The wisdom of the spiritually aged is the fullest, most profound of all because it comes out of the crucible of practical experiments with life.

The stages of spiritual growth may not correspond with physical growth. Some physical adults may be spiritual infants. Some physical children may be spiritual adults. Because time is one of the greatest factors in producing the spiritually aged, this has the best correspondence with physical development. Holding our elderly in high regard for their spiritual qualities helps to impart greater value on them, their contribution and their wisdom. Their value transcends their loss of physical abilities and any physical dependence.

Societies past and present display their priorities and standards in the way infants and the elderly are treated. A spiritual viewpoint may help to enhance and uplift societies' programs and motives with regard to children and the elderly. The recent emphasis on quality of life factors, and the fight against dehumanization are attempts to move in a more spiritual direction.

Spiritual growth is dependent on the spiritual nutrition, spiritual work and spiritual rest factors discussed above.

## Spiritual Reproduction

The ultimate in self-perpetuation, the highest level of leaving the essence of your person in other people is in the spirit you engender in other people. How much of your drive, and optimism, and caring, and happiness, and peace, and security, and love, faith, hope, compassion, kindness, gentleness, tolerance, gratefulness, altruism, patience and joy is left as a part of someone else?

Reproducing these qualities — helping others to cultivate these qualities — is a byproduct of genuine friendships and honest relationships, not a matter of preaching or counseling or prescribing — just a matter of living the spiritual life.

The second level of spiritual reproduction is settling the question of immortality. What happens to the spirit when the body dies? Is there life beyond this life? Does a part of what comprises our humanity survive death and live on forever? Ultimate reproduction is to be part of the universe for all future time. How does your belief system answer this question?

As molecules composing the physical body, you remain part of the universe. Is there another level of immortality? Reincarnation? Becoming like angels? Becoming a god? Becoming a perfect, incorruptible human not subject to illness and disease? What do you believe?

## The Major Spiritual Health Problems

The major spiritual health problems are related to negative states having to do with the absence or the corruption of love, faith and hope. These negative states are the basis for anxieties, fears, doubts, intolerance, lack of empathy, hatred, anger, low value of life and unconcern for others.

Low capacity to love, or unclear programming of what love is and how to love, may be the root cause of all the others. Some experts tell us that we function by internal scripts that get written in the brain as we grow. If the script for love is poorly written (because of poor spiritual nutrition and retarded spiritual growth), our capacity to show love and to receive love is diminished.

This diminished capacity expresses itself in self-seeking, self-absorption and

*If the script for love is poorly written, our capacity to show love and to receive love is diminished.*

unconcern for the suffering of others. The more destructive form of this condition is self-hate and hatred for others which leads to aggression, and hurt, and war, and killing and precipitation of untold human suffering. Our history is replete with hurt perpetrated on others by those who didn't know how to love.

The great paradox is when the suffering is inflicted either in the name of a loving God, or as a means to "improve" the human condition.

The lack of hope and faith leaves the human spirit weak and insecure. Doubts and anxieties reduce productivity and output of the whole person. When hopelessness, meaninglessness, purposelessness and faithlessness dominate the human spirit, is life worth living? This is a point of giving up, wanting out — out of a relationship, out of life itself.

By this time, some astute reader is asking for the statistics. Where is the scientific evidence? Where is the data? The data is within us. This is the part of our function that is not so subject to science. However, more data gathering is being done. Observations on the lives of people who have really touched other lives for good demonstrate the power of love, faith and hope. Compare the lives of people who have been the most destructive to the lives of others who have given their all to building up humanity. Compare Hitler and Mother Theresa.

The scientific test-tube for the spirit is the crucible of the individual experience. Organized observations will support the obvious truths so clearly demonstrated in the lives of others. We have enough examples to draw from in our past and in our present. We have our own experience.

The positive effect of spirituality is to inspire self and others to live the best life possible here and to settle the question of what's next. Inspiration is the mind function that provides spiritual fuel to life. It may be the capacity to transcend our known limitations, reach out to higher powers, communicate with other forces in the cosmos, dream the impossible dream. What the exact force or higher being is differs with the personal belief. What the impossible dream is, is for you to know, to define and to go after — to bring it into reality.

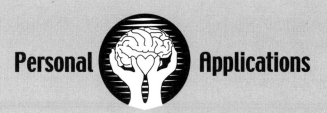

# Personal Applications

## Directions:

Complete the self-examination exercise in section A. Look at the other sections for items that may interest you at this time in your life. Select a few of the writing exercises and see what the mind creates.

**A. Self-Examination IV — The Spiritual Dimension**

Check the most appropriate answer. Note that for each item your answer will be somewhere on the line between "T" for mostly true or "F" for mostly false. If you don't know the answer, check the "Don't Know" box. Check the "Don't Care" box if you believe that an item is not important to your personal health. Give the answers that you honestly think apply — not what you would like to be true..

# Spiritual Health Factors

| | True or False | Don't Know | Don't Care |
|---|---|---|---|
| 1. I feel a deep sense of harmony and fulfillment. | T———F | | |
| 2. I always look for good to come out of every bad. | T———F | | |
| 3. I have a definite core of positive values. | T———F | | |
| 4. I am generally optimistic about life and myself. | T———F | | |
| 5. I experience positive emotions such as joy and hope. | T———F | | |
| 6. I experience negative emotions such as anger. | T———F | | |
| 7. I experience more positive than negative emotions. | T———F | | |
| 8. I know what my important, core beliefs are. | T———F | | |
| 9. I have a strong sense of meaning and purpose. | T———F | | |
| 10. I find joy in beauty, truth and freedom. | T———F | | |
| 11. I feel that there is always hope for a better future. | T———F | | |
| 12. I know that I experience spiritual growth. | T———F | | |
| 13. I feel connected to powers higher than me. | T———F | | |
| 14. I have a sense of inner peace and security. | T———F | | |
| 15. I admire people who help others without reward. | T———F | | |
| 16. I can cry when it is appropriate for me. | T———F | | |
| 17. I have no great or abnormal fear of death. | T———F | | |
| 18. I accept life's uncertainties. | T———F | | |
| 19. I have strong patriotic feelings. | T———F | | |
| 20. I feel I am living the best life possible. | T———F | | |
| 21. I know the pain of loss and the joy of recovery. | T———F | | |
| 22. I appreciate music, poetry and meditation. | T———F | | |
| 23. I strive to make realistic dreams come true. | T———F | | |
| 24. I generally fight on against all discouragement. | T———F | | |
| 25. My spiritual pleasures outweigh my pain. | T———F | | |

B. Write short definitions/descriptions for the following:

1. My purpose in life

2. The most beautiful scenery I have encountered thus far in life

3. Things I want to be liberated from

4. Inhibitions I have overcome

5. People whose lives I have touched for good

6. Feeling "sinful," feeling "righteous"

7. Basis of my people preferences

8. How and why I talk to God

9. My life after this life

10. Love, faith and hope

11. My core beliefs and values

12. The effects of religion on my life

C. Write an essay describing the perfect life in a perfect world (conditions, responsibilities, relationships, work, leisure, emotions, mental and physical abilities).

D. Over the next few days, try this experiment:

1. Ask three people you know well, "What do you think of all this talk about spiritual health and wellness?"

2. Ask the same question to three total strangers.

3. Summarize the reactions, the ideas and the overall experience in a short essay.

E. If you were to die tomorrow:

1. What important things will you leave unfinished?

2. What would be your greatest regret?

3. What would you point to as the greatest accomplishment of your life?

4. Whom will you feel sorry for the most?

5. Who will take your departure the hardest?

6. Whom will it be most difficult for you to leave?

7. What do you think is "on the other side" of this life?

F. Describe the most beautiful person you know.

G. Write an essay titled: "My Pursuit of Happiness."

# Reflections

There is more being written and researched every day about the human spirit. I think that data gathering is helpful. I think that research is fine. But the scientific method has its limitations. The spirit is the part of us where we have the most freedom for personal experiment and personal answers.

You examine your belief system, seek experiences that build up the positive emotions within your make-up and seek experiences that control or suppress the negative ones. The test of the outcome is how you affect the lives of the other people with whom you have contact and how it makes you feel about yourself.

Take a belief — any belief — a belief about how things ought to be, what we ought to do, how we ought to live, what is right, what is wrong, what is proper, what is improper. What does that belief lead you to do? What actions does it require or precipitate? What are the effects on others? What are the effects on you?

The effects on yourself or on others may be constructive or destructive. How do you evaluate the action? The feeling alone is not the full evaluation. The effect must be taken into account.

At the height of his power, Hitler must have felt very successful, fulfilled and powerful as a leader of a great nation. Evaluated only by feelings and effects on self, he was probably right. What were the effects on people's lives? That is the other half of the equation for fulfillment and satisfaction with life.

*At the height of his power, Hitler must have felt very successful, fulfilled and powerful as a leader of a great nation.*

Larry Chapman wrote one of the most thought-provoking journal articles on spiritual health that I came across early in this exploration. The title was "Developing a Useful Perspective on Spiritual Health: Well-Being, Spiritual Potential and the Search for Meaning" (*American Journal of Health Promotion*, Winter 1987, pp. 31-39). It contains very helpful definitions, an assessment questionnaire and several deeply probing questions.

For the purposes of this book, I avoid questionnaires that score, categorize or label. My aim is to stimulate general introspection and to lead to action.

The area of life where I see the need for the greatest application of spiritual wellness is how we, as members of the human family, treat one another. Consider four bases for discrimination and devaluation of people: race, religion, gender and size.

Race and ethnicity come down, primarily, to physical differences: color of skin, shape of features, texture of hair. Behavior seems to be secondary.

Why is it that darker skin pigmentation, higher melanin content, has been associated with less value in most parts of the world?

When I was in the Philippines in 1991, one of the leading articles in the papers was about mercury poisoning from a compound people rubbed on their skin to make it of a lighter color. How do people separate value from color?

Religious differences are based on teachings, rituals and traditions, the entity worshipped and the form of worship. Why do people who believe in higher beings who are mostly protective, kind and helpful to humans hurt and kill one another in the name of religion?

The causes are deeply rooted in beliefs about who is right and who is wrong, and about whose ancestors wronged whom in the past. Valuations and feelings run deep. The call for justice, revenge and retribution — human directed or ordained by higher beings — leads the emotions to involve generation after generation. Sometimes, after the other reasons are blurred, it comes down to possession of property.

Gender differences are based on reproductive physiology. The female of the species has borne the brunt of lower value, harder tasks and less reward. As if that is not enough, abuse and punishment have been much of our past history.

Size prejudice is based on physique — short/tall, fat/skinny. Larger persons many times have been treated as if they are morally weaker, less desirable and of less consequence in the scheme of things. People of smaller stature have been socially stigmatized and less valued than taller people. Why these valuations?

It would take a whole book to review and analyze the history, implications and current state of affairs of how we treat one another in these aspects of differences. The important point here is the personal applications.

How do I feel towards other people of different race, religion, gender and size? Many factors enter into these feelings of valuation — background, experiences, exposure and belief. Do I feel superior, inferior or equal to others? Do I treat others as superior, inferior or equal based on race, religion, gender and size?

Some of the reasons we contrive to justify our positions on some of these matters are ridiculous when looked at objectively. For example, a church organization was caught up in the debate of whether to ordain women to its clergy. One argument by a group of men was that women shouldn't be ordained because they may have to participate in the service of the sacraments at the time of the monthly menstrual flow. This, in some way, made them unclean or increased the possibility of their contaminating the emblems. Yet men have been seen going to the bathroom before participating in the same service!

If hand washing can be effective after defecation, what is the concern about contamination from taking care of other physiologic needs? If bacterial contamination is the concern, the greater possibility is from the function common to both men and women.

The mind-set is deeper than just hygiene and physiology. It goes back to teachings about the state of being "unclean" as classified by old ritual laws. It has taken thousands of years to progress beyond these ceremonial proscriptions and the lower value they placed on women.

The above argument is understandable, but not defensible, when you consider that some people with the above beliefs also hold that many cases of Down's syndrome result because the children are conceived on a holy day during which intercourse is wrong, if not outright sinful.

Coming back to interracial marriages, what is the basis of the valuations made and the advice given? If the advice is to avoid another difficulty in life because of how other people treat partners or children of an interracial marriage, it is good advice. In many interracial marriages, the social pressure is one additional feature to take into account.

Marriage of itself is an endeavor that requires major effort. Therefore, in the decision-making it is good to assess the additional stress, and see whether the love relationship may endure or succumb to that.

If the advice is to choose the easiest path, the couple may intellectually decide for that choice. The strength of the emotional attachment may not be so easily directed by reason. Hope, faith, belief and optimism or "blind love" may override. In this case, some expectations and preparations for discriminatory treatment would help in dealing with other people.

However, the major effect and the consequences of other people's attitudes are determined by how you let them affect you and your relationships.

Among all the racial combinations I have observed, those involving the black race seem to have had more prejudices directed at them than any other pairing. It does seem that the bigoted structure of valuation puts blacks at the bottom of the stratification — and the blacker, the lower the classification. I have observed children of such marriages who have had little or no problems feeling good about themselves, and others who have been psychologically impaired.

The important difference seems to be the reaction of the parents and caregivers to the differences in the child and the value the parents and caregiver impart to the child.

How we value other human beings is a part of our spiritual nature, and change or growth in acceptance of others involves spiritual insight, spiritual nurture and spiritual growth. I believe that value and acceptance of other human beings also involve knowledge, decision-making and psychological factors. But the spiritual factors may be of the greatest importance. Solutions may lie chiefly in our spiritual dimension.

Some final reflections are on the effects of one's core beliefs. Instead of trying to philosophize, let me illustrate what I mean with examples from the life that I know best. I share these thoughts knowing that they are very personal, may leave me open to ridicule, and with the advice that before you share similar private aspects of your life, you consider how it may make you feel, how it may make others feel and what is the purpose to be served. My purpose justifies this sharing.

I do not encourage others to be as free with their private lives unless they have given some careful thought to it. I have given considerable thought to this over the years, and feel it is the right thing to do, in the right place, at the right time. I am comfortable with the risks.

I share these thoughts, not as an example of what people ought to think or believe, but as an honest, real-life example of how growth in wellness leads to answering questions about life that involve clarification of core beliefs. This, I think, is the crux of spiritual wellness. It is growth that has no limits. It is the process of becoming more authentic and living with personal confidence in your purpose in life.

Here goes — my essay is "Seven Core Beliefs Examined and Evaluated."

1. **I used to believe that my purpose in life was to help convert everyone I met to my brand of Christianity.**

I now believe that I do not have the responsibility to convert or actively proselytize anyone to anything. I have the responsibility to live the best life possible, to ask questions and share what answers I have, to make no apologies for what I believe and to be unafraid about the hereafter.

**Background and Insight**

At eleven years of age, my purpose in life was clear. I wanted to become an evangelist to help convert the rest of the world to my brand of Christianity, so that the end of the world could happen in no more than five years from that day.

That was in 1957. As I walked out of the baptismal pool, I felt perfect and clean and holy and good. I was ready for heaven.

My parents, teachers, all the adults in my world had told me that "Jesus is coming in five years, no more. You have to be perfectly good. Anything you do wrong will be recorded in a book in heaven. If you are bad, your time of burning in hell would last longer, the more bad things written in the book." I totally and completely believed that was the way existence on earth was programmed.

The teenage years came on and the doubts and mistakes and transgressions mounted up. At seventeen, I again experienced another "conversion." Now I had the original purpose with the additional charge to tell people everywhere what they were doing wrong. The belief was, "What I am doing wrong, what every other Christian is doing wrong, is delaying the coming of Christ and extending the reign of sin." I again promised God to work harder and be good and more perfect.

I struggled valiantly to be perfect, always worried that I'd make a mistake, always feeling less than perfect, if not downright sinful. It was much later that I understood the human condition of imperfection and the fruitlessness of struggling to perform right acts. So I gave up the struggle. Goodness and rightness must be affirmed in context of the personal belief system and not left to be judged by an occasional misdeed or good deed.

I now believe that I don't have to be any one thing. I should find work that is interesting, challenging and provides an income matched with my qualifications and the lifestyle I realistically desire, with regard for maintaining health of body and mind for as long as possible.

My goal to be an evangelist was not just to hold a clergyman's job with the church. I came to that conclusion, not as a career aspiration, but as a contract with heaven — as a destiny, a holy appointment.

Entering college at twenty-one, my purpose in life was unclear. I had become disillusioned with the certainty and prediction of specific events, had no personal goal for earning, standard of living or desirable lifestyle. I was trying to fulfill other people's goals for me.

In fact, I felt that by maintaining an attitude of lack of concern for material things like housing and good clothes and higher standard of living, I was somehow earning points on someone's scale of value for self-denial.

I tried unsuccessfully to get into medical school to fulfill the goals of my parents to have a doctor in the family. Looking back on the effort, I can see a lack of drive and passion. It was not a heartfelt desire. My parents had the right to wish that at least one of their ten children should be in the highest regarded profession they knew. But it was not in my make-up.

It took a long time to arrive at goals for lifestyle and comfort and leisure and security. I can now share my insights of not having a clear purpose in life with others who may or may not benefit from any of it.

Everyone has his or her own time frame. In retrospect, I think that my indecision about lifestyle and career meant I made choices by default. It led to a lack of inspiration in pursuit of goals. Pursuit of higher education was a path of drudgery and self-flagellation to get things done because it had to be done to get to the next level.

It could have been caused by a combination of physiologic tendencies to neurotic behavior, overregulation under religious rules, extreme self-consciousness and a sensitive spirit. Things that move me emotionally call forth more drive and direction than things that are purely intellectual decisions. I should have been in a combination of philosophy, counseling and writing, rather than in a hard-core science field.

Now, in the field of wellness, associated with people highly motivated to help bring about the changes and transitions for people to pursue personal wellness, I feel comfortable and fulfilled. Every part of my background contributes to what I now do — the research, the writing and the facilitation of group workshops.

Working through this belief adjustment, I feel I was afflicted by the "Jonah Syndrome." In fact, if I were to believe in reincarnation, I would be the reincarnation of Jonah — the Jonah who spent three days in the belly of a whale! Such was the intensity of the early belief.

2. **I used to believe that God had a detailed, specific blueprint for my life, and my duty was to find that blueprint and follow it to the letter. This included whom I should marry, what I should do for a living and how I should spend my time and effort. As part of this plan, God had an angel assigned to be with me all the time, recording every thought, deed and — especially — frivolous conversation.**

I now believe that God and I are partners in finding an enjoyable way of living this life. I should make the decisions according to the best information I have, with the summation of instincts and emotions that are part of my individual make-up, hold conversations with God about these things and move ahead with the tasks at hand — with no intention to hurt others, and with motives to bring about good for self and others.

This freedom to take risks and make mistakes will be compensated for by some help and direction God gives through inspired insights and through other people. If things happen that seem difficult to understand, I'll get all the answers to life's questions when I will walk and talk with God in a different life.

## Background and Insight

From early childhood, I had a definite idea of how a relationship with God worked. Every thought, word and action was constantly being evaluated and judged as sin and not sin. My task was to do everything not sin, and keep strict regulation and control of my behavior so that I committed no sin.

Sin included making decisions that turned out to be not the best decision. The thought was, "If I really find out the will of God, I will make only the decisions He wants me to make, and things will always turn out right."

I saw things happen in my life that conscious planning, expert decision-making and foresight cannot explain — both good things and bad things.

Life is like that. The question of how we interact with the higher being we believe in is one of the anchors of life. This core belief, for any believer in any religion, generates the following questions:

1. Does the higher being (God) lead your life?
2. How is God's will for your life revealed?
3. How do you know this will?
4. How do you know when you are following or not following this will?
5. What are the consequences of not following this will?
6. How does God control human lives?

These are good questions for personal reflection for anyone — Buddhist, Christian, Confucianist, Hindu, Jew, Muslim or non-religionist. The human spirit has common, universal needs met in many different ways. Is there one final common path? Is there one final common goal? Is there one final common answer? Each one settles these questions through a personal quest.

3. **I used to believe that people were good or bad, more valuable or less valuable, according to their behavior and their physical attributes. For example, people who smoke were on a lower scale of value than those who don't. People who were unattractive were of less value to society than those who were beautiful. People with dark skin and coarse hair were of a lower social order than those with fair skin and straight hair.**

I now believe that the value of people is not tied to health or other behavior, to skin color or to hair texture. My children helped to reshape my beliefs and attitudes.

## Background and Insight

My daughter was in a predominantly black high school. As she got to be fifteen, sixteen, I wanted her to switch to a predominantly white high school so that she would have social exposure to predominantly white and Indian males. The hypocrisy of the situation was that I was a member of the board at the school she was attending. I felt it was my right to act according to my beliefs.

My daughter and her brothers helped to reshape my thinking over several months of questions and answers. Considering I had

*The human spirit has common, universal needs met in many different ways.*

fought against such attitudes before when they were directed at me, it left me to wonder about how difficult it is to adjust beliefs and attitudes.

I believe that was my deepest vestige of negative valuation of others based on physical differences. I now understand my people preferences and continue the spiritual work of purifying any residual effects of my life experience in dealing with differences.

4. **I used to believe that my church was the ultimate religious power on earth, and every other religion, sect, denomination or belief system was inferior.**

I now believe that my church is one among many agencies on earth for carrying out specific portions of God's interaction with human beings. Other entities have their specific roles in a cosmic plan for this world order.

### Background and Insight

This belief led to treating people of other belief systems as of lesser value and importance, and some as intrinsically evil. Catholics were particularly regarded as evil because of what I had learned about the inquisition and burning people at the stake because of their beliefs. The Pope was the anti-Christ and would play a major role in organizing a series of events in which a certain class of believers would be slated for extinction.

The US government would have an equal role in the conspiracy with the Vatican to destroy a large number of people around the world because of their different beliefs and resistance to the pressure to change those beliefs.

Wow! What a heavy load of baggage for a young adult to carry around! Getting to know people of different belief systems, and learning to understand why they believe as they do, and being willing to learn from the past has led to a reevaluation of these attitudes.

They are not the important aspects of dealing with other people. Sharing common goals of promoting good here on earth and freedom to let each other practice according to personal belief, and a readiness to give an answer to a question that may arise, these now guide my interaction instead of past or predicted conflicts.

Some of these differences among religious groups and belief systems come together in a story shared by a friend of the family.

He was at one of the busiest airports in India waiting for a connecting flight. Suddenly, the whole multitude of people fell silent and prayerful. Mother Theresa, weak and frail but walking with sure steps and unafraid, accompanied by two nuns, was passing through the terminal.

Shortly afterwards, the leader of a small Protestant denomination with bodyguards, press secretary and a translator came into the terminal. No one paid attention. Very few knew who he was.

After reading the book *Mother Theresa: The Spirit and the Work*, by Eileen Eagan, I felt convinced that only the Catholic system of beliefs and practices could produce a Mother Theresa.

5. **I used to believe that there is a life after death, and that in that life I would be productive and aware and active, and find out the answers to the greatest mysteries of the universe.**

I still believe that. However, if I throw out my beliefs in the real meaning of Christmas and Easter, I think that belief will die.

No background or insight necessary for this one. Just a plain choice to believe.

6. **I used to believe that one day of the week was so holy that I constantly worried about the sins of violating it through doing or thinking of anything that pertained to school, work, business or entertainment.**

I now believe that one day of the week is different from the others because of the rest I get from putting aside many of the activities of school, work, business or entertainment, and spending it to pay focused attention to building positive relationships with people here and beings beyond this world. There is strong, meaningful symbolism to that day.

### Background and Insight

The holiness of the day was so inviolate that if I were late getting home from work and that day began before I got home, I felt sinful. If I had thoughts or conversations about work or business or everyday affairs, I'd feel sinful. If I engaged in conversations that had any secular tones or frivolity, I was committing sin.

This, I believe, led to neurotic behaviors. I used to get angry with my kids for riding their bikes or shooting baskets with their friends during those holy hours — a holy anger, perhaps? However, I could work for pay during those hours as long as the work had something to do with caring for the sick. When I was a medical technologist, I would choose the shift to work during those holy hours because it was more convenient and was allowed.

The real question of the holiness of particular hours came to my clearest thinking on a flight out of Washington DC. It was Friday afternoon. At sunset, my holy day began. But I was boarding a flight for the West Coast. It was about ten minutes after official sunset, and I had just put down a secular magazine I was reading while the plane was waiting for clearance to take off.

But as the plane gained altitude and headed out west, there was the sun again. Suddenly, the day had changed from holy to secular for another few minutes. Should I finish the article I was reading before the holiness descended?

Did the holiness of that moment suddenly disappear to reappear again after the sun went down in my eyes for the second time that day? Holiness has to be about more than time zones and rules and regulations. How do you keep a balance without letting the pendulum of your belief swing to extremes?

7. **I used to believe in a literal seven days of creation when God brought this earth into being and went about the daily tasks of creating the various environments and life forms. This was about six to ten thousand years ago.**

I now believe in a universal act of creation that occurred hundreds of millions of years ago, and special acts of creation, which occurred in variable time frames and is even going on currently. These special creations gave rise to other worlds with beings similar to humans but without disease or death.

These beings have perfect memory, perfect health, no loss of function as they mature, perfect pleasure and perfect relationships.

### Background and Insight

In high school, we used to memorize a table of the age of the earth. The date of creation was set at 4004 BC. (I hadn't heard about the Oxford scholar who calculated that Adam was created at 9 AM, October 23, 4004 BC!) The date of the flood was 2056 BC. From that table we predicted that the end of the world as we know it would occur around 2000 AD. According to that time table, the end of the world is scheduled for next year!

After studying all the geology, geography, theories of evolution I had to; after following a lot of scholarly debates about science and religion and creation versus evolution; after seeing changes in other people's beliefs; and after contemplating Stephen Hawking's *A Brief History of Time*, I had to modify the original belief. This new belief I call "New Theory of Creation."

This theory includes a "Big Bang." But an orchestrated Big Bang hundreds of millions of years ago — so long ago that our methods of measurement of time cannot estimate the correct age.

From that eternity ago, God has been creating new worlds in many galaxies in a limitless universe, and populating them with intelligent beings who can travel about the universe and interact with one another.

Our solar system came into existence at the same time as the Big Bang. But the design was to populate one planet, earth, in the system, and have the others ready for population by the offspring from earth. Creation of the topology and atmosphere of earth occurred long after the Big Bang.

Since no one was supposed to die, reproduction would be at a slow enough pace that it would take millions of years to create life-supporting environments and populate the other planets in the solar system.

A flaw developed in the original plan. Sickness and death became part of life on earth and the plan to populate the other planets was postponed. It will one day be put back into operation, and humans from earth will be witnesses to creation of life-supporting environments on the other planets.

I can go on and on, but that would be only for my own pleasure. I'm on a roll here, and I can really get carried away. But I will stop and let you speculate on your own theory.

One of the points to consider in all this is that in some circles, I would be considered a heretic to think of or voice such a theory. It really doesn't matter. The freedom to think and theorize is individual and should not be subjected to any employer/employee, member/non-member or scientist/layperson relationship.

My New Theory of Creation is nothing when compared with my "Theory of a New Creation." I have seen people's lives suddenly changed from bad to good, from outright evil to genuine goodness promotion without therapy, self-management regimens, cognitive restructuring, or any prescribed method or formula.

What drama in wellness promotion! What examples of change of unhealthy habits and destructive behaviors. I have seen others who labor long and hard and still fight the battles of the bad habits and destructive behaviors over and over again. The Theory of a New Creation is the belief in the possibility of sudden, dramatic conversion and change in behavior.

I could review other central beliefs that affected my life — views on parenting, on how I regarded the rich, on attitude toward money or status, on holiness and sinfulness, on going to the movies (imagine going into a movie theater knowing that your angel would stay outside because you were on the devil's playground), on the process of how a guardian angel is assigned to every human being, or the sinfulness of eating pork and shellfish. But it would be boring and serve no good purpose.

The sample above is to stimulate personal thought and reflection. It is a challenge to change and keep the pendulum from swinging to the other extreme. It is pleasurable to adjust beliefs and hold on to the anchors of one's core being.

To go the distance, you have to peel back the layers of the soul.

## Carol's Turn

My thoughts on this chapter are about religion and God's guidance. Al and I grew up in the same sub-culture. This may account for some of the strengths in our relationship, given differences in racial origin and social environment.

Religion was always a burden. The rules were enforced without regard to people's feelings and value. The important thing was not to break the rules, not to make the church look bad, not to make your parents look bad.

I remember one young man who was leaving home unable to endure the constant, angry discipline he received because his behavior made his father, the church pastor, look bad in the eyes of his congregation. That was more important than the son's own value and feelings about himself.

Getting away from the strict evaluation and disapproval I felt in a church environment has been liberating. Getting away from social comparisons and intentional, and maybe unintentional put-downs has been a good feeling. Not evaluating people on whether they drank coffee or smoked or broke the Sabbath or didn't pay tithes or committed other grievous sins is a new experience.

But I miss the fellowship of my church. I miss the lift of the spirit given by music and song and formal reading of the scripture. I miss the acceptance and value I feel when friends share honest, warm greetings with friends. I miss the lofty themes of the choir anthems.

*The important thing was not to break the rules, not to make the church look bad, not to make your parents look bad.*

I miss the surge of joy when the choir director says, "You gave your best effort. You came in at the right time, the orchestra came in just when it should, it all came together as well as it could, and it was beauuuutifulll." Marianne says such things when they are appropriate. The work to get to that point is enjoyable and worth it. I must get back to the fellowship of my church. It is good for my spirit. I need it.

As I told in a previous chapter, both Al and I interpret many coincidences in life as God's leading. When he left teaching at Columbia Union College, he searched for several months before finding a job. He really did not find a job. The job found him. This is how it happened.

Our friend, Rob Abraham, took Al to meet with a cardiovascular surgeon in Washington, DC. Al was given a temporary job doing treadmill testing for cardiac patients. While at this job, the physician's assistant in the office saw his curriculum vitae. She had just gone on a job interview. She told Al, "You are the person they need for that job." This led to an eleven-year stay with the cardiac surgery practice of heart surgeons Jorge Garcia, Luis Mispireta, Paul Corso and Anjum Qazi.

When Al left that job to pursue his own business, he had one setback after another. Finally, he answered an ad for stop-smoking educators. This led to meeting Steve Kornblat who introduced him to Dr. Marc Micozzi.

The relationship with Dr. Micozzi led to getting to know Tom McMillen, CEO of Complete Wellness Centers, Inc., and former US congressman and NBA star. This led to a consulting assignment with Complete Wellness Centers, which led to a project for Celebration Health, the Walt Disney/Florida Hospital experiment at Celebration City, Florida. On this assignment, a relationship with the Koop Foundation and with Dr. Ken Hoffman of the Addictions Center at Uniformed Services University of the Health Sciences developed.

All these experiences added to the preparation for the current opportunity to be part of an education program in wellness and medical education with a worldwide vision. These relationships have led to the most fulfilling career of all. Making new friends while treasuring the old friendships has been a rich part of our lives.

Did all of this happen accidentally? Are they all coincidences? Fate? I believe in divine guidance. This gives me an outlook that accepts and understands any bad that happens along with the good. It gives me an outlook that is hopeful and optimistic about the future. We don't worry about keeping all the rules all the time. We live by some general principles, and let other people have the freedom to find their own truth.

This includes helping our children to make their choices in life according to what and how they believe — and allowing them to make their own mistakes. Now, instead of forcing the rules and our view of the right path, we give them guidelines and general principles and let them make their own choices. We may be wrong, but whatever the outcome, they are loved and valued and always welcome home. Home is where the spirit is comfortable.

To go the distance, you have to know the anchors of the soul.

*To go the distance, you have to know the anchors of the soul.*

# Examine the Environmental and Religious Factors in Your Life

*"Know yourself.*
*There are mirrors for the face,*
*but the only mirror for the*
*spirit is wise self-reflection."*

Baltasar Gracian

Nine

*Dedicated to*


**Preachers who stir our souls and to one preacher in particular, Dr. Charles Scriven, President, Columbia Union College**

*Thanks for guest lecturing in our course at University of Maryland University College, and for sermons on personal liberation.*


*and to*


**Hyveth Williams, Kendra Haloviak, James Hammond and Gary Sandman**

*Other guest lecturers who gave of their time and expertise to enhance a learning experience.*

uring the last quarter of 1995 and the first quarter of 1996, the US government was closed for business three times, for one to two weeks at a time. This came about because of budget battles between a Democratic President and a Republican controlled Congress.

Some people, who were not affected by the shutdown, felt it was a good thing to show how unimportant many government offices were. Others, who depended on government contracts or subcontracts for their livelihood, were very adversely affected. I know. I was one of them.

Apart from the personal effects on people I knew, one of the most poignant episodes of this shutdown, in my estimation, was an offer from the government of Bangladesh. One of the world's poorest countries, Bangladesh proposed to make a loan to the US government to pay the electric bills at the US embassy there!

The questions addressed in this chapter relate to how self-determined we are as individuals, how other forces outside of ourselves and out of our control affect our well-being, and whether, in our private spheres of influence, we can do anything to affect these forces and make a difference for good.

The environment in which we live affects our quality of life. Whether we have a choice or not, where we live, the political system under which we live, the system of commerce and business, the social services and civil authorities, the educational system and the religious system affect our lives and happiness. The question is, how much control can the individual have in dealing with these outside forces?

In this chapter, we can only touch on these topics briefly. This will serve to trigger personal thought and self-inquiry about the effects of these external forces.

In discussing religion, I feel it is worthwhile to present more information, since this is an area where more information can lead to greater self-understanding and to a greater understanding and acceptance of others.

## The Physical World

The Western approach to dealing with our physical environment and natural resources seems to be the Judeo-Christian injunction to "have dominion over all things." This has been applied to mean use of all natural resources for the immediate benefit and comfort of humans, regardless of the effects on the environment and other forms of life. Through scientific and technological advances, we have developed the tools to dominate and control just about everything except the weather, so far.

In each of these interactions with our environment in the past, we have done what seems to benefit humans, with less, little or no regard for other effects. Some of these interactions have adversely affected other humans. The philosophy seems to have been: "If I can make a profit, let the chips fall where they will."

It is my perception that this approach is changing, and must continue to change and will. We have become more conscious of our past errors and the future consequences of abusing our physical environment and natural resources.

There is no need to recount all the incidents and horror stories of toxic pollution of air, water and earth. A few key words would bring to mind the stories of environmental human-initiated disasters: Chernobyl, Bopal, asbestos, DDT, dioxin, chromium-6, PCB, oil spills, strip mining, acid rain, pesticides and herbicides.

We cannot escape the observation that disease and destruction have resulted from our thoughtless use of natural resources and careless disposal of waste products.

One good indicator of well-being among humans is the degree of concern and respect for other life forms in the ecological system. It is encouraging to see that in the latter part of this century, and as we begin the new century, we are making efforts to correct errors of the past and avoid mistakes in the future.

(As of June 1999, the bald eagle has been removed from the endangered species list in the US.)

This is happening because of increased awareness, increased understanding of how interrelated all life is, and how our planning can be done with foresight and long-term projection of consequences.

The great increase in knowledge and the resulting scientific and technological advances made over the past one hundred years can give us the tools and perspective to live in harmony with the life support system around us. We don't have to destroy or give up the comfort and conveniences we have gained.

Can we continue to make discoveries, invent new ways of doing things and produce more goods and services to enhance our life while maintaining balance and harmony with the environment? We have to. It is happening with the involvement of individuals, organizations and government agencies. Some sensible balance between the "doomsday alarmist" position and the "economic gains at all cost" position can be reached.

Without letting this become a matter of stress and discomfort, what can I do on the personal level to protect, preserve and enhance the environment where I live? This may be the personal wellness question to consider. Many people have considered it and are recycling. Others are making sure governments require environmental impact studies before permitting activities that change the use of land and waterways. All of us can do little things to protect, preserve and reclaim the physical life support systems we depend on so much.

## The World of Science and Technology

When America was getting ready to land men on the moon, many people's beliefs about the role of science and technology in relation to human existence and the existence of God were challenged. One argument predicting the failure of the mission was that humans were sinful and the rest of the universe was sinless. Therefore, God would not allow sinful human beings to establish a presence on the moon or any other place in the universe outside earth's sinful atmosphere.

*One good indicator of well-being among humans is the degree of concern and respect for other life forms in the ecological system.*

Space exploration has shattered that philosophy. Has the world of science and technology brought more stress and problems into our lives or has it brought more comforts and convenience? On the personal level, how do I feel about the possibility of nuclear destruction, the complexities of communication systems and the massive load of information available through so many different sources today?

I remember one of my goals in high school was to know everything. I had read somewhere that Sir Francis Bacon was proclaimed as a scholar who knew all there was to know in the era he lived. It wasn't long into my first biology course in college that I realized that it is impossible for any one person to know all there is to know. Our information load now doubles about every seven years. How can one keep up with this knowledge even in his/her own field of specialization?

Perception and beliefs can have a stressful effect when we consider the complexities of knowledge and systems developed through our science and technology. The thought of nuclear war can be frightening. But if you believe in a world view that does not include nuclear destruction as an endpoint to this world, it may be a stress escape — naive or not.

Instant news feed may bring the latest war, crime or natural disaster into our homes, but we can turn off the media or skip the news. Also, we can lobby to get broadcasters to spend less of their news time recounting the gory details of every murder and major crime, and give more time to positive, creative and life enhancing stories.

So, how do you perceive the impact of the world of science and technology on your personal life? Some people feel amazed and look forward with great anticipation to the new developments to come within the next ten years. Some people wish for the simpler times when life was less complicated and less demanding. The perception is the point of impact.

# The World of Government and Politics

Which system of government allows its people the personal freedom to pursue the development of their capabilities? Where do you find governments building walls to keep their people in? Where do you find governments with walls and regulations to keep people out because, if left unregulated, the inflow would overwhelm the resources?

So far, our history has demonstrated that a democratic form of government and a free market society seem to encourage rather than impede human growth and fulfillment. Maybe there is something else that works better. I have heard proposals that a "benevolent dictatorship" may be better than a democracy, but I do not know of such an experiment. The recent demise of communism, and the force and repression necessary to maintain dictators and self-appointed rulers, speak to the power of government of the people, by the people and for the people through openly elected leaders.

What is the role of the individual in the government and political process? Participation through the election process; speaking out against abuses and neglect;

pushing and lobbying for the rights of the poor and destitute; trying to encourage and promote fairness, compassion, morality, generosity, altruism and value of people regardless of differences; trying to discourage greed, selfishness and abuse of power; and trying to promote the well-being of the people and not just of the politicians.

The government and the people, or the people through its government, have the responsibilities to provide social services, an educational system and a justice system. How do these systems affect your life? Is college affordable anymore? What are the advantages and disadvantages of going straight from high school into college? Are you satisfied with the educational system, the jury system or the social support services for the poor? Do politicians, providers or recipients abuse these systems? How do you improve them? Is this of any personal concern?

Only 30% of citizens in the USA exercise the right to vote in national elections. Some sense of deep apathy must therefore exist. Why and how do we change this? Maybe it cannot be changed. Maybe it shouldn't be changed. It may reflect satisfaction and trust by the majority to let a minority make the decisions. How do you relate to this personally?

*Are you satisfied with the educational system, the jury system or the social support services for the poor?*

## The World of Work and Business

Most of us have to work to provide the basic things for living — food, clothes, shelter, transportation, etc. Is that all there is to work? Definitely not. We all seem to have a built-in need to have some form of feedback from our work that includes a sense of accomplishment, a sense of contribution to a larger purpose, a sense of satisfaction that we do good work or a sense of acceptance that this is the best way at the time to meet our needs.

The employer/employee, owner/ worker, supervisor/supervised, manager/managed, boss/underling relationship has been, in one way or another, the dominant model in the world of work and business. The corporate model has changed little over the years. Every few years, a new theory of management is released into the workplace to make things more efficient and more productive. TQM (Total Quality Management), CQI (Continuous Quality Improvement), BPR (Business Process Re-engineering) and Strategy Change Cycle have all had their day. Yet there is more change brewing in the corporate world.

When you consider the positives and negatives of your job, what factors seem to keep you tied to it? If you had your choice of career that would provide for all your needs, what would you do?

Many workers long for independence and self-direction in their careers. What are the risks and problems with business ownership? How can an individual start out towards business ownership? Many businesses are creating an entrepreneurial atmosphere to challenge employees to contribute to the vision and share in the returns.

Work and business, the economic system, may have given us the categories of poor, middle-class and rich. What is the mobility up and down this class structure? How do we regard each other with respect to these economic groupings? The world of work and business may be the area of greatest stress for the greatest number of people.

# The World of Religion and Philosophy

Because the majority of human beings are religious to one degree or another, and because differences in religious beliefs and practices have been involved in major acts of aggression toward one another, I believe that it is important for self-understanding and understanding of other peoples to know what the major religions believe and teach.

History has reviewed the holy wars. The Holocaust cannot be forgotten. Christian-Muslim, Jew-Muslim, Catholic-Protestant and Hindu-Muslim conflicts and aggressions with the resulting death and destruction are a part of our current world scene.

Can one basis of resolution be at the personal level where viewpoints can be turned from intolerance to tolerance? Changing people is a most difficult human endeavor. Change has to come from within and by the powers in which the individual believes. Religion claims to be a great mechanism for change. Is it? By what methods? Self-understanding and self-acceptance contribute to understanding and accepting others.

This summary of world religions is presented with no notions of changing anyone's beliefs or practices. It is presented for knowledge and review, for personal introspection.

This is a layperson's summary based on Peter Occhiogrosso's *The Joy of Sects: A Spirited Guide to the World's Religious Traditions*, John L. Esposito's *Islam: The Straight Path*, and Huston Smith's *The Religions of Man*. (This was later retitled *The World's Religions*, and an illustrated condensed version was published in 1994 as *The Illustrated World's Religions*.)

The major world religions are classified as those that have a deity that interacts with human beings, have oral traditions and sacred writings, claim to have significant historical events in their establishment and advocate some form of existence after this life. By these criteria, the religions of the world are Hinduism, Buddhism, Judaism, Christianity and Islam, in order of birth.

Huston Smith contends that Confucianism and Taosim should be included even though they are not strictly "religions." They advocate no deity central to their teachings. However, they are "such all encompassing systems of philosophies within present day societies, that they affect people's lives as religions do."

In addition to Hinduism, Buddhism, Confucianism, Taoism, Judaism, Christianity and Islam, I will briefly describe New Age Theology as a force to be encountered now and in the future. Also, the terms "eastern" and "western" as applied to religion or philosophy are defined.

"Eastern," apart from its reference to Asia and the Far East, means that there is no real meaning to human life and that the individual is not important. The greatest hope and purpose in living is to escape and unite with some universal spirit.

"Western," apart from its reference to Western Europe and the Americas, means that there is meaning to life. The hope for finding ultimate meaning depends on a deity who cares for and interacts with humans. The deity rewards the believer with perfect life after this life.

I think the following summaries are best served by a list of points and information without comment or evaluation. There is no intention to cover all the complexities and variations of religious beliefs and practices. These are bare-bones outlines for the purpose of increasing awareness and understanding of religious thought, to help us understand and accept one another as we are, and to serve as a stimulus for further reading.

# The Yogic Religions

## Hinduism

1. Hindu is the Sanskrit word for Indian. Both "Hindu" and "Indian" derive from "Sindhu," the river which is now called the Indus.
2. Hindus call their religion "Sanatana Dharma," which means the ancient and eternal religion.
3. The major Hindu scripture is the Bhagavad Gita, which means Song of God.
4. Hinduism has no founder or central historical event that marks its beginning.
5. The religion became established about 2500 BC, from a mixture of religious practices of the various peoples invading the Indus valley.
6. The oral history and sacred traditions are called the Vedas.
7. The writings, called the Upanishads, led to a more god-centered system of beliefs and three gods were established.
8. The highest godhead is Trimurti, the Trinity, consisting of three equal gods: Brahma, the creator, Vishnu, the protector, and Shiva, the destroyer.
9. The epic writings, the Bhagavad Gita, added the concept of the love of God for man, and love of man for God. Central to this epic is the story of Krishna, the God-man, the incarnation of Vishnu, the protector.
10. The Hindu's main goal is not to become a perfect human being on earth or a happy camper in heaven. The main goal is to be united with Brahman, ultimate reality. (A Hindu priest is called a Brahmin, the Hindu God, creator, is Brahma.)
11. In Brahman, there is no sense of individuality — only pure being, consciousness and bliss.
12. On the nature of humans, of which there are four general types (reflective, emotional, active and experimental):
    a. An individual, a jiva, becomes human after automatically passing through several lower forms of life in a process of upward transmigrations called samsara.
    b. As a human, further transmigration or reincarnation is no longer automatic, because self-consciousness now brings with it responsibility. The law of karma, cause and effect, now rules the destiny.
    c. In a process of personally responsible moral choices, a jiva goes through developmental stages to finally renouncing all for complete union with Atman, the hidden self or infinite center of being.

d.   To achieve complete union with Atman and thereby be united with ultimate reality, Brahman, a jiva must completely change his/her way of thinking/seeing, acquire virtues and suppress sins.

e.   One lifetime is not enough to acquire the virtues and suppress the deadly sins. Therefore, the cycle of samsara takes the soul through reincarnations according to the law of karma. Rebirth can be in the form of an animal, a man or woman of higher or lower status.

f.   Hindu society is divided into classes or castes based on the parts of the body of Brahma, the creator God. The lowest class of society is the outcasts or untouchables. Caste is hereditary, but slavery was never a part of the society.

13. An individual's full life normally passes through four stages: student (childhood to marriage); householder (marriage and career to retirement); retirement (a time for spiritual adventure, hermit life); and "sannyasin" (complete freedom from all earthly ties, life as a wandering mendicant).

14. Besides the stages of life, Hindu thought describes four aims of life (duty, material gain, pleasure — physical and sensual — and release or salvation).

15. The way to God has four paths, or yogas, to serve the four different types of humans. Yoga, a method of training leading to integration and union, is the method of actualizing humanity's fullest nature. People take different, or a combination of, paths according to their make-up. The four spiritually directed yogas (which are not exclusive) are:

a.   jnana yoga — the path of knowledge,

b.   bhakti yoga — the path of love,

c.   karma yoga — the path through work, and

d.   raja yoga — the path through psychological experiment.

16. Hinduism holds that all the major world religions are equal and alternative paths to the same God.

## Buddhism

Buddhism grew out of Hinduism through the life of Siddhartha Gautama, born around 560 BC.

The name Buddha, meaning the "enlightened one" or the "awakened one," was given to him as he traveled about teaching people how to achieve their own enlightenment.

The religion he established was based on intense self-effort. The key points are:

1.   The original quest started because of dissatisfaction with the doctrine of endless reincarnations, and the suffering and pain of life.

2.   The cycle of reincarnation could be broken if one attained the correct knowledge and the discipline to take advantage of that knowledge.

3.   The desires for pleasure, wealth, long life and happiness caused one to be reborn. The discipline required was the loss of all such earthly desires.

4.   The goal to be reached was nirvana — the end of desire — a state of freedom, inward peace and joy, where birth, age, sickness, pain and death cease to exist.

5.   The two extremes are to be avoided. Neither comforts, pleasure and passion nor deprivation, suffering and pain offered the way to enlightenment. A middle path exists, which can

lead to understanding, peace and higher wisdom.

6. The Four Noble Truths point out the middle way. The truths are:

   a. Existence contains suffering.

   b. Suffering is caused by the thirst or desire for pleasure, prosperity and continued life. This causes one to be reborn.

   c. To escape suffering and rebirth, get rid of desire.

   d. To get rid of desire, the eightfold path must be followed:

      i. right views,

      ii. right aspirations,

      iii. right speech,

      iv. right conduct or behavior,

      v. right mode of livelihood,

      vi. right effort,

      vii. right mindfulness, and

      viii. right rapture or absorption.

7. Buddha himself left no writings of his teachings.

8. Humans have no soul. Humans are free agents to choose.

9. Zen Buddhism, the Japanese form of Buddhism, means meditation that leads to insight, and is the branch of Buddhism best known to the west. It has at its center the need to transcend words and theories and dwell in experience, and to live in the here-and-now instead of the past or the future. The path of reaching the experience of nirvana (crossing life's river in the raft you have) is transmitted mind-to-mind from a teacher.

10. Tantra Buddhism, the Tibetan form of Buddhism, focuses on sex, speech, gestures and visions, giving rise to sexual art, mantras, mudras and mandalas. The Dalai Lama, unique to Tibetan Buddhism, is the incarnation of celestial compassion and mercy.

*The Four Noble Truths point out the middle way.*

## Confucianism

Confucius was born around 551 BC. His status as the "greatest single intellectual force" among the Chinese people was achieved after his death, and his teachings became regarded as the ideals to live by. The name Confucius is the Latin for K'ung-tzu or Kung Fu-tzu which means the "old master" or "first teacher."

1. The teachings and writings of Confucius addressed the social and political conditions of his time and answers to the question, "How ought we to live?"

2. He offered a system of teachings to establish deliberate traditions, as opposed to spontaneous traditions.

3. Moral standards and values were established and taught with the purpose of having them become internalized habits of daily living.

4. Proverbs, anecdotes, maxims, sayings, examples, stories (master-student exchanges) and fables became the means of transmitting standards and values.

5. "Man is by nature good," became the preamble to all teachings.

6. The content and goals of Confucius's deliberate traditions was "Wu-ch'ang," the cardinal virtues.

7. The teachings of Confucius were compiled by his disciples and are called the Analects. Another compilation is "The Doctrine of the Mean" by his grandson.

8. A version of what became known as the Golden Rule appeared in the teachings of Confucius as "Do not do unto others what you would not have them do unto you." This was taught as the highest principle of behavior.

## Taoism

1. Taoism (pronounced "Dowhism") is based on the short writings of Lao Tzu (title of respect for an aged man).

2. The small volume, *Tao Te Chin* (the way and its power), became Taoism's bible.

3. "Tao" means "the path" or "the way" and has the following meanings:
   a. the way of ultimate reality,
   b. the way of the universe, and
   c. the way humans should order their lives.

4. Different conceptions of the way of the universe led to three forms of Taoism:
   a. popular Taoism, based on magic, necromancy and sorcery;
   b. esoteric Taoism, a psychic approach to achieving perfection of mind and body; and
   c. philosophical Taosim, based on the concept that power is derived from a reflective and intuitive alignment with the power of the universe.

# The Abrahamic Religions

Judaism, Christianity and Islam have a common origin. They share the same story of creation of the earth by God, the creation of Adam and Eve, and the stories of the flood.

One of the common bonds today is the importance of Jerusalem to all three religions — to the Jews as a capital city and site of the famous temple; to Christians as part of the holy land where Jesus was born, crucified, buried, rose again and ascended to heaven; to Islam as a capital city and as the site of the Dome of the Ascension, the site from which Muhammad ascended to visit heaven.

## Judaism

The major beliefs of Judaism are:

1. There is one all-powerful, all-knowing and all-present God. The name for God in the Hebrew is Y-HW-H translated as Yahweh. The name Jehovah is thought to be a mistranslation of this name.

2. God created the earth and all that was in it at the beginning.

3. Everything was very good, and Adam and Eve were perfect until they disobeyed a specific command of God, and the consequences of sin and death ensued.

4. God promised to send a Redeemer or Messiah.

5. Human beings are the highest order of creation, have great capacities for good and bad, have the power of choice and were given dominion over all other forms of life.

6. God is actively involved in the affairs of humans and may exert direct control over people's lives and events to fit specific purposes.

7. The Ten Commandments given to Moses by God are the minimum standard of morality to guide social behavior.

8. Traditions and rituals teach the chosen people.

9. The coming of a Messiah or Chosen One would usher in a restoration of glory, triumph and fulfillment.

10. The Torah, equivalent to the first five books of the Bible, is the sacred writings of Judaism. It records the history and revelations of God to a chosen people.

11. The Talmud is a compilation of history, law, folklore and commentary.

## Christianity

1. Christianity is the most widespread of all religions. Its roots are in Judaism with the points of departure being the acceptance

*One of the common bonds today is the importance of Jerusalem to all three religions...*

of Jesus of Nazareth as the fulfillment of the promised Messiah; and the godhead, who is at the same time one and a trinity composed of God the Father; God the Son, who became incarnate Jesus; and God the Holy Spirit, who is present in the world today.

2. The reference to God is to the same God of Judaism.

3. The followers of Jesus of Nazareth were called Christians first around 35 to 40 AD.

4. Christians believe the following about Jesus of Nazareth:

    a.  He was God incarnate by miraculous conception of a virgin.

    b.  Being both fully God and fully man, He had power to heal, perform miracles, and raise the dead.

    c.  He lived a sinless life as a "second Adam."

    d.  He was crucified, died, was buried and rose again on the third day.

    e.  He ascended back to heaven to be with God the Father, and sent God the Holy Spirit to be present on earth.

    f.  He will come a second time to earth.

5. Jesus left no writings of his own.

6. The accounts of his life, the Gospels of the New Testament, and the story of the early Christians were written by his followers by the end of the first century AD. The Bible, consisting of Old and New Testaments, are the sacred writings of Christianity.

7. The greatest acts central to Christianity are the birth, ministry, crucifixion, death, burial, resurrection and second coming of Jesus to restore a perfect earth with perfect human beings.

8. The three main branches of Christianity are Roman Catholicism, Eastern Orthodoxy and Protestantism. The many denominations of Protestantism testify to the many ways in which the same teachings can be interpreted.

9. The life, crucifixion, death, burial and resurrection of Jesus were the final atonement and redemption needed because of Adam and Eve's disobedience.

10. The final reward of a right relationship with God through Jesus is eternal life in a perfect world. Liberals believe that other peoples can also have this eternal life without becoming Christian. Fundamentalists believe that it is only through belief in Jesus of Nazareth that eternal life can be obtained.

## Islam

1. The name Islam means "the perfect peace that comes when one's life is surrendered to God." "Muslim," (not "Moslem" or "Muslem") is the proper form of reference to people or things pertaining to this religion.

2. The God of Islam, Allah, is the same God of Judaism and Christianity. In fact, Muslims regard Judaism and Christianity as preceding Islam, with Islam being the final revelation; Muhammad, the final messenger or prophet; and the Quran ("Koran" is English spelling) as the final word from Allah.

3. The points of departure with Judaism and Christianity are as follows:

    a.  The sacred writings of Judaism and Christianity became corrupt. Allah dictated the Quran in Arabic to the prophet Muhammad to be the final revelation of his will.

    b.  Jews look forward to a coming Messiah. Christians believe in Jesus, God the Son, as the Messiah. Muslims believe Jesus was a good prophet, and in the same line of prophets, Allah called Muhammad as the "final messenger."

   c.  Jews observe their Sabbath, or holy day, on Saturday. Most Christians regard Sunday as their Sabbath, and Muslims observe Sabbath on Friday.

4. Muhammad was born around 570 AD, and received his call from Allah to be a prophet.

5. For Muslims, the guide to belief and practice in daily living is the Quran, regarded as Allah's revelations to Muhammad.

6. Muhammad was a reformer and revolutionary, calling his people to return to the worship of the God of Abraham, Moses and Jesus. This restoration of the true faith called for total surrender with resulting inner peace, the meaning of Islam.

7. Muhammad is called the "seal of the prophets" to designate that he is the last in the line of prophets from Abraham, Moses, John the Baptist and Jesus.

8. The Quran teaches:

   a.  Absolute monotheism, "there is no god but Allah."

   b.  Heaven, earth and hell make up the universe. Humans and spirits (angels, jinns and devils) inhabit the earth.

   c.  Islam was appointed by God to do his work of restoring moral, social and religious order and standards.

   d.  The day of judgment, the Day of Decision or Reckoning, will be a cataclysmic event when all beings will be judged by God to be rewarded with paradise or consigned to hell.

   e.  Law, "Sharia," as contained in the Quran and expanded by the schol-ars, outlines "the straight path" of requirements to govern the relationship of duties to God and duties to others. At the center of duties to God are five requirements known as the Five Pillars of Islam:

     i.  the profession of faith, "There is no God but Allah, and Muhammad is the messenger of God";

    ii.  prayer five times each day, facing in the direction of Mecca;

   iii.  almsgiving in a prescribed amount of individual worth;

   iv.  the Fast of Ramadan, a month-long fast where all who are able abstain from food, drink and sex from sunrise till sunset; and

    v.  the pilgrimage, a visit to Mecca, is expected at least once in a lifetime.

   f.  The laws regarding duties to others center around family law and social order, including diet, marriage, divorce, idolatry and inheritance.

9. The major divisions of Islam, which developed over disagreements about the rightful succession in leadership after Muhammad died, are Kharijites, Sunnis, Shiites and Sufis.

10. Among the various divisions and many sects and sub-sects of Islam, the Nation of Islam movement in America is significant. It was founded in 1930 by Wallace Fard, a salesman from Arabia, and has given rise to a Muslim population of diverse ethnic origins, numbering around three to five million.

## The New Age Movement

I think it is necessary to take a little more time to set a background for an understanding of the New Age, because it is

*At the center of duties to God are five requirements known as the Five Pillars of Is-lam.*

much more recent, diverse, inclusive and sometimes confusing to the layperson. Along with the references listed earlier in this chapter, I have summarized some of the thoughts and information from Irving Hexham and Karla Poewe's *Understanding Cults and New Religions*, Ruth Tucker's *Another Gospel: Alternative Religions and the New Age Movement*, and J. Gordon Melton, et al.'s *New Age Encyclopedia*.

I have tried to use sources that present information by academically qualified authors who expressly made an effort to avoid bias and castigation. I have attempted to present this brief summary without judgment and valuation.

Besides the books listed, I have read comments and expositions by several writers and attended lectures in the mid-1980s by such personalities as Norman Cousins (*Anatomy of an Illness...*); Viktor Frankl (*Man's Search for Ultimate Meaning*), and J. Krishnamurti, who, at the age of ninety, made one of his last speeches at the Kennedy Center in Washington, DC.

"New Age" is the term that serves as an umbrella for a host of new theology. This blends traditions of all the major religions into practices and beliefs that were rooted in the culture of the 1960s. There is no set system of beliefs and practices. It is an evolving and ever-changing collection of groups, cults and centers for everything from science to the God-status of individuals. Eastern spiritualistic and Third World occultism are blended into systems that produce personal spiritual experiences which attract millions of believers.

The rituals and traditions of the established religions are merged with alternative health and healing techniques with the catchall phrase New Age applied to them. The philosophy projects optimism and bliss that promises personal spiritual fulfillment to all who are disenchanted by loss of faith in their own traditions.

Aspects of Christianity, Judaism, Hinduism, Buddhism, Sufism, Taoism, science, science fiction, pseudoscience, astrology, tales of lost civilizations, disembodied intelligences, prophetic dreams, channeling, altered states of consciousness, paranormal experiences, out-of-body experiences, encounters with the dead, miraculous healing, shamanism, herbal remedies, homeopathy, crystallography and business are all part of the mix-and-match making up the New Age Movement.

The following points are presented to try to get across a broad overview of the structure and contents of the New Age Movement.

1. The term New Age derives from astrology with the understanding that the present age is the Piscean Age, the age of Christianity. This age is passing. Before we enter the New Age, the Age of Aquarius, there will be a dark, violent ending of the Piscean Age, followed by a millennium of love and light, "the time of the mind's true liberation."

2. The Aquarian Age, characterized by the power of the pervasive dreams of perfect health and wealth in our popular culture, will bring a Christ-like spiritual leader whose spirit will permeate the world and bring the final triumph of good over evil. In the New Age, a new universalist religion will be born.

3. The Aquarian Age will begin when the sun, at the spring equinox, will be in the sign of Aquarius. This will occur, as calculated by astrology, in about two hundred years. However, spiritual evolution may speed up the whole process.

4. Some of the major beliefs in the New Age Movement are as follows:

   a. All forms of spirituality that are not violent or harmful to self or others are acceptable. Beliefs are of lesser importance than experience.

   b. The primary goal of preaching and practice is to establish a universal religion based on the same mystical faith and to usher in the Aquarian Age.

   c. Everyone is God — the guru within, the higher self, the divine within. A guru or teacher leads one to become his/her own guru.

   d. Principles of individualism, practicality and commitment to social justice are highly recommended.

   e. "Return of Christ" means hope and the appearance of a spiritual leader who is Christ-like and will fill the world.

   f. New Age teachings reach "beyond self to include and empower others in compassionate love and social responsibility."

   g. There is a broad, eclectic approach to health, healing and spirituality.

   h. Several levels of "being" or planes of existence, all interconnected, are accepted.

   i. Mind or consciousness is the force behind the material world. The universal energy that supports life is the agent of psychic healing.

   j. The "common shared reality" is a personal, spiritual-psychological transformation.

   k. The tools of transformation include rebirth, meditation, wearing crystals, intensive seminars, sudden healing, astrology, massage, herbs and channeling.

   l. God is the unifying principle. God and the universe are one.

   m. Special people who become good channels of the universal energy to the world become manifestations of the ultimate unifying principle.

   n. Worship is meditation to find the consciousness underlying all religions.

   o. The new vision of the world is one of holism, earth awareness, social consciousness and human rights with equality for women. (Many of the thought leaders and founders of organizations are women.)

   p. The New Age will become established through networks of like-minded people as a result of "harmonic convergence."

5. Some of the events and personalities prominent in the establishment of the New Age Movement are:

   a. The Freemasons, the first to use the term "New Age" around 1914.

   b. The publication of *Cosmic Consciousness*, written by Richard M. Bucke, who theorized a new evolution of humans into a spiritual consciousness.

   c. The publication of the *East-West Journal* and the appearance of the first New Age prophet, Baba Ram Dass in 1971.

   d. David Spangler's book, *Revelation: The Birth of the New Age* and founding of the Lourian Association in 1973, and the publication of the *New Age Journal* in 1974.

*The New Age will become established through networks of like-minded people as a result of "harmonic convergence."*

*Answer this question: How can a person who believes in meekness, humility, grace, love, gentleness, patience, justice, peace and beauty inflict suffering and death to constrain someone else to change their beliefs?*

e. The publication of *The Aquarian Conspiracy* by Marilyn Ferguson, editor of *Brain/Mind Bulletin*, in 1980.

f. Shirley MacLaine's book, *Out on a Limb*, and the TV movie made from it in 1987.

g. The work of several eastern masters and their growth in the US with the founding of universities and communes. These include Maharishi Mahesh Yogi, founder of transcendental meditation, and Swami Satchidananda, who gave the invocation at the Woodstock Festival.

h. Several prominent scholars and physicians have contributed ideas and philosophies that strengthen the New Age Movement.

With this brief review of the major world religions, we need only to recall our history and current day events to see how religion is intricately woven into human lives. The beliefs and the emotions directed and triggered by religious teachings and practices are open to observation and study. Think about the crusades (the Holy Wars), the Holocaust, the Inquisition, the Ireland conflict, the Middle East conflict, the Indian Hindu-Muslim or Sikh question, or the American slave trade.

Answer this question: How can a person who believes in meekness, humility, grace, love, gentleness, patience, justice, peace and beauty inflict suffering and death to constrain someone else to change their beliefs?

# Personal 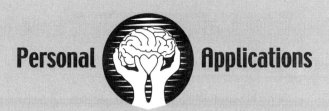 Applications

## Directions:

Think about the following questions and write down the first thoughts that come to mind. Select a few topics of personal interest and develop longer essays.

1. What do you do to contribute to the preservation and protection of natural resources and the quality of water, air and soil?

2. How do you relate to the election process for local and national government leaders?

3. How do the economic conditions under which you live affect your well-being? How satisfied are you with your present job?

4. What scientific and technological developments contribute most to your comfort and well-being?

5. Are there any aspects of the educational or justice systems that you think should and can be changed?

6. How has religion affected your life?

7. What is the biggest obstacle outside of your personal control that affects your well-being the most (environmental, economic and business, political and social, or religious)?

# Reflections

Of the factors discussed in this chapter, many things seem to be outside an individual's control. Is that really the case? What choice do we have in where we live, how we earn a living, how we relate to "the establishment," what rituals and traditions we accept, and how we express our beliefs? What factors guide us to where we are at a given place and time?

The purpose of this chapter is to present cues to the evaluation of the quality of relationship we have with the total environment. With respect to the physical world, how do we affect natural resources, other life forms and the future of these systems?

With respect to the structures and systems in our society, what voice do we have in their quality, policies and effects on people? With respect to our communities, how do we relate to people of a different race, class, economic status or religion?

These questions generally stimulate lengthy discussions. One of the activities that help to focus these discussions is essay writing. The essay that generates the best stories is "How Has Religion Affected Your Life?" From these essays I have read tales of disappointment, horror and fear, and tales of peace, comfort and joy.

Over the years, I have had atheist, Hindu, Buddhist, Muslim, New Age, Jewish, Catholic and Protestant students in my classes. Our discussions have always created and maintained an atmosphere of mutual respect, understanding and acceptance.

The old adage "If you want to keep friends, don't discuss politics or religion," is probably good advice. But for personal understanding, it seems that politics, religion, society's class structures, conservation, and work environment are appropriate topics for examination. One student's comments on this idea are worth sharing:

*In fact, this adage, in my opinion, has been a hindrance to spiritual and other progress. How can we move forward if we prohibit ourselves from discussing the very topics that are central to our lives? Because we haven't talked about them, we haven't given ourselves the opportunity to develop the skills to discuss such topics with respect and ease. (Sandra Fischer, class of '92)*

With reference to the outside forces and their effects on well-being, one experience comes to mind. Here's the story:

• • • • •

Our older son, Mike, was attending college in a small town in Michigan. He was pulled over for speeding, and the officer asked to see his driver's license.

Mike worked as a lifeguard the summer before going to college, and his license had fallen into the pool. The lamination was broken and the officer gave him a citation for "being in possession of a damaged official document." He explained that he would get it replaced during the Thanksgiving break when he went home to Maryland. The officer wouldn't allow that. He confiscated Mike's driver's license. It seemed as if he was determined to make the most serious charge possible.

Mike was summoned to appear in court. At the hearing, the charge on the docket was now "tampering with an official document." It seemed that the severity of the charge increased as it progressed from officer to precinct command to prosecutor.

After explaining to the judge his understanding of the original charge and the more serious charge of "tampering," Mike was given three choices: (a) contest the charges, get a lawyer and come back to court at a later date; (b) plead guilty and pay the fines and/or serve jail time; and (c) plead no contest and pay the fines and/or serve jail time.

After examining the options, he decided to plead "no contest." He was sentenced to twelve days in jail or one hundred and some dollars in fines. We paid the fine and hurried out of Michigan wondering how a simple condition escalated so quickly to jail time for a young man who had had no problems with the law, except for a speeding ticket.

•　•　•　•　•

Can the justice system have some preventive alternatives before they sweep young people into the punishment process? Sometimes, just a little common sense would make a big difference. For example, could the officer have given Mike the benefit of the doubt, taken him to the station, made a copy of his driver's license, had him sign a promise to get it replaced by a certain date, and had him return to the station to show that he had complied?

That would have left a much better feeling and respect on our part towards the whole system. But there is no such provision in the law. As it was, it seemed that the greatest interest was to see how severe the charge could be made and how much punishment could be handed down. What can an individual citizen do to help bring more sensitivity to our justice system? Probably not much except to tell a story, and exercise voting rights.

Time and energy may not allow for much involvement in the process, but even small protests, letters to editors and calls to congressional representatives are steps that can be taken. How many of us take the time and make the effort to contribute to changing what we don't like?

To go the distance, you have to seek to understand your fellow travelers.

## Carol's Turn

I will be very brief with the few thoughts I have on this subject of external forces and their influence on well-being.

Two things come to mind. One is the economic stress on a family trying to provide adequate housing and education for three children. I am the one who handles the family's finances, and sometimes I feel like we live under an economic slavery system. You never seem to get ahead. Prices of everything seem to increase faster than income.

It makes you really examine the whole system to see what alternatives there are to working for an hourly wage, how to earn more, keep more of what you earn, and use more of your creative energies to build some future financial security for re-

*To go the dis-
tance, it helps to be
brief and to the point.
(I'm trying to get Al
to believe this one!)*

tirement. It makes you really weigh the risks and the possible payoffs carefully.

The other comment I have is about political involvement. I was never interested in taking part in elections till the year we had a house for sale, and the mortgage interest rates went up to 16%. I blamed the political party in power for inflationary policies and voted against it. It left me feeling that my political decisions are influenced more by emotions than any persuasive arguments on the part of politicians. Don't they all exaggerate and lie anyway?

I will suppress my urge to tell about our attempts at recycling, growing vegetables without pesticides, keeping dandelions in our yard and my feelings about religion. I did promise to be brief.

To go the distance, it helps to be brief and to the point. (I'm trying to get Al to believe this one!)

# UNDERSTAND COGNITION, EMOTIONS AND MOTIVATION

*"When we do the best that we can,*

*we never know what miracle*

*is wrought in our life, or*

*in the life of another."*

Helen Keller

*10* Ten

*Dedicated to*

**Storytellers everywhere,**

*but especially to*

**Pastor I.K. Moses,** *the most humorous man of wisdom we know who, at the age of ninety-three, is keen of mind, sharp of wit and still fiddles.*

*and to*

**Cliff Okuno,** *who at his seventieth birthday party demonstrated how to kick his hand held parallel to his shoulder.*

*That was nineteen years ago, Cliff, and we will always treasure the association we shared in Charlottesville, VA. You are one of those exceptional storytellers.*

Once upon a time, a stork was returning from an early morning delivery. His flight-path took him across a field with an old well. The baby he had just delivered was a ten-pounder, and the stork was tired and thirsty. He decided to stop at the well, quench his thirst and rest a while.

The water level in the well was low. He hopped in. Too late to undo his mistake, he realized that the well got narrower as he went down, and that the water was further down than he thought. "Oh, well," he said to himself. "I might as well stay in this well, quench my thirst and rest. Well, well, well."

The water was bitter, but it quenched his thirst. He rested for a while, then began to figure a way out. The well was too narrow for him to spread his wings. He couldn't claw his way up the wall. But there was enough room so that if he could get a pole of some kind to step onto, he would reach the rim and pull himself out.

Just then, he heard a noise at the top of the well. A fox had stopped by to get a drink. "Is someone up there?" the stork shouted.

"Yeah, I'm up here," the fox answered. The engines in their respective brains were running in high gear. The stork was thinking, "How could I get him to pull me out without being eaten?"

The fox was thinking, "Wow, water for my thirst and a stork for my hunger. How lucky can a fellow be on a Monday morning!"

The fox was first to start putting his plan into action. "How's the water down there?"

"Water is great. Couldn't be bitter — I mean better. You should come down and taste for yourself."

"Is there enough room for both of us down there?"

"Lots of room. It's so roomy and the water is so good I hate to leave. I think I will take the day off and stay down here for a well deserved rest."

The fox thought for a while. "Any tricks, here?" he mused. "No, it's just a dumb stork. I'm the sly one. He can't put anything over on me."

"I'm coming in," he shouted. "Make room."

"Come on down," the stork shouted back. "But slide down the side of the wall to control your fall. It's further than you think."

The fox slid down. As he came within a few feet of him, the stork saw his chance. By quickly hopping up and putting one foot on the head of the fox, he could reach up to grasp the rim of the well and so pulled himself up.

"Thanks, Mr. Fox," said the stork as he started on his way.

"Oh, thanks, Mr. Stork," said the fox to the stork in as cheerful a tone as he could muster. "This water is great." And to himself, "How in the name of the place where the devil lives am I going to get out of this well?"

Just then, another stork landed on the rim of the well. It had been a busy night for delivering babies.

. . . . .

The fable "The Fox and the Stork" was in one of my grade school readers. I have never forgotten it, and, of course, it got embellished over the years. I see "fox and stork" games among people all the time.

Why do we do what we do in the way we do it? Psychologists tell us it has to do with motives and drives and needs fulfillment. From a layperson's perspective, I see motivation as the integrated output of the four dimensions of human function.

The physiology contributes biologic drives, seemingly based on the hedonic principles of pleasure seeking and pain avoidance. The mental/intellectual capacity of the brain contributes knowledge from which wisdom, need for consistency and conscience develop. The psyche contributes feelings of value about self and others. The spirit contributes the capacity for love, faith, hope and inspiration.

The integrated output is a mix of the four dimensions — the pleasure and pain balance in which we feel comfortable, the sense of accomplishment and achievement we believe we should reach, the factors that shape the personality and the belief system that sets a sense of meaning and purpose.

The integration of the four dimensions set the motives, drives, desires and energy level with which an individual faces the demands and challenges of life. Debate and research have tried to determine whether there is a single motive or multiple motives for human behavior. The research seems to support multiple motives, but a review of the theories is not the point here.

Lawrence Pervin, in his recent book *The Science of Personality*, reviews the theories including the "Jackass" theory of motivation.

My goal here is to explore what seems to work to help me get done what I am capable of doing — what I feel I need, should and want to do, but what seems to not get done. How do I harness my abilities to address the mundane as well as the inspirational tasks that I believe are mine to fulfill?

How do I take my cognitive skills, mix them with my beliefs and generate the emotions that feed the energy and determination to do the work? As Pervin notes, "People may not be pushed by pitchforks or pulled by carrots, but that doesn't make them jackasses either."

A good summary of the current understanding of motivation and getting things accomplished is found in Daniel Goleman's book, *Emotional Intelligence*. This should be prescribed reading for every adult.

Here are twenty-five summary points from Dr. Goleman:

1. IQ, or the intelligence quotient, a measure of thinking, reasoning and learning skills, is only part of what directs behavior, capabilities and accomplishments.
2. EQ, emotional intelligence, "which includes self-control, zeal and persistence,

*I see fox and stork games among people all the time.*

and the ability to motivate oneself" is the other, more important factor in determining success and happiness in life.

3. Both IQ and EQ can be cultivated and expanded, but the most critical stages for development are childhood and adolescence.

4. "Deficiencies in emotional intelligence heighten a spectrum of risks, from depression or a life of violence to eating disorders and drug abuse."

5. The present generation of children is more troubled emotionally than the last; they are "more lonely and depressed, more angry and unruly, more nervous and prone to worry, more impulsive and aggressive."

6. There are about eight main emotions, each at the center of a family of related feeling states. The major eight are anger, sadness, fear, enjoyment, love, surprise, disgust and shame. Moods and temperaments are expressions of the basic emotions.

7. Each basic emotion has a different pattern of physiologic arousal.

8. The emotional centers in the brain are triggered before the rational centers, especially when there is a perceived threat.

9. Academic intelligence, being able to deal with large amounts of information, contributes about 20% to the factors that determine success in life.

10. Emotional intelligence, which includes abilities like self-motivation, persistence, impulse control, delaying gratification, mood regulation, empathy and hope, plays a large part in the other 80% of the factors determining success. Luck and social class are other success factors.

11. Emotional intelligence is different from just being emotional or expressing emotions. It involves skills that should be taught, cultivated and practiced.

12. In cultivating emotional intelligence, the major skills are: self-awareness, personal decision-making, managing feelings and moods, managing stress, developing empathy, effective communication, sensitive self-disclosure, insight, self-acceptance, personal responsibility, appropriate assertiveness, understanding group dynamics and conflict resolution.

13. The skills in number 12 should, and can be, an integral part of the educational process from kindergarten onwards.

14. Negative emotions such as anger, rage, anxiety, melancholy, fear, doubt and shame can be managed constructively.

15. Motivation to get things done involves personal characteristics that contribute to the desire to put in the necessary work to develop the expertise needed for accomplishing a goal. Enthusiasm and persistence are high on that list of characteristics.

16. Accomplishments are related to how well mental abilities are harnessed with positive emotions and how well negative emotions are controlled.

17. Good moods, such as lightheartedness and mirth, enhance the ability to think clearly.

18. Hope and optimism are greater motivators when combined with realistic appraisal of capabilities and competencies.

19. Hope and optimism can be learned.

20. The state of high performance, when the best abilities are in high gear and work is being accomplished with relish and enjoyment with what appears to be "automatic output," is called "flow" or "being in the zone." This state can be cultivated.

21. To cultivate flow:
    a.  Learn to focus attention on one task.
    b.  Set a level of demand that is

higher than average but not overwhelming — not too difficult, not too easy.

   c. Review the pleasure of the end product and the personal competencies to accomplish the goal.

   d. Select an environment that is least conducive to distractions or interruptions. (Tell your junior high student it's false that you can watch TV and do the best job of studying at the same time!)

   e. The pleasure of the task accomplishment should be the ultimate reward, not the fame or the wealth or other possibilities.

22. Being in flow generates pleasure that leads to craving the state again and again. But to maintain flow requires that a challenge be present. Thus, the mind moves on to greater and greater heights of accomplishment, self-generated, internally motivated.

23. To get into flow, people must like what they have to do and have the basic skill to do it.

24. Children can be taught to develop the capacity of getting into flow and other emotion management skills.

25. Basic life skills such as controlling anger, resolving conflicts positively, developing empathy, controlling impulse and developing "character" should be integrated into mainstream education.

Being in flow, or operating in the zone, is a state to relish. Take an athlete who is operating in the zone during the most important game of the season. It's like being on autopilot. Everything is in synch. Reflexes and anticipation of the action put her in the right place at the right time for the right moves to make the shot, score the point, run the race or jump the hurdles.

Is it possible to meet life's demands with greater pleasure by being in flow more often?

From Dr. Goleman's review of the current research and from an understanding of brain chemistry in whole-person function, a picture emerges that makes sense to me in light of the framework with which we began this book. It is a simplified concept of how the brain works, and why many of us have a hard time getting things done when we have the capabilities and opportunities. It is purely an idea of synthesis and mental adventure, not proven research.

The picture is as follows:

1. There are four major electrical circuits that work together to integrate the person and fulfill an individual's potential. These are:

   a. the physiologic circuit, consisting of the sympathetic and parasympathetic nervous systems, and the hormonal and nervous control of muscle and the internal organs;

   b. the mental/intellectual circuit, consisting of sensory processing, to bring information into the brain to serve as food for learning, reasoning and decision-making;

   c. the psychosocial circuit, which sets levels of value and comfort about the knowledge of self in relationships with others; and

   d. the spiritual circuit, which deals with meta-needs and meta-values, sets and checks the fit with purpose and meaning and higher powers.

These four circuits interact and intertwine and affect each other as depicted in the diagram below:

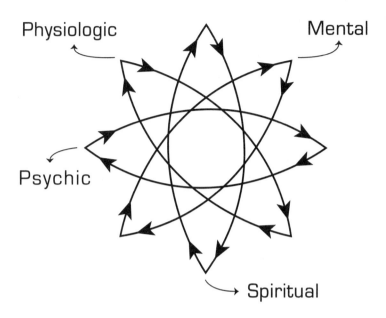

Physiologic          Mental

Psychic

Spiritual

2. Abnormal life events and biologic deficits, especially in early childhood, establish bizarre circuits, which interfere with the smooth interplay of the four major circuits. This makes it difficult for the normal circuitry to execute properly. The result is sabotage of motivation and difficulty in getting into flow. The resulting behavior may range from mildly dysfunctional to severely pathological.

3. Examples of events that establish bizarre circuits are physical, sexual or psychological abuse; trauma; abandonment; poor parenting; addictions; lack of a moral code; rejections; gross mistakes or self-perceived major failures; religious fanaticism; and lack of structure and organization. The bizarre circuit may impinge more on any one of the four major circuits, but the effect is on the whole person.

4. The more intense and concentrated the events that establish bizarre circuits, the harder and longer it takes to counteract their effects. Much can be done with self-help processes and personal growth over time, but many times the help of appropriate therapists is needed.

5. Help does not always arrive, or therapy is ineffective; and the damaged mind never recovers, never reaches acceptance, never fulfills its potential and ends in unhappiness, unfulfillment and misery, cut short sometimes by suicide.

6. The belief that the mind can heal itself through its own struggle against bizarre circuits with or without the collaboration of any other higher power (according to the individual belief system) is part of what has become mind/body/spirit medicine.

7. Every stage of life offers the opportunity to cleanse the mind of bizarre circuits, and thus promote growth and reproduction.

8. The recently evolving science of energy medicine will shed light on the role of bizarre circuits (including abnormal levels or lack of certain neurochemicals) in human behavior.

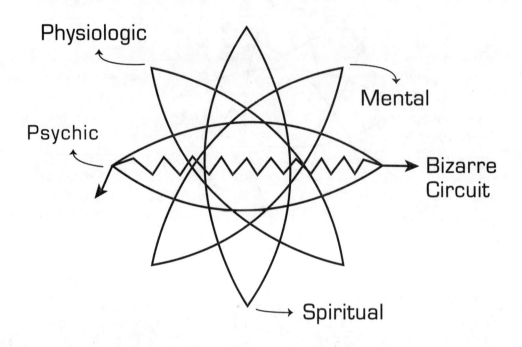

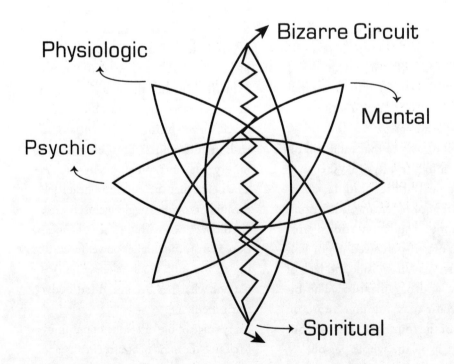

How does one untangle bizarre circuits and promote getting into flow? Over the last fifty years, many formulas have been tried. Sometimes we seem to expect that science will come up with a magic bullet for motivational disorders in the same way it did with the magic bullets of antibiotics. I believe that we have enough knowledge and insight and means to solve our major problems, if we would just put in the work.

Here is what I recommend:

1. Review your life history and examine your core beliefs. Which ones are real anchors? Which are other people's beliefs forced into you? Which ones contribute meaning and purpose to your existence? How spiritual a person are you?

2. As this self-examination leads to self-understanding and greater self-acceptance, do a futuring exercise to see what you want to celebrate with your life over the next few years. I've heard it said that most people on their deathbeds think about family, love, friendships and contribution rather than their career or possessions or money. This exercise leads to goal clarification and goal setting.

3. Make some decisions to use self-management strategies to bring about the future you really believe is possible for you and those you love. See what it takes to get into flow in your job or other pursuits. If you can't get into flow, examine the fit between you and the job. If you really hate your job or other responsibilities, examine your options. Take steps to change what you can with acceptable risks, or come to terms with the things you can't change.

4. Happiness and self-actualization will take care of themselves as byproducts of a purposeful life.

I believe that the spiritual capacity of human beings is the highest and most important dimension. It is the spirit and the spiritual connection with other beings, according to the belief system, that provide the best strengths and drive and highest pleasures in life.

It is in the dimension of spirit that we can come to the conclusion that all humans have intrinsic worth and that the categories of separation such as male/female, black/white, rich/poor, young/old, fat/skinny, religious/non-religious, creationist/evolutionist, educated/uneducated, exceptional/ordinary or other types of stratification can be transcended. This is the key to tolerance, value of life, respect and true equality. This, I believe, is the key to addressing some of the most critical needs in our lives — to stop the brutalization of one another in body and mind.

Some of the barriers to the above actions are strong bizarre circuits established by genetic factors, personality, lack of opportunity, delusions of grandeur and plain inertia — laziness. Life is short. If you think you got a lemon, get about the business of making the best possible lemonade.

Encouragement and inspiration can come from what other people use or recommend to get things done. Summary philosophy and practical approaches by prominent figures or writers serve to give us hope and insight for our own struggle.

Colin Powell, former Chairman of the Joint Chiefs of Staff under President Bush, in his book, *My American Journey*, gives a list of thirteen guidelines for a fulfilling career. He titled the list "Colin Powell's Rules."

1. It ain't as bad as you think. It will look better in the morning.
2. Get mad, then get over it.
3. Avoid having your ego so close to your position that when your position falls, your ego goes with it.
4. It can be done!
5. Be careful what you choose. You may get it.
6. Don't let adverse facts stand in the way of a good decision.
7. You can't make someone else's choices. You shouldn't let someone else make yours.
8. Check small things.
9. Share credit.
10. Remain calm. Be kind.
11. Have a vision. Be demanding.
12. Don't take counsel of your fears or naysayers.
13. Perpetual optimism is a force multiplier.

Here is what Lee Iacocca recommends to help manage self and other people if you are in a management position. And most of us are in management positions most of the time at some level, whether at home or at work, even though the job description may not say so.

In the chapter "The Key to Management" in his autobiography, *Iacocca*, one of the most successful managers in modern business poses three questions that people should ask of themselves and of the people they manage:

1. What are your objectives for the next ninety days?
2. What are your plans, your priorities, your hopes?
3. How do you intend to go about achieving them?

One of the other great business minds of this century is Tom Peters, whose 1992 book, *Liberation Management: Necessary Disorganization for the Nanosecond Nineties*, brings another factor into the milieu of factors by which people get things done. Peters talks about the luck factor this way:

Our numerous winning entrepreneurs, despite what passes for analysis in their after-the-fact autobiographies, are more or less lucky finalists in the business start-up version of Malkiel's Wall Street coin-toss.

Malkiel's Wall Street coin-toss is the description by economist Burton Malkiel about how the laws of chance alone influence careers and bring great honor and respect. The example, given earlier by Peters, is this:

The contest begins and 1,000 contestants flip coins. Just as would be expected by chance, 500 of them flip heads and these winners are allowed to advance to the second stage of the contest and flip again. As might be expected, 250 flip heads. Operating under the laws of chance, there will be 125 winners in the third round, 63 in the fourth round, 31 in the fifth, 16 in the sixth and 8 in the seventh. By this time crowds start to gather to witness the surprising ability of these expert coin-tossers. The winners are celebrated as geniuses in the art of coin tossing — their biographies are written and people urgently seek their advice. After all, there were 1,000 contestants, and only eight could consistently flip heads.

On the individual level, luck and chance are not to be discounted in whatever gets accomplished. It is the interpretation of what luck or chance is that makes the individual difference — what other factors influence the process. The belief about the situation is the key. Harnessing the strength of belief is one factor in getting into flow.

Another factor discussed by Tom Peters is the role of making mistakes. He notes that at one time in the business world, a job applicant was evaluated negatively if, among other factors, he had made major career or judgment mistakes. Now, in the nineties, people who have made mistakes are considered to have increased value for having gone through the experience and learned some things that don't work. Most scientific experiments result in showing something that doesn't work. Failures are part of the process of learning.

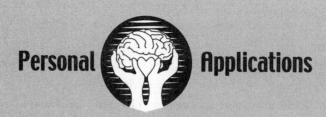

# Personal Applications

## Directions:

As you read the following, write down the first thoughts that come to mind. Go back and develop any of the ideas into longer essays.

1.  What motivational/inspirational sayings or proverbs have you memorized and can now recall?

2.  Relate a humorous story — true or concocted.

3.  Do you enjoy your present job? Have you ever done a job suitability or job satisfaction analysis?

4.  What are the major stories of your life? If you were to write a book titled *The Story of My Life*, what incident would you relate first?

5.  Relate some examples of your being in flow.

# Reflections

Once upon a time, a lamb strayed away from the flock and got lost. He wandered around for a while trying to find a way back. Suddenly, he heard a loud voice from above the clouds saying, "A lion and a lamb will find each other and show the rest of the animals something new that's really something old."

"So that's it," the lamb said to himself. "That's the reason I got lost. I must go find that lion." Immediately, his panic about being lost disappeared.

"I will find the lion," he thought, "then I will come back to the flock. They will bless me for bringing this special lion to meet them."

The lamb wandered across the hills down to the grasslands. He saw two animals coming towards him. When he recognized their shape and their wooly coats, he ran towards them. Could it be that they were also looking for the lion?

As he got closer, he could see something different about these two. They were not like any members of the flock he had left behind. One circled back of him. One blocked his way. Suddenly, they lunged for him. He sprang out of the way, leaving his attackers with only a mouthful of wool from his backside. This was his first encounter with wolves in sheep's clothing.

Further along, he heard loud, bellowing noises. An angry bull elephant was tearing off the boughs of trees and tossing them down. Roughly pushing the other elephants out of the way, defending his territory, the angry bull charged at the lamb.

It was easy for the little lamb to find shelter among the roots of a large tree where the elephant couldn't reach him. The elephant gave up the attempt, and the lamb went on his way.

In turn, the lamb met a fox whom he outwitted; a sheepdog from whom he escaped; a shark (yes, a shark, a grassland shark, maybe?) with whom he knew he couldn't swim; and a laughing hyena.

The hyena was the highlight of his second year of wandering around looking for his lion. The hyena had a theory that whenever he felt angry, or whenever things were not just exactly as he wanted them, he would rant and rave and curse and spew obnoxious gases into the atmosphere. This the hyena called "venting." It was his stress management technique. The lamb kept his distance and moved on.

He came upon a flock of sheep. He went to the leader. "There is a lion that I must find and there is something good that we must do together, and..."

   •   •   •   •   •

How would you finish the above story? As an exercise in creative writing or storytelling, develop the rest of the story of the lamb and the lion.

My Dad used to tell stories, all kinds of stories — ghost stories, stories with moral lessons and tales of adventure. His Nancy stories always had a moral lesson connected to them. As far as I can figure out, Nancy was a spider.

One of Dad's favorites was about two friends. In honor of Dad's eighty-third birthday, I want to include his favorite story titled "Braggart and Cricket."

. . . . .

These two friends went walking in the woods one day. Braggart was always out front. "Don't be afraid, Cricket," he kept saying. "I know where we're going. If anything tries to harm us, I will protect you. Even if a bear should attack, I will fight the bear for both of us. I am strong and tough. I am a western thinker. I have fought great battles and I always win."

Suddenly, a bear appeared. Without one thought for his weaker, slower friend, Braggart scampered up the largest tree, out of reach of the bear.

Cricket didn't have time to run to safety. The bear was upon him. He had heard it said that a bear would not attack a person who was or appeared to be dead. He fell to the ground and held his breath.

The bear came up to Cricket and sniffed at his head and neck, then turned and walked back into the deep woods.

When it was safe again, Braggart came down to join his friend. To make light of the situation, he slapped his friend on the shoulder and said, "So what was the bear saying when he was sniffing in your ears?"

"The bear was telling me," Cricket answered, "never to trust a boaster like you."

. . . . .

Simple stories carry some powerful lessons. Motivational and inspirational sayings have an impact on the mind to push,

pull or just add a little fuel to the engine that gets things done.

We can make use of anything that helps us accomplish what we know we are capable of doing. We can use rituals, meditation, prayer, positive thinking, the placebo effect —whatever helps the body, mind, psyche or spirit. If there is potential of hurt or damage, we must weigh the risks and benefits, make a decision and get on with pursuing realistic dreams.

We can't wait for a magic formula — not from science, not from others, not from outside. The answer lies in our belief system in combination with the other powers operating in our lives.

Hans Selye, the founder of stress physiology research put it this way in his 1956 work, *The Stress of Life*:

One of the main points of this whole discussion is that there is no ready-made success formula which would suit everybody. We are all different. The only thing we have in common is our obedience to certain fundamental biologic laws which govern all men (persons). I think the best the professional investigator of stress can do is to explain the mechanism of stress as far as he can understand it; then, to outline the way he thinks this knowledge could be applied to problems of daily life; and, finally, as a kind of laboratory demonstration, to describe the way he himself can apply it successfully to his own problems.

Maybe all that we can do is to tell our own stories — both the personal story of our lives and the anecdotes that illustrate important facets of life. What would the story of your life be? What are the anecdotes, the stories and the real-life histories of the heroes you admire? How do these affect you?

• • • • •

As a challenge to the group who took our course in the spring of 1997, we asked them to write an ending to the story of the "Lion and the Lamb That Was Lost." We offered to include one ending in the published text. Here it is with permission from Judith Hamer:

The lion that the lamb found was exceptionally strong with a loud roar and a bearing that said, "I am king of all beasts." The other animals warned the lamb about this frightening lion. The lion made winds from his roar, and he made the ground shake.

The lamb kept thinking about his many travels to locate this lion and all his experiences with different animals. He had years to learn from these practical experiences. He remembered the voice from the clouds that said, "A lion and a lamb will find each other and show the rest of the animals something new that's really something old." He pondered what the voice meant. How was this lamb going to get this lion to go back with him to his flock?

The lamb believed in the spirit of the clouds. He noticed how alone the lion seemed. The lion never had another animal around him because the animals were frightened of him. The lamb decided to talk to the lion and found that the lion's roar was loud because none of the other animals had ever explained how frightening it was, especially when it made the ground shake.

The lion asked why the lamb was covered with wool and why he followed the voice from the cloud on faith. The lion thought the lamb was intelligent until he said he followed on faith.

The lamb explained. "My intuition led me to you, my friend, and I used my intellect to convince you to go with me to my flock. I found that you needed a friend and I needed to take you with me to my flock."

The lion went with the lamb to his flock, arriving on a cloudy day, the first of March. The winds were howling from the lion's roar. By the end of March the lamb's friendship calmed the lion's roar. This produced the saying, "March comes in like a lion and goes out like a lamb." The something old, the lion's loud roar, had changed to something new based on faith, spirit and intellect.

## Carol's Turn

Maybe I should turn this around and tell some of Al's stories. I haven't had the chance to spend much time getting to know my father-in-law, but I have heard many of the stories. Like his dad, Al likes to tell his own stories, and many fond memories for our family are the times we sit around listening to the stories of his childhood on the island of St. Vincent.

These stories seem to have an impact on the children. Lessons about life seem to get passed on as stories when teaching the principle alone is not effective. Maybe this is part of emotional intelligence. I don't know. I just know that stories give pleasure.

*To go the distance, a storyteller in the crowd makes for a lighter journey.*

One of Al's favorite stories is about two duck hunters. As they planned a hunt, one hunter followed the principle that he should line up all his ducks in a row before he shot. The other believed that if he jumped in among the ducks, he would have a chance at shooting some as they got startled and began to fly in all directions. When the hunt ended, both hunters had the same number of ducks, but different stories to tell.

My view on all this is that whatever the combination of reasons that keeps us from getting things done, and whatever the combination of things that helps us in getting things done, it has to be worked out personally. I am still working out that understanding for myself. There is always something to hope for and work towards.

To go the distance, a storyteller in the crowd makes for a lighter journey.

# CLARIFY YOUR PURSUIT OF HAPPINESS

*"The point of reflecting*

*on happiness is to learn*

*how to be happy, and*

*perhaps to remind us that*

*we are luckier than we realize."*

Leroy S. Rouner

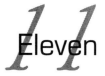
Eleven

*Dedicated to*

**Kaitlyn, our granddaughter**

*You exponentially multiply and integrate our happiness.*
*(Grandpa will explain this on your way to kindergarten!)*


*and to*


**All our future grandchildren**

There seems to be a lot of confusion about what happiness means. Is it just hedonic pleasure? Is it feelings? Is it virtue? Is it deep-down satisfaction? It seems that many of us are actively searching to clarify the meaning of happiness.

The search involves both laypersons and professionals. It is a personal pursuit, a personal definition. But are there common principles, common pathways? Do we have to wait to stumble into happiness accidentally, or is there a way to chart a path to happiness?

Some say that happiness is based on illusion. Some, that self-reports of happiness are self-deceptions. Is there an answer to satisfy the part of our humanity that seems to desire happiness?

What did Thomas Jefferson mean by "happiness" when he included the statement enshrined in the Declaration of Independence that "the pursuit of happiness" is one of the inalienable rights of citizens?

What did the French mean by the word "happiness" when, in 1789, the French Declaration of the Rights of Man and of the Citizen said, "The goal of society is common happiness?"

More to the point, what do individuals mean when they say they are happy or unhappy? Is there happiness in a world that has produced two world wars, the nuclear bomb, the Holocaust, suppression of peoples and forced suffering?

In the past fifteen years, the philosophical literature and sociological research has taken up the subject with new vigor. The resulting reappraisal of this state of the human condition has led to some interesting research and some very illuminating discussions.

Let me again voice my disclaimer. I am not an expert or scholar of the social sciences. I see my role as a layperson, facilitator of thinking and self-examination because I have come to a particular place in history at a particular time when there is academic freedom and encouragement to do so. To this task I bring a particular synthesis of ideas and personal experiences.

My goal is to stimulate personal introspection to promote personal wellness. In doing so, I must be aware of the discussions and ideas of the experts, and share that in a synthesis that is compatible with a model that addresses the needs of the total person.

The following sources have reinforced the need to address this subject and provided perspectives and ideas with which to fulfill the task. I recommend a careful reading of these three books. They give a broad survey of the philosophical roots of our definition of happiness, and summarize the current research on happy people and the reasons they are happy.

1. *In Pursuit of Happiness*, published by the University of Notre Dame Press in 1995, is a collection of lectures in the series "Boston University Studies in Philosophy and Religion." This is a joint project between the Boston University Institute for Philosophy and Religion and the University of Notre Dame Press.

In their very readable, thought-provoking styles, philosophers like Charles Griswold of Boston University, Margaret Miles of Harvard Divinity School, Huston Smith of Syracuse University and Tu Wei-Ming of Harvard University give their definitions of happiness and the ramifications for personal living. This volume must be digested slowly. It is pleasure reading of a high order — solid mental nutrition.

Here are some definitions and summaries of the discussion:

a. Long-term happiness is tranquillity — not emptiness but a dynamic rest, which has overcome deep anxieties about life's greatest questions.

b. Happiness is desire and delight in the interconnectedness of all things in an immensely generous universe.

c. Happiness is not just pleasure but a blessedness where paradoxical states like happiness and unhappiness are blended together in a "peace that passes all understanding," with the positive absorbing the negative state.

d. Joy is not quite happiness for "joy is a sensation which surges through us when we are doing especially well at what we are good at doing."

e. Happiness is joyful performance of God's will, integrating spiritual joy and enlightenment with selfless altruistic concern for the happiness of others.

f. Happiness is satisfaction derived from gaining one's humanity where harmony with nature and with heaven leads to participatory joy in building up the community.

g. Leroy S. Rouner, the editor of this volume, writes a closing to the introduction which paraphrasing or summarizing would destroy. So I quote two paragraphs from page 9, and hope that this qualifies for fair use and more publicity for this volume, which has been a delight for me to read. I quote:

All of which reminds us that the point of reflecting on happiness is to learn how to be happy, and perhaps to remind us that we are luckier than we realize. At the least, we all have brief moments of joy. And we all have the reflective opportunity, which Charles Griswold celebrates, for a rationally ordered life in which we take responsibility for our choices, and have the satisfaction of trust that we have chosen well. Those of us who are religious have had moments of God-given ecstasy; and, most of all, we know something of Huston Smith's deep assurance that nothing in heaven or earth can finally separate us from the love of God, and that we are therefore truly among the blessed.

And even for those who are not religious, but who are sensitive to the life of the world around them, there is what Margaret Miles has called the Great Beauty, the realization that the world in its benign generosity can be lovely beyond any singing of it. In these times of tragedy and trouble, that alone is enough to give us an Augustinian "glimpse" of what it means to be truly happy.

2. *Happiness and the Limits of Satisfaction,* written by Deal W. Hudson (Rowman & Littlefield Publishers, Inc., 1996), is a concise review of the philosophical evolution of the meaning of happiness. Dr. Hudson, a former associate professor of philosophy at Fordham Univer-

sity, is currently editor of *Crisis* magazine of Washington, DC. He takes a strong stand against the popular, common definition of happiness in terms of feelings alone, and reviews the traditional meanings which seem to have been lost from the definition and from modern life.

Dr. Hudson calls today's definition of happiness "well-feeling," which is a subjective, self-reported psychological state, subject to misinterpretation and self-deception. He passionately argues for the re-inclusion of "eudaimonia," from the Greek word for happiness, which carries the meaning of "moral virtue in a life capable of objective signs of happiness — objective in terms of being observable and desirable by others."

"Happiness," he writes, "belongs to those who, given their humanity and their circumstances, have distinguished themselves to their friends by their steadfast and successful commitment to the life they envision."

A few chapter titles may entice you to read this book. Again, it is pleasure of a higher, slower order — high nutritive value for the mind. In chapters such as "Popular Views of Happiness," "The Rejection of Psychological Happiness," "The Enigma of Jefferson's Pursuit," "Happiness and Pain" and "The Passion for Happiness," Hudson reasons the reader into an evaluation of definitions and personal applications of happiness.

"Well-being," or "the state of our lives taken as a whole," is distinguished from "well-feeling," which is "momentary and passing states of feeling."

There is a minimum moral code of behavior that must be included in the happy life, or that is necessary to produce the happy life. Responsibilities may not produce immediate feelings of psychological happiness, but they are part of a happy life.

Hudson presents a much-appreciated review of philosophy from Aristotle, Locke, Aquinas and others. His quote from Aristotle is telling of his viewpoint. "Happiness is the final end for the sake of which everything else is done."

He takes to task the preachers of positive thinking and visualization of "the good life" for recommending the "immediacy of feelings" over moral virtue which produces longer lasting feelings.

Some major points of Dr. Hudson's treatise are:
a.  Ambiguity about what happiness is, is caused by ambiguity about human nature.
b.  The human desire for happiness cannot be avoided — it is "an intractable fact of human nature."
c.  Happiness involves internal consistency, maintenance of a stable character, a reason to live and a vision of the best possible life.
d.  Subjective talk and appraisal of happiness may be escapist and self-deceiving, and are complicated by mood, tactics of avoidance and denial, and "the angle of self-scrutiny."
e.  Happiness consists of more than feelings. The legacy of the moral philosophers argue for inclusion of:
    i.   **eudaimonia** — moral virtue;

ii. **euthumia** — joy, gladness, cheerfulness and good-heartedness;

iii. **ataraxia** — freedom from disturbance or pain; and

iv. **beatitudo and felicitas** — tranquility and peace; deep-down feelings of delight and satisfaction.

The happy moment must be distinguished from the happy life. Earthly happiness must be distinguished from transcendental happiness.

f. Pain is a teacher in the school of happiness, providing the opportunity for growth. But the wise do not seek out pain. When it comes, pain is recognized as an opportunity for self-mastery.

g. Jefferson's philosophy was based on the Christian ideal of God's will for humans to be happy, since God made humans with the nature to desire happiness. But this happiness is also a call to moral virtue, leisure, freedom and lack of ill will towards others.

3. *The Pursuit of Happiness: Who Is Happy — and Why* is written by David G. Myers, Ph.D., a social psychologist at Hope College in Michigan. He summarizes much of the current research about well-being, life satisfaction and quality of life studies. Here are twenty-five items from this discussion. See whether your experience or knowledge agrees with these conclusions based on happiness research.

a. Well-being is subjective. But it is more than "well-feeling." It is "sometimes called 'subjective well-being' to emphasize the point — a pervasive sense that life is good. Well-being outlasts yesterday's moment of elation, today's buoyant mood, and tomorrow's hard time; it is an ongoing perception that this time in one's life, or even life as a whole, is fulfilling, meaningful and pleasant."

b. More people report being happier than was previously estimated. Earlier estimates were that 20% of Americans were happy. Actual reports show more like 80% are happy.

c. College students in the eighties and nineties rated financial success as more important than developing a meaningful life philosophy.

d. Above a certain basic need, higher income has little or no effect on increased happiness.

e. The attitude about income and possessions is more important than the absolute amount.

f. The proportion of reported happiness did not increase as personal wealth increased nationally in the USA between 1930 and 1991.

g. What we say influences what we think and feel; positive talk promotes positive attitudes.

h. Happiness is at a core level of living between the highs and the lows that are the norm of human life.

i. One of the conscious efforts we can make to build our core level of happiness is to manage our expectations and comparisons. Traditions and rituals that encourage self-denial and sacrifice seem to contribute to this.

j. From teens to over sixty-five years of age, the same percentage of the population (80%) in sixteen nations report being satisfied with life.

k. The popular notions of unhappiness due to post-menopausal and "empty-nest syndrome" factors in women, as well as the instability of men in "mid-life crisis" are not supported by large-scale research.

l. Older people report just as much happiness and satisfaction with life as younger people.

m. The happiest senior citizens are those who are actively religious, enjoy close relationships, have sufficient health, income and motivation to enjoy a variety of activities.

n. Whether you are a housewife, corporate CEO, construction worker or file clerk, career happiness is having work that is compatible with your interests and abilities and provides a sense of competence and accomplishment.

o. Women are twice as likely as men to suffer bouts of depression and to feel worried or frightened, but women more often than men report intense joy or intense sadness.

p. Women attempt suicide more often than men, but men are two to three times more likely to succeed.

q. Men, as compared to women, are five times more likely to become alcoholic and eight times more likely to commit violent crimes.

r. Differences in race, education, parenthood and where you live have very little effect on reported well-being.

s. Minority groups (ethnic, disabled, women) in America have similar levels of self-esteem as do white males.

t. Fire walking and astrology have only placebo effects.

u. High self-esteem, a sense of personal control, optimism and extroversion are the inner traits that correspond to positive mental attitudes and greater well-being. These can be learned.

v. Setting goals, getting immersed in an activity, paying attention to what is happening and savoring the immediate experience make work and life more enjoyable.

w. A social support system consisting of close relationships, comfortable companionship and an inner circle of loyal intimacy promotes well-being and happiness.

x. The ingredients of a happy marriage are sex (quality over quantity), intimacy, equity and growth.

y. A belief system that engenders something larger and outside of self; that provides something meaningful to share in connectedness with others; that challenges altruistic responses to human needs; that offers a deep sense of purpose, peace and acceptance; that provides vision and courage to live in the present; and that generates hope that reaches beyond the life-span, is a great contributor to coping, to well-being and to happiness. Empirical science cannot study it all, or prove or disprove it.

The above brief summaries should serve to whet the appetite for more of this kind of reading. I am looking forward to the next Boston University Studies in Philosophy and Religion volume, *The Longing for Home*.

In light of the framework we have used to examine wellness, there is not much more that can be said about happiness. However, a restatement may be useful.

On the physiologic level, we must learn to optimize health functions, prevent diseases, promote health, engage in enjoyable leisure activities, obtain treatments and undergo rehabilitation to maintain the capacities to function without pain and restriction for as long as possible. This contributes to happiness.

On the mental level, we develop our capacity to learn. We make decisions and choices. We accept codes of conduct and virtue. We develop self-discipline and practice self-management. We set goals and vision positive outcomes. We work. We play. We create, and we think. This gets work done, brings mental pleasures and contributes to happiness.

On the psychosocial level, we take our sense of our own value, and we evaluate it and seek to increase it. We grow. We relate in interdependent circles. We deal with other people and value them in ways consistent with our belief and value systems. We become part of other people's lives. We participate in shared pleasure and help soothe one another's pain. We contribute to other people's happiness and enrich our own.

On the spiritual level, we define our purpose in life. We choose our meaning. We believe or do not believe in powers much greater and higher and more powerful than anything we have known or experienced. We transcend ourselves and hope to transcend everything earthly. We find answers to life's deepest questions. We find happiness, shared happiness for self, others and the community of human beings.

On a whole, humans tend to be optimistic about happiness. So much so that in the face of hardships, discouragement, loss, wars, crimes, violence, hurt and neglect, we can still find happiness.

Our capacity for happiness may be related to our capacity for love. Usually, we can't dictate falling in love. It happens. The early "maps;" programming of the brain; pheromones; and mental, psychosocial and spiritual codes and beliefs set us up for falling in love.

Maybe, there is something similar for falling into happiness. Most of the philosophers I read agree that if happiness is seen as a state to strive for, a state to grasp, it may remain out of reach. It is a byproduct of effort in life and grace — effort that matches abilities, and grace that fits with the personal belief system.

Some other thoughts, doubtless stimulated by the reading I have been doing over the past weeks, seem to beg to be included:

1. Happiness involves fighting to grow in goodness and to extinguish badness. To come to the end of life, whenever that might be, and believe "I have fought a good fight" is a happy summary. But it has to be an authentic fight — not a feigned battle.

2. Experimentation with life has a curious combination of excitement and deeply grounded happiness. Any experiment has certain risks of failure. Nevertheless, a personal "experiment with truth" as Gandhi said, is worth the risk of failure. Then, whatever the outcome, it is acceptable.

3. The ends and the means, the destination and the journey, personal virtue

and public responsibility, individualism and the community in balance are necessary for happiness.

4. It seems that a lot of current lifestyles, in the words of Deal Hudson, "are wrapped up in self-consuming decadence and disdain for public responsibility... Happiness is surrendered for the trappings." These thoughts remind me of the story "The Dog and His Shadow."

．　．　．　．　．

It seems that a smart dog would go to a butcher shop everyday to receive a bone from the butcher. He had to cross a bridge to get to the shop. He had made the trip many times without mishap.

One day, he stopped on the bridge to look over into the water below. He saw his reflection holding a bone that looked larger than what he had.

All of a sudden, he dropped his bone, and plunged into the water to snatch the larger bone from the shadow in the water. The real bone floated downstream out of reach. This smart dog spent many days searching for the shadow he saw in the water, even forgetting about the butcher shop close by.

．　．　．　．　．

The "trivialization of happiness," as Hudson puts it, "is only a shadow of the real thing."

To go the distance, it helps to know when and why you are happy.

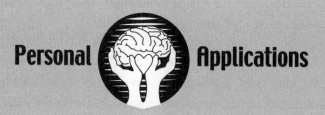

# Personal Applications

## Directions:

Write down the first ideas that come to mind as you read the following assignments. Select one or more items to expand into a longer essay.

1.  Make an outline of what you will say to a group of teenagers about your definition of happiness and your evaluation of your own life as a happy life.

2.  Watch the movie, " It's a Wonderful Life." If you have seen it before, it will stand the repeat. Don't wait to watch it on broadcast TV with all the distracting commercials. After viewing it, write a short summary.

3.  Describe the happiest people you know.

4.  Make a list of "the things that make me happy."

5.  Write an ending to the story of "The Dog and His Shadow."

6.  Make a list of "things I cannot afford to lose." What will happen if you lose any of them?

## Reflections

After writing this chapter, I had the pleasure of visiting with Dr. Hudson in his Washington, DC, office. This is the first time I have had an opportunity to meet privately with the author of a book I really enjoyed and ask questions and share ideas on the subject.

Occasions such as these expand the mind. We talked about wellness and happiness and our role in getting across the deeper meanings of pleasure, enjoyment of life and lasting happiness to a world in need of getting beyond superficial feelings. We discussed definitions of high self-esteem and the true meaning of humility.

I hope we get the chance to collaborate on the obvious next topic: "Wellness and the True Meaning of Happiness." It is a joy just to contemplate this idea and discuss the content of such a book. It is an even greater joy as I reflect on how people touch one another's lives at particular moments in time, unaware of the personal effects and the private needs being met.

Happiness has more to do with relationships than with things.

## Carol's Turn

"Are we having fun yet?" is on the coffee mug I usually drink from. But the cat in the drawing is all tense and stiff trying hard to have fun. It seems to be saying, "The harder I try, the more difficult it is to be happy."

Happiness and fun are different. Fun is part of a happy life, but it is not the full experience. Some of the happiest occasions in my life have been simple acts of reaching out to someone in need.

I tell these experiences not to boast about doing good. It is rather a tribute to our friends who have been so kind and helpful to us during some difficult times — times when it seemed that our decisions had ruined our present happiness and set us and our children up for future unhappiness.

I know that these friends would prefer that I not use their names. They know who they are. It seems that we have been on the receiving end of their help and kindness more than we wanted to be, but they gave graciously without expecting anything in return.

During those times, we also got to know the feeling of helping and giving of the little we had. It is a much happier feeling to give than to receive. I relate these because they seem to be out of the ordinary. Here are the incidents I recall with pleasure.

．　．　．　．　．

One night in 1987, we received a call at around two o'clock in the morning. A friend from a nearby community was on the phone telling about his friend whom we didn't know. This friend of our friend had been stopped by the police and was caught driving with an expired registration. He was in jail and would only be let out by posting a bond, which neither of them could raise.

We drove over to the bank and raided the checking account through automatic teller machine withdrawal. It was uplifting and pleasure producing to help.

*Happiness has more to do with relationships than with things.*

It was even better to continue to build a relationship with our friend, who felt that in whatever his circumstances, we would try to help. The joy of the immediate experience seemed to contribute to the longer term happiness with the friendship. Analyzing it now seems okay, but at the time it was the experience that was creating the good memory. It just happened.

· · · · ·

The other incident is also about a friend in jail. This was in 1990. Looking back now, we wonder why we were the ones called on by people in jail. We don't think it happens to many people we know. Does it say something about the company we keep? I'm just kidding. I don't worry about it.

We got the call about six o'clock one Sunday morning. We usually sleep in on Sundays. But this brought us wide awake. A woman's voice. She had been on a date and was stopped for speeding. A gun was found in the car, and she and her date were in jail. Without money for bail, they would have to remain there till a hearing could be arranged.

Al and I knew we couldn't say no. There was no one else to ask. Could we borrow to help them? We called American Express, and they raised our credit card limit to cover the amount needed. We didn't stop to think about repayment then. The desperation in the voice was beyond weighing options. We just had to find a way.

· · · · ·

Helping other people is one of the keys to happiness. A community that helps and provides opportunities to help is a growing community.

Other keys to happiness are like the rooms of a house. This illustration goes over well in the classes I've attended. Each room of the house contributes factors to happiness: the bedroom, the kitchen, the den, the recreation room, the living room, the family room, the basement. Having friends visit (limited to the appropriate rooms!) is a special pleasure.

One of our recent outreach to others that is very meaningful to me is the time we invited a single, teenage mother with her newborn to share our home. To see a young person rise to the challenges of life's circumstances, and to see a young child prosper in an atmosphere of love and support, bring warm feelings and deep-down satisfaction to me.

I relate the above incidents only as examples of what I believe contribute to happiness for me. People who help others find this to be true. There is a lot of kindness and concern in our world, in spite of the bad and the evil we see and hear of everyday. If more people would be open to take the opportunities to help where they can (and millions do), our world would only be better for it.

There may not be any specific formulas or keys to happiness, but we do know a lot about it. It is part of what pulls us to live the best life possible. Each of us defines and refines it according to our own beliefs and rules.

To go the distance, you have to help somebody.

# Examine Your Reasons for Procrastination

## (The Top Ten Reasons It Took Fifteen Years to Write This Book)

*"They call you mad. Wait for tomorrow and keep silent. They throw dust upon your head. Wait for tomorrow. They will bring you flowers."*

Rabindranath Tagore

*"I keep stringing and unstringing my instrument, but I have not yet sung the song I came to sing."*

Rabindranath Tagore

*Dedicated to*

**Each other**

*How sweet it is!*

*How rough the way!*

*Lemonade, anyone?*

*P*rocrastination is defined as putting off doing something that a person wants to do, is capable of doing and is trying to do. If the thing gets done, it is late, or it doesn't get done at all. The effects of this condition ranges from mild effects on behavior and productivity to severe, chronic, paralyzing disruption of major life goals.

In researching the literature on procrastination, I came across the names of two experts who have been asked to edit a special issue of the *Journal of Social Behavior and Personality* to be published in the summer of 1999. The issue is titled "Procrastination: Current Issues and New Directions." The experts are Dr. Joseph Ferrari in the Department of Psychology at DePaul University, Chicago, and Dr. Timothy A. Pychyl in the Department of Psychology at Carleton University in Ottawa.

The power of the Internet was very helpful in this survey because these two experts, their students and research colleagues run a website which gives excellent summaries of the professional and self-help literature on procrastination. The address of this site is http://www.carleton.ca/~tpychyl/index.html.

In my estimation, this is a very credible and valuable site, which will continue to grow as a source of education in the new field of procrastination research and treatment. The following summary statements should serve as an introduction to reading this site for an excellent discussion of the subject. In the items below, **IT** stands for procrastination, and **THEY** for procrastinators.

1. IT was once regarded as a sin.
2. THEY represent about 40% of the population and experience loss (of productivity, opportunity, income, credibility, etc.).
3. About 25% of people experience IT as a chronic, debilitating condition.
4. The causes of IT can be on the physiologic/genetic level, the cognitive, behavioral and emotional levels, or the subconscious level.
5. Behaviorally, IT is a bad habit that has been reinforced.
6. IT is unrelated to ability or intelligence.
7. THEY often have perfectionist expectations and are overconscientious.
8. THEY may display an irrational fear of success or failure, which leads to neurotic avoidance.
9. IT is related to fear of failure, lack of conscientiousness and high impulsiveness.
10. IT is related to a lack of self-efficacy, low self-esteem, high self-consciousness and exaggerated self-criticism.
11. IT is related to high sensitivity to criticism and rejection.
12. THEY may be unable to delay gratification of pleasure.
13. THEY may lack self-control.
14. THEY may be anti-authoritarian.
15. THEY may lack motivation, energy or organizational abilities.
16. IT may be related to childhood trauma or faulty parenting.
17. IT may be a "learned helplessness" reaction as an adaptive coping mechanism.
18. IT may be related to other psychological disorders such as narcissism, borderline antisocial personality disorder, passive personality disorder, obsessive/compulsive disorder, phobias and neurotic behavior.

19. Some of the behavioral traits include indecisiveness, doubt, perfectionism and inflexibility.

20. IT is a maladaptive coping syndrome, which needs to be regarded seriously and treated.

21. IT can be treated by strategies that include cognitive/behavioral techniques, psychodynamic approaches, relaxation techniques and drugs.

22. Self-help sources for IT include *Doing It Now: A 12-Step Program for Curing Procrastination and Achieving Your Goals* by E. Bliss. (Scribner, 1983), and *Do It Now: How to Stop Procrastinating* by W.J. Knauss. (Wiley & Sons, 1997.)

23. IT is summarized (theory, research and treatment) in a book by Dr. Ferrari and his colleagues who describe five cognitive distortions THEY may have:
    a. overestimation of time left to perform tasks,
    b. underestimation of time required to complete tasks,
    c. overestimation of future motivational states,
    d. misreliance on the necessity of emotional congruence to succeed at a task, and
    e. belief that working when not in the mood to work is suboptimal.

24. If THEY are college students troubled by academic procrastination, Dr. Ferrari and colleagues recommend the following steps:
    a. Make a list of everything you have to do.
    b. Write an intention statement.
    c. Set realistic goals.
    d. Break down goals into sub-goals.
    e. Make the task meaningful.
    f. Promise yourself a reward.
    g. Eliminate tasks you never plan to do.
    h. Estimate the amount of time you think it will take to complete a task and double it.

25. IT is a whole-person problem and can be addressed in terms of whole-person healing.

That's enough to help us see what we are talking about and to use our experience in producing this book as an example of some of the procrastination factors we have had to deal with. One question that comes to mind is about the balance that exists between factors that are under a person's control and factors that are not. Do the personal beliefs (such as in a God that is actively involved in a person's life-plan) play a role in understanding procrastination?

Beginning with reason number 10, here is how we see a project we started in 1984 coming to completion in 1999.

**#10.** *Al*: My style of writing was too scientific. We started writing this book in 1984. The main ideas, the chapter titles and an outline were completed by the time the course was offered for the first time at the University of Maryland, fall semester 1984.

All my writing experience up to that time was for scientific journals. The paper I had done the most work on, with the help of Dr. Steve Ely, was published in the *American Journal of Physiology, Cardiovascular Section* in 1982. I was still in that mode, and by the time the first version of this book was well on the way, it read like a scientific paper. We discarded it. I started and abandoned three other versions before this one came into existence. The chapter titles were changed each time we revised the contents.

This reason for procrastination seems to be lack of confidence that we were reaching the right audience in the style we thought we should.

**#9.** *Carol & Al*: We believed there were enough books on health and wellness on the market during the mid-1980s. High level wellness was becoming a popular topic, and self-help books of all kinds were flooding the market. Yet we couldn't find one with the scope of coverage that we needed. We tried a couple of different ones as the text for the course, but none of them stood by themselves. So we continued to write, yet dissatisfied with the product.

This reason for procrastination seems to be lack of belief that we had something different and useful to offer.

**#8.** *Al*: I didn't understand the process of writing a book until I took a course from an author. The only writing instruction I had in school was freshman composition. I attended one writer's workshop at the Review and Herald Publishing Association in the early 1990s.

I really came to understand the book writing and publication process in 1993, when I took a short course at The Writer's Center in Bethesda, MD. Mariah Burton Nelson, author of *Are We Winning Yet: How Women Are Changing Sports and Sports Are Changing Women*, brought to the course her experience and encouragement. She showed the class copies of her book proposals and an actual publisher's contract. Her techniques were direct and effective. I sometimes wonder if I'm the last one from her class to finish the project we all started or re-started then.

A quote from Mariah's class, which has stuck with me, is: "Remember, the editor is your first reader. If your manuscript does not please your first reader, you may not get another."

(Mariah, the Women's World Cup Soccer Finals on July 10, 1999, showed how women are changing sports!)

This reason for procrastination seems to be lack of specialized knowledge.

**#7.** *Carol & Al*: We had visions of making a business out of the book instead of just writing a book. We were learning to desktop publish, and planning spin-off businesses, and doing the illustrations, and setting up a marketing strategy for the book, workbook and course. These were distractions. We spread ourselves too thinly to be effective at a demanding task.

This reason for procrastination seems to be lack of focus and looking at the tangible outcome instead of concentrating on the process.

**#6.** *Al*: For eleven of the fifteen years of writing, I was absorbed full time in work and subject matter that drained my energies and left me unmotivated to put in the effort necessary to get this job done. I didn't like or enjoy my full-time job. This was used as an excuse until I saw it as an obstacle to get around.

This reason for procrastination seems to be consuming distraction and lack of fit between philosophical interests and work necessary to make a living.

**#5. *Carol & Al*:** The subject matter had to mature in our minds and in our experience. Crossing the middle-age line into the realm of senior citizens has been good seasoning for the content of this book.

This reason for procrastination seems to be just a needed maturation process. Some things mature more slowly.

**#4. *Carol & Al*:** Some aspects of our personality and behavioral style needed time to grow and adjust. We had to overcome fear of success, fear of failure, dealing with rejection and redefining perfection. We had rejections from three journals for a concept article, and about seven publishers for the book. Each rejection would push us into a depression from which it took some time to recover.

*When the right time meets the right preparation, good things happen.*

We also didn't appreciate how difficult it is to change human behaviors — our own as the prime example.

This reason for procrastination seems to be a lack of understanding of human behavior.

**#3. *Carol*:** We needed to test what we were teaching in our own lives. Dealing with the ups and downs of life goes beyond theory and classroom discussions. My weight control struggle was a major test. If I couldn't settle on a lifestyle plan that worked, how could I teach these principles?

Certain experiences gave a richer context for this material. Wisdom — personal wisdom and shareable wisdom — develop only with time and experience. This is part of the experiment with life.

This reason for procrastination is that experiments in life take time.

Could the time have been shortened by greater discipline?

**#2. *Carol & Al*:** Our entire life experience is wrapped up in this approach to Wellness — how we understand ourselves as individuals, as a couple, as parents, as children, as friends, as members of several communities, as siblings, as co-workers, as business associates, as professionals. That is not easy to summarize and put into perspective.

This reason for procrastination might be that we were overwhelmed with the breadth of the concepts we had synthesized.

**#1. *Carol & Al*:** It's time had not yet come. When the right time meets the right preparation, good things happen. This timing in our lives we think of as divine direction. This is our life on the cosmic level. Do you think we are deluding ourselves?

On the mundane level, we were two damaged psyches in search of healing. We found each other, and the struggle to heal as whole persons has been a time-consuming process. But with healing comes the right time for sharing. We have shared for fifteen years in the classroom and now comes the time to share to the world.

This reason goes beyond our personal reasons and looks to fit within a cosmic plan. The fifteen years were necessary preparation for a work that has been appointed for us to do — a work to spread a message of hope, love, inclusiveness, tolerance and understanding of self and others.

To go the distance, we needed to experience whole-person healing.

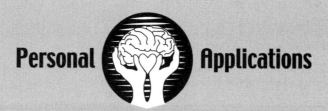

## **Personal Applications**

### **Directions:**

Write the first thoughts that come to your mind when you read the following suggested activities.

1.  Write a letter to your parents (whether they are alive or not), reviewing their feelings and your feelings about the dreams they had for you.

2.  Think about something you have always wanted to do planned to do, or started to do but never completed. Write down the top ten reasons that that something is not yet done.

3.  Rent a copy of the movie "Field of Dreams." After viewing it, write down what may apply to your life as answers to the following questions:

    a.   What must you build and who will come?

    b.   Ease whose pain? Why?

    c.   Go what distance? How?

    d.   Did you hear the voice too? What voice?

    e.   If who was much of a friend, he would have given you the directions himself?

f.  I want whom to stop looking to me for answers?

g.  I want whom to think for themselves?

h.  If you could do anything you wanted, what would it be?

i.  Is there enough magic out there in the moonlight to make such a dream come true?

j.  If you had gotten what you might have stayed where?

k.  Do you ever find yourself looking for "low and away," but getting "in your ear"?

l.  What people will come? From where? For what?

m.  Have you done everything you were asked to do?

n.  What's in it for me?

o.  Do you know something about which you can say, "What a story it will make?"

p.  You can't go back to what?

q.  What do you say to someone who is now worn down with life and you didn't have the chance to let him/her know how you feel?

r.  What is heaven?

## Reflections

This movie, "Field of Dreams," speaks to me of parent-child relationships, and dreams for one another.

* * * * *

The spring and summer after I graduated from high school, and before I started teaching at the same high school, I spent about six months with my dad, planting and harvesting a crop of cabbage. Among the seven of us brothers, I believe that I was the only one who had a chance to spend such concentrated one-on-one time with our dad.

Dad and I never got as close as I now feel with my sons, but those were different times with different psychological factors operating in parent-child relationships. For his eightieth birthday, I had a chance to spend some quiet time with Dad and Mom.

They shared the stories of how they met and fell in love, how they weathered a hurricane together, what their greatest hopes and dreams were for their ten children, and how they thought things had turned out.

They held high hopes for all of us. They never understood why each of us was always at the top of our class through high school, but none of us became a doctor. That was their greatest dream — it seems the dream of every Indian family to have a child who is a physician. I tell them, "If I had gotten a hit, I might have stayed in the game of scientific medicine."

The pain of such a disappointment is not hard to deal with. They are getting over it — especially now that one granddaughter is a physician and one grandson has just started medical school. They have dealt with an even greater disappointment. They never expected to live this long. They didn't expect to die, either.

We talked about their core beliefs and how they had to adjust their beliefs to reality. "It's all part of life," Dad said. "Even though your faith may give you assurances of certain things and certain events, you can never know for sure how things will turn out. The future only God can see accurately."

They shared with me some of the special events of my life. This was the time I felt the closest to my parents. We really were communicating, reaching into each other's heart and soul to touch the individual there. Yet it was not emotionally draining. It was casual conversation. They were just sharing memories.

They told again of how the one-and-one-half-year-old brother before me died of pneumonia before Dad could get back from the doctor's with the medicine needed. They had no car, and Dad rode a donkey the ten miles to the doctor's office. It was too late by the time he got back.

The death of a child has to be the most traumatic of life's events. But with time and other demands of life, you put it into perspective and move on.

According to their understanding of world events, all their children were supposed to be translated from this world into the next without experiencing death. They worked hard for that to happen. They tried to be perfect parents and perfect believers as best they knew how.

With only a fifth grade education, Dad developed preaching abilities that were worthy of a seminarian. Mom never went to school, and it was interesting to see my younger sisters teach her to read.

Mom and Dad did their best with what they had. With hard work and faithful attention to live what they believed, they raised a family of ten.

Education had a great emphasis in their plans, and among us all there are two going on three doctorates, at least nine master's degrees, ten bachelor's degrees and middle-class lifestyles (except for the poor writer!)

Among the grandchildren, there is one physician (another in the making), two lawyers, several holders of master's degrees and everyone will at least graduate from college. They have a lot to be proud of and thankful for.

The few days of quality time I spent with them in April 1996 was one of the treasured times of life. When they die, I don't think I will grieve in any inordinate way. We believe it will be better if Mom goes first, since she is so dependent on Dad. But who knows what will happen? "It's in Gods hands," Mom says. They are prepared to die.

They have no fears or uneasiness when planning for it, but it doesn't occupy any unusual portion of their time and thinking. They have fought a good fight. They are accepting and resigned to how things have turned out.

• • • • •

Mom and Dad, this one's for you. It should ease anything that's left of the pain. Heaven begins here on earth. Maybe this closeness and acceptance we feel now is heaven?

## Carol's Turn

Our children used to poke fun at their father for watching movies like "Field of Dreams," "The Gods Must Be Crazy" and "A Brief History of Time."

How can dead baseball players come back and be seen only by some people?

How can a coke bottle falling from the sky change people so much?

How can humans know what black holes and dying stars look like?

Now they understand. Occasionally, they join him to watch movies along those lines. "If you build it"? Maybe? What have we built for our children? We have more to build.

It takes time to build. Quick fixes, fad diets and weekend seminars can't do it. It has to be a whole-person lifestyle effort. In the process, the mind heals itself, the shattered psyche recovers and whole-person redemption is experienced. We have learned a lot about dealing with depression.

Our heaven on earth is the love and closeness we feel with our three children and our three-year-old granddaughter. We have to share them with other families now, and that enlarges our heaven. Heaven on earth is in the hearts of those with whom you share unconditional love.

To go the distance, it makes a big difference to know and feel the healing power of unconditional love.

# REFLECT ON WHAT HUMANS NEED AND WHAT WE OUGHT TO DO

*"I don't know what your destiny will be, but one thing I know. The only ones among you who will be really happy are those who will have sought and found how to serve."*

Albert Schweitzer

*"In my judgment, it is philosophy, not science, which should be uppermost in any culture or civilization, simply because the questions it can answer are more important for human life."*

Mortimer Adler

*"God grant that not only the love of liberty but a thorough knowledge of the rights of man may pervade all the nations of the earth, so that a philosopher may set foot anywhere on its surface and say: 'This is my country!'"*

Benjamin Franklin

Thirteen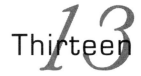

*Dedicated to*

All the students who have taken the HLTH 498P course at University of Maryland University College since it was first offered in 1984. Your input has been extremely valuable in preparing this material for the broader audience.

Special thanks and recognition to **Sandra Fischer**, class of '92, who read the manuscript thoroughly and offered very valuable insights. I felt honored to be mentioned in your class president's address at your graduation ceremony.

Special thanks also to **Judith Hamer**, class of '97, who saw the fit between the course materials and the high school curriculum she was developing at the time.

In the spring of 1967, I spent a weekend with two of my younger brothers on the beautiful island of Bequia. We had a rowboat at our disposal, but our rowing skills were not the greatest — less than average, I'd say.

We decided to cross from one side of the calm, quiet harbor of Port Elizabeth over to the other side just for the fun of it. We knew where we wanted to go, and started out for that spot in a straight line.

As we headed out across the harbor, we realized we were drifting out to sea. We struggled hard to pull against the current, but it was stronger than we were. To complicate matters, the boat sprang a leak. On the verge of panic, we saw a sailboat from the harbor coming towards us.

Some of our friends had seen our predicament and came to the rescue. I still see the strong, muscular sailor twirling the rope over his head as he prepared to toss it over to us. What a feeling of relief as we were towed to the safety of the calm waters of the bay.

. . . . .

It may sound somewhat presumptuous for a physiologist/health educator to tell people what humans need. That is the province of theologians, social scientists, philosophers and, heaven help us, politicians.

My point of view is that those who have taken the time and made the effort to really understand themselves and other people; those who have examined their lives in terms of wellness, fulfillment, happiness and service to humanity; those who seek to integrate body, mind and spirit into a dy-

namic, functional whole have some ideas about what humans need. People's needs are the same everywhere. We share a common nature. We all have solutions in which we believe. Few of us get the chance to share them beyond our most intimate circle.

As a teenager growing up without television or movies, I used to read voraciously. My two favorite sources were the numerous books by E.G. White and Perry Mason novels.

The conflict was that reading E. G. White was approved and encouraged by my parents and my church, while Perry Mason novels were not. So I would read E. G. White (probably fifteen books altogether) in the open, and Perry Mason novels under the covers at night with a flashlight. (I wonder now what effects that had on the development of neurotic behaviors!)

I'm telling this to make a point. Both sources had something to say about what the world needs. Perry Mason always ended his cases by getting a key witness to confess to a truth, which was suppressed all along. Perry Mason would say, then, that the world needs people to tell the truth as they have experienced it firsthand.

A quote from E.G. White, which we memorized in grade school, addresses specifically the "want of the world." It began with " The greatest want of the world is the want of men…"

The entire quote is insightful and may be the reason the title of this chapter came to mind, so I include it here:

The greatest want of the world is the want of men — men who will not be bought or sold, men who in their inmost souls are true and honest, men who do not fear to call sin by its right name, men whose conscience is as true to duty as the needle to the pole, men who will stand for the right though the heavens fall. (Education, p. 57)

## Spirituality and Healing

In emphasizing the role of spirituality in health and happiness, it may seem that I have left the world of science behind and landed in the world of philosophy and theology. I may have. But at this point, I don't believe in separate worlds.

As an individual who seeks personal integration of the best of health, the best of fulfillment, yes, the best of life, I have to use my science, my philosophy, my theology and anything else I have to optimize health and happiness.

It is encouraging to see that science is slowly catching up and moving in the direction of demonstrating that spirituality may have a more primary role in life. It also costs a whole lot less than the scientific, biomedical treatments we have come to rely on. And that might be the crux of the problem of meeting needs. Economic goals may not be the best goals to guide the fulfillment of these needs.

What the world needs now is not more technology for healing the body. The world needs more spirituality for healing the mind and thus enabling and empowering health of the body. It doesn't mean dis-

*What the world needs now is not more technology for healing the body.*

carding science. It means using science, the best of science, to promote the fullest understanding of human needs and to address those needs in an integrated effort.

In 1983-84 when Dr. Burt and I discussed the ideas that led to establishment of the course and this book, it seemed to me that there was only a small, weak voice in academia that called for health education/promotion to address the deeper, more spiritual needs of humankind.

That small voice has now grown into a loud, resounding ground swell. The research is being done with strong scientific design to demonstrate the role of spiritual factors in dealing with the major diseases — heart disease and cancer.

In 1991, I attended the First National Conference on Eliminating Coronary Artery Disease, sponsored by the Caldwell B. Esselstyn Foundation in association with the Cleveland Clinic.

I heard Dr. Dean Ornish present his work in reversing coronary artery disease. This conference was a major statement in applying a total lifestyle approach to the prevention, control and reversal of heart disease and cancer.

But conferences don't change lifestyles.

I recall that I made a one-sentence report on this conference to the group of heart surgeons who sponsored my attendance. "We don't have to worry about the business of coronary artery bypass surgery being affected, because the lifestyle changes required are demanding enough that it would take another twenty years before the general population embraces them." The surgeons continued to do more coronary bypass surgery each year.

Now I believe that the impact is beginning to be felt. The statistics are showing it. Deaths from heart disease have declined over the past five years. In the next fifteen years, the impact of lifestyle changes and any improving techniques at disease management will be far greater. There is a swell of support and a clamor to address felt needs. It is now beginning to make economic sense. That seems to be when things change.

What gives me this optimism is that the pioneers, such as Dean Ornish, are being joined by others from various disciplines in promoting the integrated lifestyle approach that is shown to affect disease processes. They are joined by a mass movement of laypeople who are openly expressing their dissatisfactions with the older biomedical approach to health and healing. The people are voting with their pocketbooks.

In the process, however, we cannot discard sound science. Science is providing support for the role of spirituality in health and happiness.

Steve Hawks of Utah State University presented a review of three major studies that give evidence in this direction. These studies should provide ammunition to push the practice of medicine towards inclusion of spiritual factors and less dependence on expensive technology.

In "Review of Spiritual Health: Definition, Role and Intervention Strategies in Health Promotion" (*American Journal of Health Promotion*, May/June 1995, Vol. 9,

No. 5), Dr. Hawks summarizes the methods and results of three major studies. These are the Ornish study on patients with coronary artery disease, the Spiegel study on patients with breast cancer and the Kabat-Zinn study on stress.

The perspective of his review is to examine the related spirituality factors.

## 1. Ornish on Coronary Heart Disease:

**Methods:** 41 patients with angiographically demonstrated coronary artery disease were assigned randomly to the treatment group (low fat vegetarian diet, stress management training and moderate exercise) or the usual-care group.

**Results and Interpretation:** Significant heart disease reversal was seen in 82% of participants in the treatment group after one year. Patients receiving traditional care continued to worsen. Cost of the treatment was about one-tenth the cost of a single bypass surgery.

Dr. Hawks' interpretation is important:

The major premise behind the lifestyle heart trial's approach to the treatment of coronary heart disease is that the earlier you intervene in the multi-causal chain of illness, the more beneficial the effects. Rather than the biomedical approach of treating the later causal factors of heart disease with surgery, aggressive drug therapy, or both, the heart trial program attempts to emphasize the earliest links in the chain of heart disease.

*It doesn't mean discarding science. It means using science, the best of science, to promote the fullest understanding of human needs and to address those needs in an integrated effort.*

According to the lead researcher, Dr. Dean Ornish, this philosophy reflects the view that a lack of emotional and spiritual health is the most elemental cause of heart disease, because the stress that results from poor emotional and spiritual health influences the development of negative health behaviors that then place the individual at risk for heart disease developing.

He goes on to point out that the program was "intentionally designed to help participants enhance their emotional and spiritual well-being through increased connectedness to self, others and a higher power." This represents "an internal, spiritually-based motivation for lifestyle change rather than an external, risk-reduction (fear)-based motivation."

*How do you teach patients to "live life as fully as possible?"*

To be advocating an internal, spiritually based motivation in comparison to an external risk-reduction or fear-based motivation, is a radical change in approaching heart disease.

## 2. Spiegel on Breast Cancer

**Methods:** 86 patients with metastatic breast cancer were randomly assigned to a treatment group or a usual-care group. Treatment consisted of weekly 90-minute discussion sessions.

"The focus of the program was on living life as fully as possible, and the sessions revolved around seven themes (many of which seem related to components of spiritual health as defined above): encouraging mutual support, coping with dying, developing a life project, realigning social networks, working through doctor-patient problems, enhancing family support and pain control. Each session was composed of members sharing their fears, learning coping strategies for dealing with death, grieving the loss of members, helping each other, learning to savor the preciousness of life, facing disease directly and practicing self-hypnosis for pain control."

**Results and Interpretation:** "At 10-year follow-up, analysis of death certificates indicated that the experimental group had lived approximately twice as long as subjects in the control group who received traditional care only. Additionally, intervention subjects reported only half the pain sensation of control subjects...

"Finally, repeated measures from the Profile of Mood States taken at 4-month intervals showed that control subjects had a substantial worsening of mood, including anxiety, depression, fatigue, confusion, and loss of vigor. Treatment subjects, on the other hand, showed significant improvement in the same mood states during the course of the intervention."

How do you teach patients to "live life as fully as possible"? How might this regimen become incorporated into conventional medical practice?

## 3. Kabat-Zinn on Stress Reduction.

The specific studies are not reviewed. The stress reduction clinic program in general is described and commented on as follows:

"The primary practice of the clinic is group-based mindfulness meditation that includes formal 'sitting' meditation and yoga, as well as informal techniques such as walking meditation and daily mindfulness.

"Participants are encouraged to adopt an attitude of commitment to the program while avoiding a 'goal' orientation. Instead, the attitudes of acceptance and nonjudgment help them find internal, holistic healing through greater self-awareness followed by self-acceptance.

"Like the psychosocial intervention for cancer, the stress reduction clinic does not have a stated goal for enhancing spiritual well-being. Yet, some spiritual health components seem to be targeted such as rearranging priorities to find new meaning and purpose in life, finding a greater sense of connectedness with others, and especially finding more connectedness with self."

## World Needs

So what does the world need? I believe that scientific studies such as those cited above should go on. They show that the greater need in the world is not the need for newer and more expensive technology and drugs and surgery. The greater need now is to integrate and incorporate what we already know — what we have known all along — that spirituality is a key to health, healing and happiness. And the world needs spiritual interventions to address the root causes of the major problems of the human condition.

So here is my list of the top seven needs of the world, and what we ought to do about them.

## The World Needs Integration

This means integration on the individual level, family, community, national and international. Integration on the individual level involves self-understanding, acceptance of personal responsibility to make a positive difference in the world, and to demonstrate a life directed by love.

This then leads to better families where aims and goals are directed toward producing other happy people. Happy people, happy with themselves, produce integrated communities where the value of different peoples is not based on race, gender, size, religion, personality or wealth.

To get to this point, a spiritual renewal on the personal level is the only way. In combination with any higher power in which the individual believes, personal effort at self-understanding and self-management may yield this integration. The challenge is to test as a personal experiment.

America has had a great experiment with integration. The visible fight has been through racial, ethnic and class integration. Everything has not been resolved. It never will be. The government has made positive strides, especially after being forced to do it, but there is still more to be done.

However, most of what is left to be accomplished is in the heart of the individual — respect for diversity and just willingness not to use differences to get in each other's way towards personal integration and wellness. Is that too much to ask of our fellow citizens? No.

But the government can't legislate how you should love me and allow me to be myself. You have to believe that that is right and good to do (even before the research data proves it).

The greatness of integration is that it makes everyone feel a part of the whole — with respect and honor for diversity, individuality and differences. Diversity, more than just strengthening the gene pool, produces greater strength than just the sum of the parts. Integration is more than summation. (That's all I remember from calculus!) The whole is greater, stronger and accomplishes more than the sum of the parts.

Another frontline of integration is the healthcare field. I observed first hand how class and ego and behavioral style get in the way of necessary progress in integration among related specialties. It provided a good contrast to being in the thick of the current effort to integrate complementary and alternative therapies into mainstream medicine. Integration of healthcare is fascinating and exciting work. But it is subject matter for another discourse.

I believe that efforts to integrate on any level in any branch of human endeavor are facilitated when individuals seek personal integration and feel integrated within themselves. What do you see as the personal contribution you are making towards greater integration?

## The World Needs Love

Love means dealing with one another for mutual good, perpetrating no willful hurts and seeking to contribute to the happiness of other than oneself alone. This is what love directs on the personal level, the communal, the national and the international. How do we arrive at this state? Love must be understood and practiced first on the personal level.

Individuals and communities that have love don't victimize one another. There is enough inevitable suffering among human beings without willfully perpetrating more.

A victimizer, moved by love, seeks to make right what can be made right, and apologizes to the victim. A victim, restored by love, moves on with life regardless of what the victimizer does or doesn't do. Love, not sentimentality, is the most positive force for good in the world, but, as Leo Buscaglia said in his book, *Love*, "to love others you must first love yourself."

We ought to ask ourselves how do we understand, demonstrate and practice love? Love in business transactions? Nonsense? Love on our highways? Love at the worksite? Without appropriate love, what respect, tolerance, sensitivity, honesty and integrity mean?

## The World Needs Peace

Peace means inner calm on the personal level, the communal level, the national and the international levels. Peacemakers are people who know how to love and specialize in the practice of the calming effects of love in action.

Peace must begin in your own soul. Peace that says there are anchors to this soul regardless of what is happening around it. Peace that looks for ways to find answers.

It is Utopian to think that everybody wants peace, but if more individuals desire, and lovingly agitate for, and work towards peace in their small corner, what will happen to peace on earth?

## The World Needs Faith

Faith is belief in possibilities and in making impossibilities real. Faith helps us to hang on to the possibilities that love and peace can grow and become a rule of life rather than an ideal of philosophers and religionists. It is a strong abiding faith in the desire for goodness and laying hold of a way to that desirable goodness.

It is a faith to dream impossible dreams about integration, world peace and harmony. The world needs people of faith. Faith grows and is strengthened by exercise.

We ought to examine and define the basis of our own faith and assurance in the eventual triumph of goodness over badness, of life over death and of righteousness over evil. This, I believe, is what drives the human spirit to hope and work towards positive goals with optimism about the outcome.

## The World Needs Hope

Hope means to have something, even a small thing, that indicates that things will get better, that something will work out, that there will be an end to unnecessary pain, somehow, somewhere. Hope draws the human spirit to rise above and transcend today's setbacks and tomorrow's obstacles and forge ahead with the tasks of growing love and peace and faith.

We ought to examine and lay firm hold on and share the hope that is within us, according to our own beliefs.

## The World Needs Liberation

I once heard a series of sermons by a preacher, one of my favorite preachers. His titles, "Liberating Solitude," "Liberating Freedom," and "Liberating Action," gave serious food for thought.

Personal liberation may mean liberation from our own fears, our missed opportunities and our blunders large or small. To forgive oneself and move on to try another time is liberating. To examine one's capabilities and strengthen what needs to be strengthened, to accomplish what is to be accomplished, is liberating. To break the bonds of self-doubt and claim "can do" with realistic appraisal of challenges is liberating. To be free of the stigma of classification based on externals is liberating.

And personal liberation is enhanced and optimized by societal liberation. To answer our own prayers, we must be vigilant to safeguard our freedoms and insist on free, democratic nations to safeguard the freedoms of the world. We have to be active and involved in liberating peoples who are oppressed. We each have a role to play in spreading freedom.

## The World Needs Restoration

Personal restoration is to lift up the fellow citizen when he/she is down. The act may only be in the mind, through recognition of each other's dignity and equality.

Restoration calls for sensitivity to one another's needs, desire for community, for fellowship, for participation, regardless of past mistakes or willful neglect. Acts of restoration reach into and strengthen our capacity to forgive and be gracious.

Restoration on the personal level and restoration on the communal, national and international levels — what does it all mean?

The restorer and the restored both have roles to play — both have responsibilities in the process. On a one-on-one basis, on an institutional level, on a societal level, how do we view forgiveness, punishment, acceptance, penance and restoration?

Families need to be restored. Some family ties need to be built where the opportunity to build was not there before, or was missed. The world and the individual need restoration.

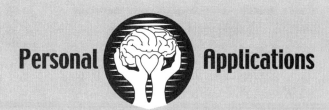

# Personal Applications

## Directions:

Write down the first answers that come to mind as you read the following questions.

1. What do you think the world needs?

2. Who is the most optimistic person you know?

3. Who is the most loving and accepting person you know?

4. Who is the person you know most likely to be an active promoter of peace and harmony?

5. What trouble spots on earth do you know of and what were the original causes of the trouble?

6. Who is the historical figure you dislike the most?

7. Who is the historical figure you admire the most?

# Reflections

So what ought we to do? We have to learn and seek to become better integrators, more effective lovers, risk-taking peacemakers, grounded faith builders, optimistic hope sharers, determined liberators and adventuresome restorers. To this is what personal wellness and self-realization lead.

I would be intellectually dishonest if I concluded this discourse without revealing what, in my belief system, is the final solution. In my belief system, the answer is in the Christ of Christianity. The rules and the doctrines and the rituals are secondary, but my happiness, my wellness and self-realization would be different if I were to throw out Christmas and Easter, the baby and the sacrifice.

During a twelve-week mind/body skills group at the Center for Mind/Body Medicine in Washington, DC, I had the opportunity to examine how all the skills we were practicing connected with our deepest beliefs. In my experience, as I entered into the use of the meditation, guided imagery, mindfulness and spirit-guide processes, I noticed that they tend to reach for an anchor in my belief system. The most effective connection I could make was with the once deeply held religious beliefs.

In the Christ of Christianity, I see a practical example of a life promoting integration, spreading love, making peace, growing faith, inspiring hope, promoting liberation and effecting restoration, for the most people for the longest time.

You may not share this belief. I accept you as equal in your position and respect your belief system as much as I hold to mine. I ask the same respect as a person with a different belief system from yours.

I encourage you to be intellectually honest about your beliefs and propose solutions to the world's greatest needs. We don't have to believe exactly the same, but we can work together to build up each other and a better world. We don't have more time to act. We have less time with each passing hour.

Together, we can find solutions to the things that divide us. That's what the world needs, and that's how we ought to live — with personal wellness and self-realization.

I believe that ultimate personal wellness and self-realization is to settle the question of how the transcendent connection between ourselves and the rest of the cosmos is effected. This is the private anchor from which we then deal with one another to promote health, well-being, wellness and happiness.

If this sounds like bringing religion into the center of the discussion, it is not off the mark. But I like to think of it as spirituality, a spirituality that is promoting an integration of all the meaningful experiences that affect health.

The spiritual dimension transmits energy and life enhancing drives to build up the psyche, bolster the information processor of the mind and rejuvenate the physiology. Much of this is beginning to be understood by our scientific methods, but a lot of it is outside of those techniques.

The debate has been intensified by the recent publication of a paper titled

"Religion, Spirituality, and Medicine" in the prestigious medical journal, *The Lancet*. In a February 1999 issue, Sloan, Bagiella and Powell present a review of the literature from which they conclude that the evidence for positive health effects of spirituality is weak and caution against overzealous inclusion in the medical interaction.

In a special commentary in his journal, *Alternative Therapies in Health and Medicine* (May 1999, Vol.5, No.3), Larry Dossey examines the *Lancet* article and points out that the whole evidence is stronger than the *Lancet* authors determined, and there are good reasons and proper ways for spirituality to be part of the medical encounter. This debate will and should continue. Part of what the world needs is discussion and examination of the evidence.

So now we see non-scientists and scientists, professionals and laypersons, teachers and students, physicians and patients, employers and employees, Third World and First World citizens collaborating to find solutions to what the world needs.

Utopia is an unrealistic place. The reality as we face a new century is that change takes time and work. The time is now, and the work is to promote integration, love, peace, faith, hope, liberation and restoration. We each must find our piece of the work as we look for our piece of the pie.

Brian de Alwis, author of a series of booklets called "Bullock-Cart Theology," quoted the famous Indian poet, Rabindranath Tagore:

*I keep stringing and unstringing my instrument. But I have not yet sung the song I came to sing.*

To find your song, to sing in freedom, to know your instrument — this is personal wellness and self-realization.

So here's my version of the ending to the story with which I began the Preface:

· · · · ·

The young woman had composed an original piece of music which she played on her reed-flute everyday. On one visit to the seashore to celebrate an exceptionally beautiful sunrise, she was caught up in contemplating the horizon. What was beyond? Who was out there? What music was being played by other women in other countries?

She had heard about a land of great freedom and opportunity beyond belief.

She wondered about her people back in the mountain village. Would they believe her report of the beauty of the sunrise? Should she go back to tell them, to convince them to travel to the plains and see for themselves? Would they laugh at her story?

She went down to the docks and bought passage to the land of opportunity.

· · · · ·

The ultimate goal of being human is to go the longest distance for the longest time.

*To find your song, to sing in freedom, to know your instrument — this is personal wellness and self-realization.*

## Carol's Turn

I don't pretend to know what the world needs. I can't address what the world needs. I can only see what people around me need, and I believe that it is love and acceptance for self and others.

I also believe that real-life examples of the struggle with life mean more to me than all the scientific data in all the books and journals. Al keeps reminding me that we must have both.

I hope that our attempt to share our life experiences and insights does not present us as "bleeding hearts." We are not looking for sympathy. We are only sharing what we believe are self-examined lives and humbly suggest that you try the same, in your own way, in your own time.

To go the distance, it helps to be energized by realistic idealism.

# EXPERIMENT WITH PERSONAL WELLNESS

*"Broken bones heal strongest."*

Kenneth Pelletier

Fourteen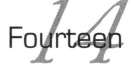

*Dedicated to*


*Two special couples:*


**Gnanaraj and Pam Moses**

*Your support and advice was always timely and very helpful. E.G., you have been a loyal friend and worthy confidante. Pam, sharing the same birthday with our daughter, Annette, has been special to us and we hope she will become the strong, gentle woman you are.*


*and*


**Joseph and Juanita Gurubatham**

*Your example and loving encouragement has made a big difference in our lives — including teaching me a kinder, gentler game of racquetball!*

The chapter titled "Pathways to Love and Intimacy" in Dean Ornish's book *Love & Survival*, begins this way: "There are many pathways to love and intimacy. In the continuing process of learning to open my heart…"

That's what we have been learning over these fifteen years in a classroom on the campus of the University of Maryland — to open the heart. To see this type of learning take place has been rewarding. To feel the level of intimacy built after twenty-five strangers have met for three hours each week for sixteen weeks is transforming. We learn intellectually and fulfill academic requirements. But we learn more about the human condition and how we each endeavor to live authentic lives. We share ourselves with one another not in an emotional, sappy mode, but in honesty and a dignified comfort level that is nurturing.

The idea of this chapter is to point out a few ways in which I have tested in my own life some of the concepts I try to get other people to consider. The time, place and forum for "opening up the heart" will differ for each one. Much of this discussion may feel "squishy" to you if you were expecting science. This is one form of the science of intimacy.

## Experiment #1
# To Stop Eating When I'm Comfortably Full

## Hypothesis

I can be successful at controlling the craving for food and the amount I eat, especially when the eating is for pleasure and delight rather than nutrition.

## Background and Methods

The reason for the effort is the belief that even though I enjoy food so much, in excess, it has the potential to produce long-term pain by precipitating physiologic diseases. My major cravings are for meat and fish — dishes such as Carol's beef stroganoff, Mike's beef balangee (eggplant), Vimala's fish curry, Sue's lamb, goat and chicken byriani and Tom's goat curry. At special occasions for celebrations, I get accused of taking a third helping as my dessert.

My experiment consists of reducing the amount I eat at one time, spreading out the occasions when I have these meals and skipping the dessert. I find that if I eat my salad without dressing, my craving for more is reduced. I also try to increase my exercise during the week following the feast. That is easy for me to do — an extra game of racquetball.

## Results and Discussion

I manage about 75% of the time to keep things in balance. When I overeat, I compensate in the days following. I have been successful in keeping my weight at a fairly constant level for the past twenty-five years and my cholesterol level below 190 mg/dl.

I keep trying to become a vegetarian, which I think is the ideal, but it is a difficult transition for me. Eating loses a lot of its pleasure in vegetarian fare, I find. However, I have increased the amount of fruits and vegetables I consume, and I eat mostly fruits and salads the day after a major feast.

*This is one form of the science of intimacy.*

I pay attention to my overall intake of fat and animal protein to reduce the risks I believe are associated with a diet of animal products. I have been able to reduce the proportion of red meats by using more chicken and fish.

Maybe as I grow spiritually, I will acquire the loss of desire for these pleasures. Or maybe, with enough effort, self-discipline and self-denial, I will acquire the control needed to overcome these cravings for the foods that titillate my palate. Maybe, I will go on the "Hallelujah Diet" and gain those marvelous results people report.

It would be good to get to the point where I have overcome my craving (addiction) for my "soul food," and be able to enjoy a strict vegetarian diet. This, I think, is the ideal. As I contemplate this ideal, I balance my risks, keep tabs on the indicators of imbalance and continue the personal experiment.

## Experiment #2
# To Obtain Regular, Enjoyable Exercise

## Hypothesis

I can be successful at maintaining a regular exercise program with workouts at least three times per week.

## Background and Methods

My temperament, disposition, make-up, call it what you will, is such that I have never been able to stick to any workout routine that does not involve a competitive sport. If I try to jog, run or do aero-bics, I get exhausted in a short time — ten to fifteen minutes.

However, if I play soccer or racquetball, I can last for two hours at close to maximum output. At that point, I experience the "exercise high" — hot and sweaty and deliciously exhausted.

Over the years, I have tried to build into my routine enjoyable activity that gives me the exercise benefit I believe contributes to overall health and well-being. For a time, we had family soccer games on Sundays. This lasted for a few years, but the game became too risky on the knees, ankles and shins, and it was only once a week. So I quit.

Then I made the discovery of a lifetime — racquetball. It is so simple a game to learn, easy to play, and it gives a steady workout with pleasurable exhaustion at the end — whether you win or lose. (But more enjoyable when you win!) This led to a regular exercise program which I have been able to continue for the last fifteen years, and I look forward to keeping it up for the next fifty.

## Results and Discussion

Racquetball takes total concentration. When the mind is thus absorbed, no stressful concerns about work or other problems occupy the consciousness. The body seems to function on reflexes. You do a "dance with the ball," falling into its rhythm of unpredictable bounces and angles off the wall for which you develop reflexive anticipation.

The delicious state of heat and sweat and exhaustion at the end of sixty to ninety minutes of walloping the little blue or green ball is addictive. Especially so when you play studs twenty years younger than you are, and you win more than your fair share of games.

Over a seven-year period, Chuck, Rob and I maintained a standing schedule of playing three times per week. On these mornings, I would awake before the alarm, and, fair weather or not, there was always a feeling of anticipatory excitement on the way to the game.

It was fun while it lasted, but changes inevitably occur, and it came to an end. Now, access to racquetball will be on the list of priorities as we look for our next home.

It helps to maintain a workout schedule with commitment to at least one other person. Some people can discipline themselves to exercise alone or do so in non-competitive activities. For me, I need the "thrill of the competition and the agony of defeat." I imagine as I age I will play a slower game, but I see racquetball in the rest of my future.

## Experiment #3
# To Optimize Sexuality and Sex Education

## Hypothesis

I can actively contribute to building an optimum sex life as one of the mainstays of our marriage and help our children develop a wholesome attitude towards human sexuality.

## Background and Methods

Even though I am a physiologist by training, I used to feel uncomfortable talking about the human side of sexuality as compared to the science. I was pleasantly surprised to find in Mahatma Gandhi's autobiography a discussion of his views on sexuality and the practical application of his beliefs on his family life. This gave me a launching point for discussions on the practical aspects of sex in its social context.

My approach to discussions about optimum sex addresses the subject on four dimensions of function:

1. The physiologic features such as frequency, duration, intensity, positions, gymnastics, G-spots and pleasure centers, nerve traffic, the delicious total nervous system discharge of the sexual climax and the contribution of non-genital nerve centers. (Remember, I flunked my reproductive physiology comprehensive exam on the first try. So I had to study real hard since there was only one more chance.)

2. The mental features such as decision-making, moral codes of behavior, time and place, choice of partner, readiness, family planning, risk-taking, celibacy, monogamy and phase of the life cycle.

3. The psychosocial features such as value of the sex partner, social responsibility, reputation, self-esteem, gender sensitivity and homosexuality.

4. The spiritual features such as whole-person caring and love, appreciation of the gift of sexual pleasure by whomever you believe created sexual reproduction as the method for humans to bond and

procreate, and any transcendent lessons and values imparted by the marriage relationship.

The most experimentation we have been involved in is the sex education of our children. We decided not to leave this up to the schools, their friends or other influences, so we set out a strategy to impart values and information about human sexuality with age-appropriateness. The older children were always involved in preparation for the next child. Questions were always answered matter of factly.

We tried to be the first ones to explain the physiology of human sexuality by setting aside a special weekend for a one-on-one with each child. When we believed the time was right, around eight or nine years of age, I had each boy plan a weekend camp-out for just the two of us. Carol did a similar thing for our daughter. By this time, they had enough background information from everyday life, friends, books, school and TV, to be ready to have a father-son, mother-daughter lesson on this whole area of knowledge. (I think we got that idea from one of Dr. James Dobson's books.)

We shared our values about premarital sex, homosexuality and marriage, but we promised each child that after they were eighteen, we would not carry the responsibility for their choices. We would not keep constant tabs on where they were, what they did or whom they saw. We would trust them to take care of themselves and act responsibly.

Our responsibility for their personal conduct would be over, and they were to have the control to act according to their beliefs and values. We were willing to risk their making mistakes. We let them know explicitly that no matter what happens, they will always be loved and cherished, and nothing they can do will ever cause us to love them less.

## Results and Discussion

The weekend campouts with my boys are fond memories. We have pictures of fishing and boating. The anatomy and physiology book we briefly surveyed included all the organ systems, and I felt special to realize that I was the primary source of this kind of information for my sons. Even so, one question caught me by surprise: "So how do the sperm and the egg find each other to start the single cell that becomes a full-grown baby?" I felt good to be the first to share that piece of information and to set it within the context of a commitment in marriage.

We believe a home atmosphere in which human sexuality is comfortably discussed is important to adolescent adjustment to life and adult responsibilities. However, like other human beings, young adults make mistakes regardless of how much you try to help them avoid it. The two main objectives of parenting on the subject of sexuality are to impart a comfortable attitude towards sex and marriage, and to be prepared to demonstrate how to handle mistakes that young adults make in spite of education.

## Experiment #4
# To Learn to Love a Dog

## Hypothesis

I can learn to love and accept a dog in our home.

## Background and Methods

I grew up in a culture where dogs were kept as watchdogs, slept outside the house, got better on their own when they were sick, and if they got lost or died, it was no big deal.

Carol grew up in a culture where dogs and cats were like members of the family and were loved and cared for as children — including visits to the vet and treatments at all cost. She had a cocker spaniel, Billyboy, for fifteen years!

As the kids came along, they seemed to have inherited their Mom's affinity for dogs, and from the time they could talk, they wanted one. I resisted for over twenty years. Finally, for our twenty-fifth anniversary, the family won my vote to get a dog for Mom. We bought a black American cocker whom David named Apache, after the army helicopter. Carol was more pleased than if she had gotten diamonds!

## Results and Discussions

I was sure to make it clear that I wouldn't clean up after the dog, give him baths, take him on walks, train him or take him to the vet. Apache brought an extra realm of activities to our home. Carol had an additional level of caring to give.

Shortly after Apache became part of the family, my business ventures went sour and we lost our home. Apache was a better anti-depressant for Carol than any prescription. He became so attached to her and she to him that I was drawn into the relationship.

For the first time in my life, I felt an emotional connection to a pet. He is affectionate, protective and playful. I never thought the day would come when I would sit on a couch with a dog beside me with his head in my lap, and I would fondly stroke his head. But it has, and I feel I have grown in a new direction.

## Experiment #5
# To Love a Spouse Who Is Overweight

## Hypothesis

I can be successful at maintaining a healthy relationship with my wife and recognize that other qualities and attributes are more important than her physical shape.

## Background and Methods

As a teenager, I was very idealistic. One of my conclusions about mate selection was that I would not place physique at the top of the list of qualities I would look for in a woman. I would first get to know the person and assess shared goals and dreams and spiritual fit before physical characteristics were factored in.

I have had a chance to see how those ideals play out. In a culture that places great emphasis on physical appearance, being the husband of an overweight woman is a stigma second only to being an overweight woman. Some of the feelings associated with this relationship result from my sensitivity, self-esteem and temperament, and the acceptance and support of the social group in which I am comfortable.

The "problem" was only very mild at the beginning of the relationship, and I believed that we would each contribute to helping each other reach and maintain good physical shape. We were both in medical work, yet we didn't have any understanding or ideals of health promotion. Consequently, our health promotion goals were not explicit.

## Results and Discussion

One of the situations I have studied is the feeling that comes with walking into a room full of people with one of the larger women in the crowd on my arm. It takes an act of mental discipline to deal with the self-consciousness and brush aside the obvious interpretation of people's stares. It is most likely compounded by the difference in skin color — brown man and white woman. It took many years to develop the reflexes to quiet these uncomfortable feelings.

Some other sensitive men know the feeling of which I speak. You make the best of these occasions. You try to not feel the way you feel, but you cannot shut off the feelings. They seem to be programmed. You take cognitive control, rationalize and try to get absorbed in the occasion.

But afterwards, you gently remind her of the current weight loss and conditioning plan she is working on. You lovingly say, "Is there anything more I can do to be of help? You know I only want this for your health. But you must get to

the place where you want it for yourself so strongly that it becomes your priority. You do that in your own time. Regardless of what happens, I will always be here for you."

Then you examine your own feelings, and you see the truth that health, her health is a good reason, but at the top of your list is her looks — the conformance to fashion that you idealistically tried to ignore. You have now capitulated to the culture.

So you think about gentle love and tough love. How do you really help? You see the struggle and you conclude that the simple equations of input, output and energy expenditure are skewed. There has to be something more. She seeks medical help. They offer drugs. She refuses. You agree.

So you encourage and hope. You count the good qualities, and you conclude that everything else is right and good but for this one thing. And you continue to love with faith and hope and attitude adjustment to counterbalance walking into the next social affair with feelings of discomfort.

To every overweight person, smoker, alcoholic, short person, bald person, untanned or overtanned person, whatever the reason for your feelings of being inadequate, unattractive, self-conscious or unaccepted, may you have someone to love and support your efforts to be comfortable with yourself, wherever that may lead.

To those who love and live with people with various health risks, may you and I grow to a comfortable acceptance of ourselves as we are, accept others for what they are, and offer love and support without the mental oppression we sometimes exert.

## Experiment #6
## To Practice "Other-worldly" Consciousness

### Hypothesis

I can develop the spiritual dimension of my life by practicing certain rituals and rites that make me feel connected to higher powers on a daily basis.

### Background and Methods

As a teenager, I took my religion seriously. I believed that it was a good thing to practice the presence of God — develop a sense of being where you are always with the highest power in which you believe.

The method of cultivating this was to have formal, kneel-down prayers three times each day, to say grace before every meal and to read a selected portion of scripture or religious writing each day. So I kept up the effort for as long as it felt functional to my well-being, and as long as it remained part of my belief as a requirement for spiritual growth.

### Results and Discussion

When a ritual or routine is fresh, it seems to be very enjoyable, stimulating and functional. When it becomes overused and just a mechanical, scheduled, an out-of-obligation-or-fear event, it loses its enjoyment and purpose and becomes a burden.

Over the past thirty years, I have had many reasons to reflect and adjust my religious rituals, practices and beliefs. The one that I think remains intact in mind, but not in outward behavior, is the practice of God-consciousness. It has matured to a place where I believe it is more functional now, yet stripped of the outward signs, schedules and obligatory practices.

## Experiment #7
## To Rob God

### Hypothesis

I can restructure my belief about what it means to rob God, and maintain comfort and peace with my conscience.

### Background and Methods

I was indoctrinated very early in life with the belief that it was a requirement of serving God to pay at least 10% of total income to the church as "the tithe." Additional offerings were required but the tithe was holy, and any failure to pay a full tithe was robbing God.

Seeing the affluence and what I thought of as fiscal mismanagement in the church in America, I decided to send my tithe back home to the Caribbean. Then, when my local church had financial difficulties, I reassigned my tithe to local budget instead of the prescribed channel. Later, when my family had financial difficulties, I quit paying the tithe altogether.

### Results and Discussion

Part of the personal debate with this practice depends on the belief about the relationship between self and God, the question of sin and guilt, the question of forgiveness and repayment, the authority of the church, and the best way to stimulate reform. This is an experiment in progress. It is an experiment of a higher order for the soul since it touches on the deepest relationships of human lives — self, authority, sin, guilt and righteousness, and, of course, money and God.

After several years of disregard, I have renewed the vow of my earlier conviction. How do I affect change and help balance inequities yet maintain a comfortable conscience? It is an experiment in progress.

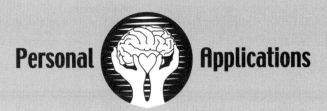

# Personal Applications

## Directions:

Review your experience to identify areas where you feel you have experimented with important questions about life, health and wellness, and evaluate the results or outcomes.

Some of the parameters to consider are:

1. We all experiment with life. Life on earth may be the biggest experiment in the universe.
2. One person's experiments may be another person's self-evident, simple, everyday truth.
3. Safety in experimentation is the experimenter's responsibility. Experimentation with obviously risky possibilities should be carefully evaluated.
4. There is a background of information necessary for every experiment. Sometimes there is insufficient information, and it may be prudent to wait before experimenting. A recent example of insufficient information, in my opinion (and I've heard some experts agree), is on DHEA (dehydroepiandrosterone), a steroid hormone, and Melatonin, a hormone that regulates the sleep-wake cycle. In my opinion, these drugs were sold to the public as non-prescription items before there was sufficient information about their effects, especially long-term effects. With this belief, I have not been willing to experiment with these products.
5. Moderation, the middle road, is most often the safer course in many areas, especially where there is a lack of clear evidence.
6. Check with the experts. There is a lot of good information, and there is a lot of bad information, out there on many subjects. The best experts are those who are dedicated to uncovering knowledge without the possible biases of the profit motive. I like to check with university-based researchers.
7. Check out the experts. Some experts have had major impact on our beliefs and practices, but their "scientific findings" were later determined to be flawed. The examples that come to mind are the Kinsey reports on sexuality published as *Sexual Behavior in the Human Male* (1948) and *Sexual Behavior in the Human Female* (1953).

Rachel Wildavsky, Senior Staff Editor at *Reader's Digest*, in a recent article on "Sex, Lies and the Kinsey Reports" (*Reader's Digest*, April 1997), explains several of the biases and flaws in the methods and background that led Alfred Kinsey to the conclusions he made from his data. A most interesting point for me was "Kinsey believed that sex was a simple, biologic reaction to stimuli with no moral, spiritual or psychological dimension." His work had a profound impact on the sexual revolution of the sixties.

The Hite Report on sexuality was also flawed in its research methodology. The sample was skewed, yet the results were accepted as practices of the general population.

## Reflections

The format of the above experiments is only a device to promote thinking about lifestyle changes and evaluation. The confounding problem is that there is so much good information and so much mis-information out there that sometimes we feel confused. One of the responsibilities for parents and educators is to help children build a belief system that promotes healthy pleasures in all dimensions.

Citing the above personal experiments is a means of bringing to the reader's attention examples of adventures in personal wellness. There is no attempt to value one belief over another, or to suggest that these exact experiences and experiments are relevant to anyone else. They may be, but that is not the purpose of relating them.

The purpose of sharing them (at some personal risk) is for illustration of what wellness encourages. This is the nature of wellness. It is unique to the individual's beliefs, life experiences, concept of natural and supernatural forces and relationships. What I hope to accomplish by these rather private disclosures is to challenge the reader to try the process.

It would be naive of me to think that this is a new idea. From what my students tell me, many individuals are engaged to some degree in testing and evaluating life experiences in a similar fashion. It is not the stuff of general conversation. It is part of the private quest for fulfillment. Yet it is to be encouraged when someone else is open enough to share his/her private quest in a serious forum.

This chapter brings me full circle in the discussions from physiology to spirituality. The integrated whole is the fully functioning person. Regardless of limits or challenges or deficits or loss, every person is a whole person, the unit of wellness and self-realization.

To go the distance, intimacy is rocket fuel.

## Carol's Turn

Experiments in family life add a sense of challenge and fun. I recall Al describing his first experience with Yoga when he was at the University of Maryland in 1984. At the time, he was concerned about how the church leaders would view such out-of-the-mainstream practices. Now, he talks about how to adapt useful practices with less concern for what others think about it.

Another experiment that produced practical benefits for our family was a relaxation technique. It included a taped visualization and a back massage that ended with the "feather-light touch." The kids thought it was very effective, but it led to a habit where they wanted this "back rub" very often.

My personal experiment has been with weight control. It is an everyday battle. The physiology and the psychology of obesity are not simple. I am now learning, from an expert who worked as a physician in the Ohio State University weight management program, about the hormonal factors in severe obesity. Some of this new information offers hope for dealing with this problem on a long-term basis.

This experiment has been a lot of struggle with periods of hope and discouragement, failures and successes, and challenge to rise above stigmatization. It is mostly hard work.

My most recent experiment with weight was use of a combination meal replacement and an herbal extract. This was a physician-supervised study. It worked well enough that I lost fifteen pounds in three months. But I got tired of the taste. It was making me nauseous to use it twice each day. I know some people who enjoyed it. Is there something wrong with me? Why can't the same thing that someone else uses successfully work for me? Could my depression at the time affect my body so differently? I believe it did. One participant in the same study lost forty-five pounds in six months. I accept my individual difference and experiment with something else.

One of the most enjoyable experiments I undertook was learning the techniques of whole-body massage. Al began to experiment with this during the year he spent in the Department of Health Education at the University of Maryland. He explained the physiology of deep receptor stimulation and superficial receptor stimulation. We bought a book on massage therapy and learned some techniques.

It is now interesting to see that massage therapy is being merged into mainstream healthcare.

Other experiments we have tried have to do with the following:

1. Nutritional supplements — we both have a serving of Spirulina in skim milk every morning, and it has made a big difference in our joint pains, which were getting worse after forty. (Note: this is personal experiment, not science.)
2. Pain control without drugs — we have tried natural methods of pain control and less dependence on over-the-counter or prescription drugs. Relaxation techniques seem to have very good effects.
3. Daily gratitude list — I think this came from Oprah Winfrey. She encourages her viewers each day to make a list of things for which they are grateful. It also fits with the philosophy of Hans Selye, who talked about the other side of gratitude — to do things to earn other people's gratitude without expecting anything in return.
4. Music as a spiritual experience — music like Handel's "Messiah" and Brahms's "Requiem," Rutter's "Gloria" and the spirituals like "Nobody Knows the Troubles I've Seen" are soul-inspiring. More so when you sing with a choir than if you just listen to them. It is so uplifting and deeply spiritual. I don't see popular music having the same effect.

   One of the best experiments we have tried was to get a group of college students together, practice some easy but enjoyable pieces in four-part harmony, and travel around to churches to sing and give motivational talks. I miss this. Maybe someday, we can do this again.
5. My experiment for the future is to find a way to work with children — here or in India. I believe to give love and caring in the early years of life is the most fulfilling thing a human being can do.

The best experiment about health and wellness I know is how to find joy in life despite all the hassles. It seems to involve the simple, everyday things.

To go the distance, I must look for the joy that fuels the struggle.

*Life goes on. There is always hope for renewal.*

# CONTEMPLATE THE FUTURE OF HEALTHCARE: INTEGRATIVE MEDICINE?

*"When health is absent, wisdom cannot reveal itself, art cannot become manifest, strength cannot be exerted, health becomes useless and reason is powerless."*

Herophilus

*Mark Twain calls on some new neighbors: "My name is Clemens, Sam Clemens. We ought to have called on you before, and I beg your pardon for intruding now in this informal way, but your house is on fire."*

Mark Twain

*"Above all," the doctor said, "you must eat more fruits, and particularly the skin of the fruit. The skin contains all the vitamins. What is your favorite fruit?" The patient looked confused and discouraged. "Coconuts," he said.*

Toastmaster's Treasure Chest

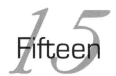

*Dedicated to*

*Two groups that are memorable examples of comfortable integration:*

*Rockville Full Life Fellowship*

*and*

**The Summer '99 Mind/Body Skills Group** *at the Center for Mind/Body Medicine, Washington, DC (Nancy, Jerry, Judy, Edith, Louise, Barbara, Rachel, Lori, Al & Maria).*

The goal of this chapter is to present a very brief overview of the current efforts to integrate healthcare, and to paint a picture of what a healthcare system of the future may offer. This brings the framework for personal wellness promotion full circle — person-centered with supporting systems.

We started out in Chapter 1 with a conceptual framework that took the eighteenth century model of knowledge and healthcare as a starting point, reviewed the changes brought about by scientific medicine and noted the progression of models that led to the Health Promotion Model. Personal wellness and personal responsibility is the core of this new model. We cannot rely on the conventional healthcare system for our entire healthcare needs.

Where are we today and where are we headed? How do we integrate the many options into a cooperative system where the consumer, not economics or technology, is the main object of care?

My thoughts on this subject were greatly influenced by the book *Fundamentals of Complementary and Alternative Medicine*, edited by Marc Micozzi, MD, PhD. It was my first exposure to a comprehensive source within mainstream science- and medicine on the various therapies and practices which, as a hard-core science trained individual, I had regarded as quackery or second-class medicine.

More than the book, the personal relationship with Dr. Micozzi led to my serious evaluation of the newest trend in healthcare — the move towards integration. I was privileged to have close contact with practitioners from several specialties in healthcare, and to study the models of integration that are even now in the process of development.

Exposure to other books followed. Along with reviewing the books, conversations with the authors were most helpful. I am particularly indebted to those among the following who sent me copies of their work and who took the time to discuss the subject:

1. Adrianne Fugh-Berman, MD. Dr. Fugh-Berman, author of *Alternative Medicine: What Works* (1996), is a medical officer with the National Institute of Child Health and Human Development, a practitioner in alternative and complementary medicine at clinics in Washington, DC, and President of the National Women's Health Network. Her book is a concise review of the science (pro and con), history and practice of alternative therapies.

2. Mary Morton and Michael Morton, PhD. Dr. and Mrs. Morton have co-authored, *Five Steps in Selecting the Best in Alternative Medicine: A Guide to Complementary & Integrative Health Care* (1996). Mary tells of her personal experience in reversing her severe scoliosis through the process of partnering with an expert practitioner of the deep tissue bodywork technique known as Hellerwork. Michael relates the process of searching that led him to find an approved treatment for prostate cancer that was available in Canada and Europe but not in the USA. Using that treatment and the new outlook of hope and inspiration that resulted from the process, his dad lived seven years longer than doctors had predicted. This volume is a guide to the process of exploration, selection and partnering with the appropriate licensed practitioners who can

complement the medical care dispensed by the conventional healthcare system.

3. Jennifer Jacobs, MD, MPH. Dr. Jacobs, consulting editor for the book *The Encyclopedia of Alternative Medicine* (1996), was a member of the program advisory council of the Office of Alternative Medicine at the National Institutes of Health (NIH). She has combined homeopathic approaches with her practice of family medicine. The book is a colorfully illustrated synopsis of the majority of the alternative therapies.

4. Don Powell, PhD. Dr. Powell, President of the American Institute for Preventive Medicine, has authored several books and booklets on self-care. He distributes materials and programs on disease prevention and lifestyle modification. His booklet, *HealthyLife: Self-Care Guide* (1997), and his book, *Health At Home: Your Complete Guide to Symptoms, Solutions and Self-Care* (1997), give practical help in applying knowledge and techniques that enable consumers to participate more confidently in the process of their healthcare.

After reviewing these sources, talking with many of the authors and other experts and laypersons, and recalling our own experiments with alternative therapies, these are the conclusions we arrived at:

1. There is a crush of information, and it is a massive headache to weed out the good from the not so good. Everyday, it seems like every newspaper, every TV station and radio program offers new information on some health subject. A person can't know everything or follow everything.

We keep an open mind to new information but wait for more information on a subject before trying anything new. We do not want to be pioneers for new treatments. Maybe, at some point of desperation, we may chose to be pioneers. Yet we are open to experimentation if the product, procedure or process has good odds not to cause harm and may be helpful.

The information overload occurs because of better consumer education and the advances in media. For example, between 1910 and 1970, it used to take about ten to twenty years for the results of many scientific studies to move from the laboratories to practitioners and consumers. The process was orderly: publish in the peer-reviewed science journal, discuss at meetings, confirm results with more research, publish in review articles, include in textbooks, teach the health practitioners, and use and educate the public.

In the 1990s, the process is reversing: release the news to the public via the competing media before the scientific journal comes off the press, and let the practitioners catch up as they can. Case in point: a study on the dangers of the appetite suppressant, fen/phen, was published in the August 18, 1997, issue of the *New England Journal of Medicine*. The results were that this weight reduction drug is associated with heart valve problems in people who had no other risk factors for valvular disease. The news of this study was released to the media in the first week of July 1997.

To deal with the information overload, we use the sources in which we have had confidence for other science and health matters. For example, when DHEA and Melatonin were popularized and available over the counter, we waited for more information. The National Institute on Aging issued a report and advised against their use. This report can be obtained free of charge from the NIA by calling 1-800-222-2225, or at http://www.nih.gov.nia.

Other good sources of information are:

a.  National Center for Alternative and Complementary Medicine at the NIH (1-888-644-6226) or website http://nccam.nih.gov.

b.  The FDA *Consumer Magazine* (1-800-532-4440 or website http://www.fda.gov); and the HealthFinder website (www.health finder.gov).

    We recently used this source to review the history and make a decision on the use of homeopathy. We received the gift of a detoxification treatment from a friend who is a pharmacist and expert in homeopathic remedies. Our natural instincts, based on our background and beliefs, were against its use. However, it came highly recommended. We found a six-page article in the *FDA Consumer Magazine* (April 1997) about homeopathy, its history and the theories on which it is based. We are still making up our minds about trying this cellular detoxification regimen.

c.  Universities with medical schools: many of the major medical schools have courses in alternative and complementary medicine. Harvard Medical School's course is titled "Alternative Medicine: Implications for Clinical Practice." Many medical schools are establishing divisions to research and teach complementary medicine. The University of Maryland Medical School has a division of Complementary Medicine within the specialty of family practice in the Department of Medicine. One of the research projects sponsored by the Office of Alternative Medicine (NIH) has to do with acupuncture.

2.  Distributors and retail merchants are not the best sources of information or recommendation of products and therapies.

3.  There is a lot of quackery out there, and if basic principles of human function are understood, it may help to avoid some of the quackery.

4.  The emerging healthcare delivery system will be a combined practice where the best of scientific medicine is practiced, where other practitioners are part of the process, where research to establish and understand alternatives is undertaken, and where the best interest of the patient as a mind/body whole is at the core of the philosophy of healthcare.

This model will include cradle-to-grave care with prevention as the primary care, use of the least invasive and least expensive measures first with progression to more intensive measures as needed. Full partnership with an educated consumer, reduction of lifestyle risks, optimization of human function and promotion of fulfillment and happiness will be part of care. Personal responsibility and cooperation with professional care will become the norm. Spirituality will play a major role and philosophy will be as important as the science.

5. The best practitioners, in our opinion, are experienced medical doctors (MD graduates of high quality medical schools) who have taken the time to become educated in nutrition, lifestyle management, alternative and complementary therapies, and who work in collaboration with licensed practitioners of these therapies with respect for each other's expertise.

Examples of the move towards integration are seen in several business models, and several insurance companies and state health departments. In most cases, medical doctors take the lead in organizing the program and coordinate care with naturopaths, nutritionists, chiropractors, acupuncturists and others. In some cases, the alternative practitioner is the lead organizer and collaborates with the MD physician. A few of these, all started in the 1990s, are:

1. American Whole Health started by David Edelberg, MD, with headquarters in Reston, VA, and centers in Bethesda (MD), Chicago, and Denver.

2. Arizona Center for Health and Medicine started by Mercy Healthcare network. Samuel Benjamin, MD, was the medical director and one of the chief architects of this program.

3. The New England Center for Integrative Health started by Robert Rufsvold, MD.

4. Columbia-Presbyterian Complementary Care Center opened in 1995 to test alternative and complementary therapies as applied to patients undergoing heart surgery. Research design and methodologies are used in structured trials of the effects of relaxation and therapeutic touch, for example. The program has expanded to include other areas of medicine such as oncology and neurology.

5. Geffen Cancer Center and Research Institute started by Jeremy Geffen, MD, in 1994, in Vero Beach, FL.

6. Complete Wellness Centers, Inc., a network of integrated clinics started by former congressman Tom McMillen in 1995. This approach starts with an existing chiropractic clinic and adds an MD, with other practitioners brought in as needed in each Complete Wellness Medical Center.

7. Celebration Health, next to Disney World in FL, is probably the most ambitious of these new approaches to the study and modeling of the new healthcare. Launched in November 1997, Celebration Health is a collaboration between the Disney Company and Florida Hospital in Orlando. One of the goals is to establish and monitor all aspects of health and well-being in a model city built under the paradigm of whole-person healthcare from cradle to grave. The programs established and studied here will be extrapolated to communities throughout the country.

The above programs combine treatment, prevention and conventional medical care with some level of alternative and complementary therapies. They deal with behavioral, psychosocial and spiritual matters as well as the physical.

HMOs are beginning to offer coverage for alternative therapies. States such as Washington and Oregon are offering services in their state-sponsored programs that include use of alternative therapies.

In the midst of all this change and discussion of change, there is a danger that some simple, basic components get neglected. For example, people seem to get excited about exotic therapies and supplements (DHEA and Melatonin, for example) and lose sight of common health promotion such as thorough hand-washing, giving up smoking, losing weight and increasing physical fitness.

I see the new paradigm aiming at:

1. increasing and maintaining the basic preventive measures;
2. using self-care and lifestyle change;
3. utilizing a stepped approach with simple, more natural (more often, less expensive) remedies tried before drugs and surgery are recommended;
4. including documentation and research to substantiate outcomes and quality of care that may shed light on the best combination of therapies; and
5. taking full advantage of the placebo effect.

The scientific method was very careful to rule out the placebo effect — to establish the intrinsic effectiveness of a product or procedure apart from the individual belief and individual variability. This is an area of debate and research. Since our belief system contributes to the physiologic responses, there seems to be a place for the therapeutic use of this effect.

The aim of this brief overview is to stimulate thoughts and actions in relation to the current trends in healthcare and to examine personal use of the new approaches that are emerging.

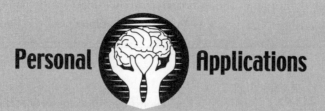

# Personal Applications

## Directions:

Write down your first thoughts as you read these questions or statements and follow up with decisions to take some action where it may help with your use of the healthcare system.

1. Have you used any alternative or complementary therapies in the past?

2. Are you currently using any alternative or complementary therapies?

3. Is your primary physician a mainstream MD or an alternative practitioner?

4. If your primary care physician is an MD and if you use alternative therapies, have you discussed that subject with your doctor?

5. What self-care practices do you use as part of your personal responsibility for your health?

6. What would you like to see happen for the improvement of healthcare services that affect you and your family?

# Reflections

The media seem to spew out articles every day on some aspect of integrating healthcare. One of the major articles to fuel the debate appeared in the *New England Journal of Medicine* in 1993. In this paper, titled "Unconventional Medicine in the United States: Prevalence, Cost and Patterns of Use," Dr. David Eisenberg and his colleagues reported that in 1990 about sixty million Americans used alternative therapies at a cost of $13.7 billion. Furthermore, the estimated number of annual visits to alternative practitioners exceeded the number of visits to all primary care physicians.

Dr. Eisenberg has followed up that paper with one that appeared in the *Annals of Internal Medicine* in July 1997. In this paper titled, "Advising Patients Who Seek Alternative Medical Therapies," a step-by-step strategy is given to guide the mainstream physician in taking the initiative to direct the course of the patient's involvement with alternative therapies. This represents a major step towards integration. The patient is the beneficiary of the process, and the case for insurance coverage of alternative services is strengthened.

A more recent survey by the Eisenberg group was reported in the *Journal of the American Medical Association* in 1998. This study showed that 42.1% of adults in the USA used some form of alternative therapies in 1997 and spent $27 billion out of pocket for these treatments.

It seems that the major influence on the move to integrate medicine is grass-roots agitation by consumers. Voting with the pocketbook gets the attention of professionals. However, there is a core of professionals who help to steer the movement. These are open-minded enough to be inclusive yet set standards to safeguard the well-being of the consumer. But the educated consumer is the key figure in the movement.

Other influences on the direction of the integration process include the following:

1. **The US Congress.** In June 1997, I had the unexpected privilege of sitting in the office of Congressman Peter DeFazio, Representative from the Fourth Congressional District of Oregon, to listen to his description of two bills he is sponsoring in Congress. One, the "Access to Medical Treatment Act," will recognize the rights of consumers to elect to be treated by any licensed health practitioner with any therapy the individual requests, as long as there is no evidence the treatment causes harm. This will broaden use of and access to alternative therapies. (This should provide an opportunity to make better use of placebos!) There are safeguards built in for informed consent and against misleading claims and false labeling.

The other bill was titled "Establishment of the National Center for Integral Medicine." This legislation is aimed at elevating the Office of Alternative Medicine in the National Institutes of Health to the status of a full center with an annual budget comparable to what is currently spent on dental research — $198 million. The current Office of Alternative Medicine has an annual budget of $12 million. The new center will have an Office of Disease Prevention, Office of Behavioral and Social

Science Research, and an Office of Dietary Supplements.

I believe that these bills are moving healthcare in the United States towards the integration that will give the consumer broader options in prevention and treatments. I support, and encourage others to support, these bills.

The Congress passed legislation in the fall of 1998 establishing the National Center for Alternative and Complementary Medicine at NIH. The Access to Medical Treatment Act is still alive and will be reintroduced in late July 1999. The Senate is currently debating the "Patient's Bill of Rights" to govern the power of Health Maintenance Organizations.

2. **Universities.** Universities are making bold advances towards integration. Case in point: the University of Bridgeport in Connecticut is in the process of opening the nation's fourth school of naturopathic medicine. According to Dr. James Sensenig, the interim Dean of the College of Naturopathic Medicine, "The naturopathic curriculum will be as rigorous and stringent as conventional medical curricula." The scientific course-work will be similar to that of conventional medical schools with courses in anatomy, physiology, microbiology and pathology. The additional course-work will include clinical nutrition, homeopathic medicine, botanical medicine, Oriental medicine, counseling and stress management. (For more information, call 203-576-4109.)

There are ten Complementary and Alternative Medicine (CAM) Research Centers which conduct research on alternative treatments. These were established at major universities with funding from the Office of Alternative Medicine at the NIH (see *Complementary and Alternative Medicine at the NIH*, Vol. IV, No. 2, April 1997, obtained free of charge by calling 1-888-644-6226). They include:

a. Bastyr University — Center for CAM Research on HIV/AIDS;

b. University of Maryland, Baltimore, Center for CAM Research on Pain;

c. University of California, Davis — Center for CAM Research on Asthma, Allergy and Immunology;

d. Stanford University — Center for CAM Research on Aging;

e. University of Texas School of Public Health — Center for CAM Research on Cancer;

f. University of Virginia School of Nursing — Center for CAM Research on Pain; and

g. Columbia University College of Physicians and Surgeons — Center for CAM Research on Women's Health.

3. **The Internet.** There is a lot of junk on the Internet. There is also a lot of good information. Websites are multiplying exponentially. A few of the sites I have used and have found excellent information and health promotion helps from both conventional and alternative perspectives are:

— www.columbia.net — This is an online health risk appraisal the page /hra/hral.html.

— www.sunsite.unc.edu — This has information on herbal medicine at the page /herbs, and a behavioral temperament evaluation known as the Keirsey Temperament Sorter at the page /jembin/mb.pl.

— www.wellweb.com and www.healthy.net — Two sites with major sections in alternative and complementary medicine.
— www.drkoop.com is an excellent place to start with any health search.
— www.discoveryhealth.com is the most recent and most comprehensive one I've come across so far.

There are many other websites that have good information if you have the time and patience to stay in front of the computer screen. I still prefer perusing the journals in the library.

4. **Andrew Weil. MD.** Dr. Weil is probably the most influential single person in popularizing the use of alternative therapies and plant medicines.

After graduating from Harvard, Weil did not take the customary internship and residencies. He spent three-plus years in South America studying medicinal plants and herbs. He then devoted his career to teaching, writing and lecturing on alternative therapies. A recent article in *Time* (May 12, 1997) gives a brief review of his work and his philosophy.

Weil writes for the popular market, and his books *Spontaneous Healing* and *8 Weeks to Optimum Health* remain on the best-seller lists.

I'll close this chapter with two reminders:

1. Beware of quackery. The *FDA Consumer Magazine* for June 1995 reported on two fraudulent medical devices. One was called the InnerQuest Brain Wave Synchronizer, which was promoted to relieve stress by altering brain waves. It consisted of an audiocassette and eyeglasses that emitted sounds and flashing lights. The only effects observed were to cause epileptic seizures in some users. In June 1993, an estimated $200,000 worth of the devices were seized by US Marshals and destroyed.

The other device was the High Genki machine for the treatment of diabetes, high blood pressure, muscular pain and arthritis. "It beeped, buzzed and gave mild electric shocks." It was seized and destroyed in November 1993.

2. The primary responsibility for health rests with the individual. The primary responsibility for illness rests with the physician. A partnership is needed to provide the best of prevention, health promotion and illness care.

My colorectal cancer screening kit sits on the desk next to my computer as I write this chapter. I received it three, maybe four, weeks ago. I am supposed to do certain things, get stool samples and mail them to the lab. This has been shown to be an effective tool in early detection of colon cancer.

I have no impetus to do this task. This is part of self-care. I know I should do it, I believe I should do it, I promise myself I would do it, but I haven't yet. Why? I shouldn't wait on "a feeling of readiness." I should just do it because it is good to do it.

*The primary responsibility for health rests with the individual. The primary responsibility for illness rests with the physician.*

I need to push myself. I need to deal with the reasons for procrastination.

It is time for another physical, so I'll call and make an appointment to see the physician. This will help to get me to do the unpleasant task of collecting a stool sample to send in for screening.

So how do you integrate self-care, alternative therapies and mind/body/spirit medicine?

The steps are:

1. Seek to understand yourself as a whole person.
2. Set up a self-management plan for preventive health in consultation with your primary care practitioner.
3. Seek credible information on the complementary and alternative therapies, and ask your primary care practitioner to incorporate these into your care plan. Share your sources of information with your primary care practitioner.
4. Learn and use a specific mind/body technique such as the Benson relaxation technique.
5. Use meditation and mental imagery that connect with your core beliefs about spirituality.
6. Experiment with wellness in everyday living.
7. Learn to let go of the past, live in the present and vision a desirable future.

To go the distance, integration on the personal, professional and social levels makes sense.

## Carol's Turn

In an effort to avoid back surgery, I took the advice of a friend and tried a chiropractor. Our friend had related his story of how he went to the chiropractor's office barely able to walk and was instantly healed by an adjustment.

I wasn't that fortunate. The roughness of the manipulation and the sudden twists and jerks on my spine seemed to make things worse. I ended up having back surgery. That was in 1983.

Since then, I have visited a different chiropractor who used gentler techniques along with massage and electrical stimulation of the muscle. I did have some positive results from this.

I still am not making the progress I desire in regaining physical fitness. I am now in discussions with a new endocrinologist who has ordered a full pituitary-thyroid-adrenal evaluation. I don't cheat on meals. I exercise. Al eats three times what I eat, and he loses; I gain.

In some areas of health promotion, I believe that psychosocial and spiritual issues may have to be dealt with before the physical issues. It may be that there is more healing in the spirit than in the body. I thought I had dealt with all my issues. Maybe I have not. I'll try that again. I am reading *Prayer Warriors* by Ron Halverson. Al says that the healing power of prayer is a topic of scientific research. Imagine that!

Last month, I attended a weekend workshop conducted by Iyanla Vanzant, author of *Yesterday, I Cried: Celebrating the Lessons of Living and Loving*. The title of the workshop was "The Wonder-Woman Weekend." What a joy to fellowship with women from all over the country who are working on letting go of the past and building an optimistic future! This type of healing has to become part of conventional healthcare.

Will the healer of the future be a praying herbalist trained at Harvard with an internship in Peking? This new breed of doctors will have to spend a long time in school. It may be better to have several of them pooling their expertise to meet the needs of each patient. But who will pay for it all?

Ouch! I feel the pinch in the pocket book. I didn't mean to end on a note of pain. This work was supposed to be about healthy pleasures!

To bring about integration, people have to be courageous. Kenneth Pelletier says in his book *Sound Mind, Sound Body*, "A courageous person is not without fear but is one who accepts the fear and proceeds against all odds."

Sometimes the odds fall against you. But when the long shot pays off, the soul is revived.

To go the distance, I travel best as part of a team.

# POSTSCRIPT –
# GOING THE DISTANCE

*"Let a man examine himself, and so let him eat…"*

St. Paul

Facilitating the course HLTH 498P at University College, University of Maryland, has been the most enjoyable and intellectually stimulating project I have undertaken thus far. Writing this book with Carol has been part of that.

As we look back, we see a number of factors that led us to this moment in time. Our core beliefs were compatible. Our dreams were similar. Our vision of and our paths to wellness, happiness and fulfillment meshed very closely. Some of our conclusions are as follows:

1. Our important beliefs, dreams, hopes and mission in life were set at an early age. An individual's mission in life does not have to be anything exotic, earth-shaking or even known to other people. However, we believe everyone can identify a reason for living, a cause to be devoted to, a mission to carry out.

2. As we came close to finishing this task, we felt that if we were to die before this book is published, we would depart with a sense of unfulfilled mission. Our task would be still incomplete. We are close — close enough to taste it, to touch it, to grasp it firmly. Close, but no cigar.

3. If we die any time after this book is published, we will depart with a sense that our lives fulfilled one of the highest purpose — living a life with honest devotion to our deepest beliefs. We have had the opportunity to share thoughts on how to take what life brings and make the best of it. We have encouraged others to fight a good fight.

4. We hope to live another fifty years, at least, and spend a lot of that time sharing these concepts and encouraging people of all ages, backgrounds and circumstances to find their own paths to wellness. There are no experts out there to substitute for personal belief and wisdom — most of this seems to come from trial and error, while acting on the available information.

5. We are not perfect in any dimension. We feel that we have failed our children in major ways thus far, but there is hope for making it up in a big way. We believe that we were too permissive and allowed too many personal choices too soon. That was a risk we were willing to take. If we erred in parenting, we believed it was better to err on the side of personal freedom as opposed to passing on the neurotic behaviors we both saw in ourselves.

6. The relationships in our lives have been the most rewarding part of living. We have always downplayed the importance of things or of wealth. We have grown into a comfortable middle course. We have hurt some people, but we harbor malice toward no one, especially not toward those who hurt us.

The people we cherish most, even if we don't communicate regularly, are those who were open and honest in accepting us as an interracial couple. Among the many, we think of Cliff and Marcie Sutherland, true and honest friends from our years at Andrews University; Dick and Dianne Raye, friends from our four years at Michigan State University; and Bob and Dianne Mitchell, friends from our three years at the University of Virginia. We have been fortunate to be always surrounded by a wonderfully supportive circle of friends everywhere we lived.

7. Everything in our lives, from childhood to finding each other and experiencing the ups and downs we have experienced together, seems to have been programmed for us to accomplish this task as our main, shared mission in life. We interpret that as a connection with the greatest, highest force for good in the universe.

8. We have been looking for an opportunity to adapt these ideas to a younger audience, because we feel that the adolescent years are the most important in laying the foundation for a happy, productive life. Besides our experiments with our children, we have connected with another opportunity as this book is in its final stages of getting ready for publication.

   One member of the class of 1997 was involved in designing a new curriculum for the magnet program in the county high school system where she is a teacher. As she read through this manuscript, which was being used as the text for the course, she said that this was the synthesis of materials she was looking for but had to use several textbooks to get. She is leading the way to adapt this material for the high school audience.

9. We don't believe that this work is exceptional. It is ordinary, straightforward, but honest. Our sharing of our lives and personal experiences is in that spirit. The combination of our viewpoints, experiences and educational levels made this our unique offering.

10. We will continue to make good music together, to restring our instruments as they need it, and to sing the song we came to sing.

In conclusion, we feel that there are two stories that need endings. We have asked readers to make up their own endings, and we feel we should offer ours. Here is the ending of "The Dog and His Shadow" from Chapter 11:

• • • • •

The butcher missed the dog's daily visit to his shop and wondered what might have happened. He inquired of his other customers, and someone mentioned seeing a dog downriver searching for something.

The butcher took one of his largest bones and came out to the bridge. Sure enough, he could see the dog downriver. He waved the bone and called to the dog. There was no response. It seemed that the dog was so absorbed in searching for the shadow of the bone he had seen in the water that he was oblivious to the butcher's offering.

After several days of coming out to the bridge and calling to the dog, the butcher was ready to give up. He came out to the bridge for one last try and did not see the dog. He turned around to go back to the shop having concluded that the dog had left or had been washed away by an overnight storm. He was so absorbed in his thoughts that he wandered over the edge of the bridge and fell into the water. He was swept downstream still holding the bone in his hand.

As he came into shallow water and gained his footing, he scrambled up onto the bank of the river still carrying this big, marrow-filled bone. A weak barking attracted his attention and out from the bushes came the most emaciated, scraggly-looking, skin-and-bones animal he had ever seen.

When the dog saw the bone in the butcher's hand, he gained new strength. The butcher reached down and gathered the dog onto his shoulder and took him home. They both had steak for dinner that night.

.  .  .  .  .

The other story that calls for an ending is the "The Lion and the Little Lamb That Was Lost" from Chapter 10. Here is our ending:

.  .  .  .  .

The little lamb did not get to finish the sentence. "You fool," the big ram, leader of the flock, yelled. "Don't you know what a lion does to sheep? You must find a lion? There is something good you must do together? How stupid can you be?"

"But the voice from the clouds said...," the lamb was trying to explain. "There is no voice in the cloud," the big ram said. "You better give up this nonsense or you will soon be eaten alive. Lion food is what you will become. Grow up, little lamb, grow up."

Little lamb decided that he couldn't stay with this flock. He left and continued his wandering. He came upon a large grassy plain with many animals. As he moved cautiously among the animals, he heard a low moan coming from a tall clump of grass off to one side. He went to investigate.

There he was — a mighty beast with long flowing mane, a kingly animal five hundred times bigger than a little lamb. "This is the lion I must find," thought little lamb. "I must introduce myself."

"I am Little Lamb," he began.

"Yes, I was expecting you. A voice from the clouds told me you would come. Don't be afraid. I am not like the other lions. I heard the voice from behind the clouds." The lion was kind and friendly.

"I must take you to meet my flock," the lamb said. "I don't know how they will react, but the voice said..."

"I know how they will react," the lion broke in. "They will run in terror as we approach. Sometimes, I wonder if the voice from the clouds really knows that much about animals."

They walked for the whole week before coming in sight of the flock — not his own flock, but the one where the big ram had told him he was stupid. There was already a lot of confusion and bleating and running in circles. It seemed that this was going on for a while. It must have started before they had come into view.

Suddenly, a large, dark mass appeared off to one side of the flock — a bear was on the attack. He had already killed several of the best warrior rams and was going after others.

The lion charged into the fray, straight for the bear. After a battle that lasted the rest of the day and all night, the lion emerged — alive but bleeding. The bear was dead because of bleeding from the wounds inflicted by the lion. Several sheep were dead because of bleeding from the wounds inflicted by the bear.

Little lamb surveyed the sight in the light of the rising sun. The lion's blood was red. The bear's blood was red. The sheep's blood was red. "This is something new to me," he said. "Blood from all animals is red."

"That's something old," the lion chimed in. "I've seen it hundreds of time. We all bleed the same, we all die the same, but we all live differently. I don't think I should stay."

Just then, the big ram, leader of the flock, came over. He had been hiding in the center of the flock to protect himself. "I saw what you did for the flock," he said extending a hand of welcome to the lion. "We want you to stay."

"No," said the lion. "My work is done. I must go back to the plains and win back my place as leader of my pride. That voice from behind the clouds must be there, all right, but I don't know if any other lion heard it. Watch out for bears, and lions too. Good luck, Little Lamb."

As the lion slowly faded from view, the big ram, leader of the flock, and the little lamb that was lost stood side by side in solemn silence. They were both thinking similar thoughts — the voice from the clouds, the lion, the bear and the lost lamb that had now found a new home.

## Carol's Turn

These thoughts came to mind as I watched two televised funeral services. One on Saturday September 6, 1997, was for Diana, Princess of Wales. The other on Saturday, September 13, 1997, was for Mother Teresa.

There has never been and maybe there will never be a woman quite like Princess Diana. She had a place at the very top of human society and was able to reach out to others at the very bottom. Her life's mission was cut short at the age of thirty-six. One of her accomplishments was to help remove some artificial class barriers and connect human beings in bonds of love and compassion.

What might have been if she were to live another fifty years! From all the clips shown of her interviews and speeches, her words that stuck in my mind are: "The biggest disease in this world today is people feeling unloved."

Mother Teresa, who died a few days after Princess Diana, was buried in a state funeral in India. Her death, at the age of eighty-seven, was expected. Her health was failing for several years. What a full life of service to others!

I believe that these two women died happy. One died suddenly with much music still left in her. The other, after a long life doing what made her happy — serving others. One died surrounded by symbols of wealth, status, pleasure and promise. The other died surrounded by conditions of abject poverty, suffering, pain and signs of hopelessness, but died with deep satisfaction.

Both died happy, I believe, because of their ability and their opportunities to love and serve. Love and service seem to be the common bond. Love in all dimensions seems to be what brings happiness and fulfillment.

The words from Mother Teresa that touched me most are: "The greatest disease in the West today is not TB or leprosy; it is being unwanted, unloved, and uncared for. We can cure physical disease with medicine, but the only cure for loneliness, despair, and hopelessness is love." (*Mother Teresa: A Simple Path*. Ballantine Books, New York, 1995, p. 79).

It so happened that on the Wednesday (September 10) between these two Saturday funerals, the front-page article of *The Washington Post* was titled "Love Conquers What Ails Teens, Study Finds." This was a report of one of the most extensive studies on teenagers. The study is titled "The National Longitudinal Study of Adolescent Health." The highlight of the report is that love and connection to parents and teachers is the best protective factor against destructive behaviors.

There must be something to love. We are talking about love more openly, studying love and living love. Am I mistaken? I believe that we will let love, patience, tolerance, gentleness, kindness, peace and hope be more common in words and deeds in the years ahead. This is personal wellness. This is self-realization.

Women of all ages have a large part to play in the practical applications of love to life. It seems that as women take on leading roles in business, science, government, social services and other areas of life, a "kinder, gentler" atmosphere develops. Am I mistaken? I don't think so. I believe that future research will support this.

Thank heaven for women like Princess Diana and Mother Teresa. Thank heaven for the millions of unknown women who successfully combine motherhood and service outside the home, each according to their own beliefs and choices. May their numbers continue to increase.

It may be that personal wellness and self-realization is really about loving and being loved.

The simple path, in the words of Mother Teresa, is this:

*The fruit of silence is prayer*
*The fruit of prayer is faith*
*The fruit of faith is love*
*The fruit of love is service*
*The fruit of service is peace.*

The message of the sixties generation, "Peace and Love" isn't just meaningless slang. Those people of the sixties generation are the fifty-something's of today. Maybe we are really taking this peace and love thing seriously, after all. But are we having fun yet?

Maybe it is by peace and love that we can go the distance. Maybe it is for peace and love that we go the distance. Whatever the challenges in life, love can win, love can conquer.

Since writing the above, I have read Dean Ornish's book, *Love & Survival: The Scientific Basis for the Healing Power of Intimacy*. This is a summary of the strong scientific evidence for the role of love in health and well-being. But love transcends science. And we don't need more scientific studies to believe in and use the power of love. It is good to have scientific support, but it is better to put principles to practical use. So how do we love? Let us find the ways.

It begins with self-examination, self-understanding, self-acceptance, self-management and self-actualization according to the personal belief system. So, go the distance, climb your mountain, make lemonade, and make love and peace and joy.

# In conclusion we offer: The Seven Precepts of Love for Going the Ultimate Distance

1. **Homeostasis:** Love with balance. (Love yourself enough to get to know yourself well, but don't take yourself too seriously. Love someone else so fully that you are willing to give your life for theirs.)

2. **Nutrition:** Love so that you nurture yourself and others. (Love is food for the soul and, if you believe Shakespeare, "Music is the food of love. And if music is the food of love, then play on.")

3. **Stress:** Love so that the "fight or flight" mechanism has armor for the fight or a place of refuge for the flight.

4. **Work:** Love your work or find work you love. And above all, work your love.

5. **Rest:** Love your way to inner peace and world peace.

6. **Growth:** Love to serve others. It's only by giving that love grows.

7. **Reproduction:** Love infinity. This is ultimate self-perpetuation, the ultimate distance.

It may sound corny, but love is the greatest recipe of all. The scientific method is beginning to prove it. Each human knows it deep down inside — the shortest distance. Each human spirit seeks to connect with it at the farthest reaches of the universe — the ultimate distance.

# SELECTED REFERENCES

Aakster, C.W. "Concepts in alternative medicine." *Social Science and Medicine*, 1986, 22(2): 265-273.

Ackerknecht, Erwin Heinz. *A Short History of Medicine*. Baltimore: Johns Hopkins University Press, 1982.

Alexander, Linda Lewis. *New Dimensions in Women's Health*. Boston: Jones and Bartlett Publishers, 1994.

Allen, R.J., and R.A. Yarian. "The domain of health." *Health Education*, 1981 July/August, 3-5.

Anspaugh, David, et al. *Wellness Concepts and Applications*. Baltimore: Mosby, 1994.

Benson, Herbert. *Timeless Healing: The Power and Biology of Belief.* New York: Simon & Schuster, 1996.

_____. *Your Maximum Mind*. New York: Times Books/Random House, 1987.

Buscaglia, Leo F. *Love*. Thorofare, NJ: C.B. Slack, 1972.

Chapman, Larry S. "Developing a useful perspective on spiritual health: well-being, spiritual potential and the search for meaning." *American Journal of Health Promotion*, Winter 1987, 31-39.

Cooper, Robert K. *Health & Fitness Excellence: The Scientific Action Plan*. Boston: Houghton Mifflin, 1989.

Covey, Stephen R. *The Seven Habits of Highly Effective People: Restoring the Character Ethic*. New York: Simon & Schuster, 1989.

_____. *First Things First: To Love, to Learn, to Leave a Legacy*. New York: Simon & Schuster, 1995.

Craik, K.H., R. Hogan and R. Wolfe, eds. *Fifty Years of Personality Psychology*. New York: Plenum Press, 1993.

Drucker, Peter F. "Managing Oneself." *Harvard Business Review*, 1999. March-April, 65-74.

Eberst, R.M. "Defining health: a multi-dimensional model." *Journal of School Health*, 1984, 54(3): 99-104.

Eisenberg, David, et al. "Unconventional medicine in the United States: prevalence, costs and patterns of use." *New England Journal of Medicine*, 1993, 328(4): 246-252.

_____. "Advising patients who seek alternative medical therapies." *Annals of Internal Medicine*, 1997, 127(1): 61-69.

_____. "Trends in alternative medicine use in the United States, 1990-1997." *Journal of the American Medical Association*, 1998, 280(18): 1569-1575.

Engel, G.L. "The need for a new medical model: a challenge for biomedicine." *Science*, 1977, 196 (4286): 129-136.

_____. "The clinical application of the biopsychosocial model." *American Journal of Psychiatry*, 1980, 137(5): 535-544.

Esposito, John L. *Islam: The Straight Path*. New York: Oxford University Press, 1998.

Eysenck, Hans Jurgen. *Fact and Fiction in Psychology*. Baltimore: Penguin Books, 1965.

Flexner, A. *Medical Education in the United States and Canada: A Report of the Carnegie Foundation for the Advancement of Teaching*. Bulletin 4. Boston, 1910.

Frankl, Viktor Emil. *Man's Search for Ultimate Meaning*. New York: Insight Books, 1997.

Fromm, Eric. *Escape from Freedom*. New York: Holt, Rhinehart & Winston, 1941.

Gandhi, Mahatma. *Autobiography: The Story of My Experiments with Truth*. Washington: Public Affairs Press, 1954.

Goleman, Daniel. *Emotional Intelligence*. New York: Bantam Books, 1995.

Gordon, J.S. "Holistic medicine: toward a new medical model." *Journal of Clinical Psychiatry*, 1981, 42(3): 114-119.

Greger, R., and U. Windhorst, eds. *Comprehensive Human Physiology: From Cellular Mechanisms to Integration*. New York: Springer, 1996.

Hawking, Stephen. *A Brief History of Time: From the Big Bang to Black Holes*. NewYork: Bantam Books, 1988.

*Healthy People 2000: Midcourse Review and 1995 Revisions*. U.S. Department of Health and Human Services, Public Health Service, 1996.

Hetzel, Basil S. *The Story of Iodine Deficiency: An International Challenge in Nutrition*. New York: Oxford University Press, 1989.

Hexam, Irving, and Karla Poewe. *Understanding Cults and New Religions*. Grand Rapids, MI: W.B. Eerdmans, 1986.

Hole, Jr. John W., *Human Anatomy and Physiology*. Dubuque: W.C. Brown Co., 1993.

Hunt, Morton M. *The Story of Psychology*. New York: Doubleday, 1993.

Iacocca, Lee A. *Iacocca: An Autobiography*. New York: Bantam Books, 1984.

Inglis, B., and R. West. *The Alternative Health Guide*. New York: Knopf, 1983.

Jain, Nem Kumar. *History of Science*. New Delhi: Oxford & IBH Pub. Co., 1982.

Jenkins, C.D. "New horizons for psychosomatic medicine." *Psychosomatic Medicine*, 1985, 47(1): 3-25.

Knaus, William J. *Do It Now: How to Stop Procrastinating*. Englewood Cliffs, NJ: Prentice-Hall, 1979.

Lewis, C.S. *The Four Loves*. New York: Harcourt Brace, 1960.

Lister, J. "Current controversy on alternative medicine." *New England Journal of Medicine*, 1983, 309(24): 1524-1527.

Melton, Gordon J., et al. *New Age Encyclopedia*. Detroit: Gale Research, 1990.

Micozzi, Marc S., ed. *Fundamentals of Complementary and Alternative Medicine*. New York: Churchill Livingstone, 1996.

Myers, David G. *The Pursuit of Happiness: Who Is Happy—and Why*. New York: W. Morrow, 1992.

Nozick, Robert. *The Examined Life: Philosophical Meditations*. New York: Simon & Schuster, 1989.

Occhiogrosso, Peter. *The Joy of Sects: A Spirited Guide to the World's Religious Traditions*. New York: Doubleday, 1994.

O'Donnell, M.P. "Definition of health promotion." *American Journal of Health Promotion*, 1986, 1(1): 4-5.

Ornish, Dean. *Love & Survival: The Scientific Basis for the Healing Power of Intimacy*. New York: HarperCollins Publishers, 1997.

Ornstein, R.E. and D. Sobel. *Healthy Pleasures:* Reading, Mass: Addison-Wesley, 1989.

Peele, Stanton. *The Meaning of Addiction: Compulsive Experience and Its Interpretation*. Lexington: Lexington Books, 1985.

_____. *The Meaning of Addiction: An Unconventional View*. San Francisco: Jossey-Bass Publishers, 1998.

Pervin, Lawrence A. *The Science of Personality*. New York: John Wiley & Sons, Inc., 1996.

Peters, Tom. *Liberation Management: Necessary Disorganization for the Nanosecond Nineties*. New York: A. A. Knopf, 1992.

Powell, Colin L. *My American Journey*. New York: Random House, 1995.

Seeburger, Francis. *Addiction and Responsibility: An Inquiry into the Addictive Mind*. New York: Crossroads, 1993.

Selye, Hans. *The Stress of Life*. New York: McGraw-Hill Book Company, 1956.

Siegel, Rudolph E. *Galen's System of Physiology and Medicine*. New York: S. Karger, 1968.

Smith, Huston. *The Religions of Man*. New York: Harper, 1958.

_____. *The World's Religions*. San Francisco: Harper, 1991.

_____. *The Illustrated World's Religions: A Guide to Our Wisdom Traditions*. San Francisco: Harper, 1994.

Smith, T. "Alternative medicine." *British Medical Journal*, 1983, 287(6388): 307.

Smuts, J.C. *Holism and Evolution*. New York: Macmillan, 1926.

Tucker, Ruth A. *Another Gospel: Alternative Religions and the New Age Movement*. Grand Rapids, MI: Academic Books, 1989.

Vanzant, Iyanla. *Yesterday, I Cried: Celebrating the Lessons of Living and Loving*. New York: Simon & Schuster, 1998.

Weil, Andrew. *Spontaneous Healing: How to Discover and Enhance Your Body's Natural Ability to Maintain and Heal Itself*. New York: Knopf, 1995.

_____. *Eight Weeks to Optimum Health: A Proven Program for Taking Full Advantage of Your Body's Natural Healing Power*. New York: Knopf, 1997.

Weiten, Wayne. *Psychology: Themes and Variations*. Pacific Grove, CO: Brooks/Cole Pub. 1998.

# INDEX